M. K. Herbert · P. Holzer · N. Roewer (Eds.)

Problems of the Gastrointestinal Tract in Anesthesia, the Perioperative Period, and Intensive Care

Springer
Berlin
Heidelberg
New York
Barcelona
Hong Kong
London
Milan
Paris
Singapore
Tokyo

M.K. Herbert · P. Holzer · N. Roewer
Editors

Problems of the Gastrointestinal Tract in Anesthesia, the Perioperative Period, and Intensive Care

International Symposium in Würzburg, Germany,
1–3 October 1998

With 82 Figures and 39 Tables

Springer

Priv.-Doz. Dr. M. K. Herbert
Universität Würzburg
Klinik für Anaesthesiologie
Josef-Schneider-Straße 2
97080 Würzburg, Germany

Professor Dr. P. Holzer
Universität Graz
Abt. für Exp. u. Klin. Pharmakologie
Universitätsplatz 4
8010 Graz, Austria

Professor Dr. N. Roewer
Universität Würzburg
Klinik für Anaesthesiologie
Josef-Schneider-Straße 2
97080 Würzburg, Germany

ISBN-13:978-3-642-64301-9 Springer-Verlag Berlin Heidelberg New York

Library of Congress Cataloging-in-Publication Data
Problems of the gastrointestinal tract in anaesthesia, the perioperative period, and intensive care : International symposium in Würzburg, October 1 to 3, 1998 / ed.: M.K. Herbert ... – Berlin ; Heidelberg ; New York ; Barcelona ; HongKong ; London ; Milan ; Paris ; Singapore ; Tokyo : Springer, 1999
ISBN-13:978-3-642-64301-9 e-ISBN-13:978-3-642-60200-9
DOI:10.1007/978-3-642-60200-9

Softcover reprint of the hardcover 1st edition 1999

Production: PRO EDIT GmbH, 69126 Heidelberg, Germany
Cover design: design & production, 69121 Heidelberg
Typesetting: Mitterweger Werksatz, 68723 Plankstadt, Germany
SPIN: 10718011 19/3133-5 4 3 2 1 0 – Printed on acid-free paper

Preface

After a long period of neglect, the gastrointestinal tract is increasingly being recognized as an important target of anesthetics and anesthesia-related processes, as well as of conditions and treatments related to peri- and postoperative period and intensive care. Drugs used in anesthesia and intensive care and physiological or pathological changes in the perioperative period affect the digestive system in its function from the pharynx to the colon. Prolonged postoperative ileus or stasis of propulsive peristalsis in the critically ill or multiply injured patient may impair enteral nutrition and give rise to complications such as sepsis or multiple organ failure.

In view of this new understanding of the clinical relevance of gut function, we felt that a book on problems of the gastrointestinal tract in anesthesia, the perioperative period, and intensive care was badly needed. The present volume is the product of an international symposium which brought together physiologists, pharmacologists, experimental and clinical anesthetists, gastroenterologists, surgeons, and intensive care physicians to discuss all major contemporary aspects of bowel function in health and under the influence of anesthesia, surgery, and intensive care.

The chapters of the book are designed to take account of the most important developments in this emerging field of gastroenterology. The topics treated in depth in the various articles cover the gamut of the physiology, pathophysiology, diagnosis, and treatment of gut-associated problems in anesthesia, the perioperative period, and intensive care. A number of chapters focus on the properties and functional aspects of gastrointestinal motility, the impairment of intestinal motility in critically ill patients and in the perioperative period, and on new therapeutic strategies to improve gastrointestinal propulsion.

New insights into the mechanisms of gastrointestinal secretion, absorption, the intestinal microflora, and the barrier function of the intestinal mucosa in health and disease have led to rational approaches for the prevention and treatment of subsequent complications by early enteral nutrition, new compositions of enteral formula diets, and supplementation with additives. Disturbances of intestinal perfusion in the perioperative period as well as under intensive care conditions promote the development of systemic inflammatory response syndrome, sepsis, and, in the worst case, multiple organ dysfunction or failure. Another section of the book deals with postoperative nausea and vomiting, a condition that is increasingly better understood as the predisposing risk factors and underlying mechanisms are revealed. The improvement of pharmacological prevention and therapy which results from these advances is likely to reduce the incidence and severity of unpleasant episodes of nausea and emesis in daily clinical practice.

Many chapters of the book have been written by leading authorities. Because of particular relevance or topicality, several communications made by the participants of the symposium have been included as short communications in order to expand the range of the book. We trust that the book meets the need to integrate the state of the knowledge on bowel function in health and under the influence of anesthesia, surgery, and intensive care. We also hope it will become the first in a series of volumes continuously updating the growing information in this emerging field. With this initial volume in print, we are very grateful to all contributors for providing so freely of their time and expertise and to Marika Stauch, Lindrun Weber and David Roseveare of Springer-Verlag for their invaluable help in guiding the book through the press.

M. K. Herbert, P. Holzer, N. Roewer

Contents

List of Contributors

PART I

Gastrointestinal Motility

INVITED ARTICLE

Properties and Functional Aspects of the Enteric Nervous System

M. Schemann · D. Reiche · M. Neunlist

Department of Physiology, School of Veterinary Medicine, Bischofsholer Damm 15, 30173 Hannover, Germany

Introduction: The Role of the Enteric Nervous System

The gut is a completely unique organ in that it has its own nervous supply. Gut functions such as motility, secretion and microcirculation are under the control of the enteric nervous system (ENS), which is embedded within the wall of the gut [5, 40, 41]. In addition there is a close interaction between the ENS and the enteric immune system; thus, neuro-immune interactions are important for the actions of many mediators of immunocompetent cells [4, 9]. The ENS is the largest accumulation of nerve cells outside the brain; in humans it consists of about 100 million neurons. They are organized into two main plexuses; the myenteric plexus located between the two muscle layers and the submucous plexus located between the circular muscle and the mucosa. In many, certainly in all large mammals, the latter consists of an inner and outer plexus. Myenteric neurons located between the longitudinal and circular muscle layers regulate mainly motility. Submucosal neurons situated between the submucosa and the mucosa are involved in the regulation of such mucosal processes as electrolyte resorption, mucus secretion, mucosal blood flow and neuro-immune interactions. In addition, both plexuses act in concert to coordinate secretion and motility.

Motor disorders are the most obvious result of dysfunction of the ENS and have been reviewed recently [13]. Lack of sphincter relaxation might be related to a loss or dysfunction of inhibitory neurons containing VIP and NO, which leads to achalasia or gastric stasis and to outlet obstruction in infantile hypertrophic pyloric stenosis. The ENS has been implicated in various gut disorders, such as Hirschsprung disease characterized by aganglionosis, von Recklinghausen's disease, microcolon disease characterized by hyperganglionosis, and a variety of inflammatory diseases, such as Crohn's disease or ulcerative colitis. Dysfunction of particular neuronal populations in the ENS might contribute to disorders of gastric contractility and emptying [12, 33, 38]. Furthermore, anaphylactic reactions or responses to toxins such as cholera or *Clostridium difficile* toxin involve neuronal pathways in the ENS [27]. A recent study demonstrated excitotoxicity in the ENS and suggests that overactivation of enteric glutamate receptors may contribute to intestinal damage associated with anoxia, ischemia and excitotoxins present in food [17]. The kind of dysmotility arising from enteric nerve damage depends on the gut region and the degree and specificity of nerve damage. Loss of inhibitory neurons would lead to hypermotility, which would also occur after a total loss of enteric neurons. Hyperactivity of inhibitory nerves or impaired function of excitatory nerves would cause loss of tone in the gut. Today, however, it is

M. K. Herbert et al. (Eds.), Problems of the Gastrointestinal Tract in Anesthesia...

still difficult to characterize the kind or degree of possible nerve damage by identification of motility disorders.

The ENS is structurally and functionally related to the central nervous system and contains afferent (sensory) neurons, interneurons and motor neurons. Afferent neurons are mechano- and/or chemosensitive. Interneurons process these signals and modulate the activity of other enteric neurons. The final pathways for the output from the ENS consist of motor neurons, which can activate or inhibit the various effector systems.

The independence of the ENS of the central nervous system was acknowledged very early and led to the idea that pathways within the ENS directly organize various motor reflexes [1, 21]. Some of the groundbreaking experiments were performed by Magnus and by Bayliss and Starling, who discovered inhibitory and excitatory motor behavior that was dependent on the integrity of the ENS and did not require any extrinsic input [1, 21]. They described the peristaltic reflex, which consists of inhibi-

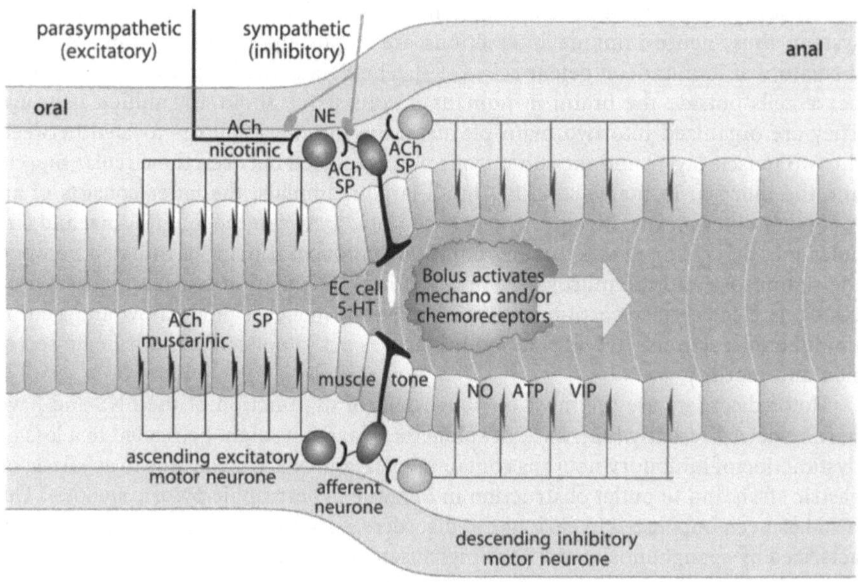

Fig. 1. A simplified model illustrating the enteric circuits in the myenteric plexus involved in the excitatory and inhibitory components of the peristaltic reflex. The peristaltic reflex is activated by a mechanical or chemical stimulus. Activation of primary afferent and motor neurons in the ENS leads first to a relaxation of the circular muscle anally and a contraction orally of the bolus, which makes the propulsion of the bolus possible. The primary afferent neuron is responding to the increase in muscle tone during distension or to mucosal stimuli involving activation of enterochromaffin cells that release 5-HT. The processes of the primary afferent neuron within the myenteric plexus now activate inhibitory motor neurons descending and excitatory motor neurons ascending to the circular muscle. Transmission of enteric primary afferent neurons to enteric motor neurons might also involve ascending and descending interneurons, which are not illustrated here. The model shows only the primary afferent neuron in the myenteric plexus and does not include the wiring for primary afferent neurons in the submucosal plexus. Parasympathetic input is mainly through activation of nicotinic receptors, whereas sympathetic input is primarily through activation of presynaptic α_2 receptors, leading to inhibition of acetylcholine release. Extrinsic afferents are not illustrated in this scheme. (Adapted from [41])

tion of the muscle anal to and excitation of the muscle oral to the site of stimulation, the stimulation being either a local distension or a local application of chemicals. These polarized motor responses are the main reason why the intestine is able to propel its content in an oral-to-anal direction (Fig. 1). Magnus reported in his paper that in most cases the relaxation preceded the contraction; thus, the relaxed segment is able to receive the bolus propelled by the contracted segment.

Besides the important role of the ENS in the peristaltic reflex other reflexes, such as secretion induced by mucosal stroking [6] or vasodilatation following mucosal stroking [8], have been shown to be due to activation of intrinsic neuronal pathways of enteric neurons.

Transmission Processes Within the ENS

The discovery that enteric neurons synthesize various putative neurotransmitters and that they are found in certain combinations led to the concept of the chemical coding of enteric neurons [7]. Thus, enteric cell populations have specific colocalization patterns of transmitters, i.e. a particular neurochemical code. Neuropharmacological studies supported the view that plurichemical transmission is as important for communication between enteric neurons as it is for control of the effector systems by enteric neurons.

Thus, it is not surprising that over the last two decades electrophysiologists have discovered that the enteric nervous system contains the entire synaptic repertoire for evoking fast and slow postsynaptic inhibition and excitation. In addition, it has been shown that synapses are a target for many neurotransmitters that presynaptically inhibit or facilitate transmission. These synaptic events are the basis for interneuronal communications and reflect the various mechanisms for inhibition and activation within the ENS. The list of putative transmitters and neuromodulators is still growing, and those given below are a selection of some of the most relevant ones.

One of the primary transmission modes depends on fast excitatory postsynaptic potentials (fast EPSPs). They are responsible for the rapid and short-lasting activation (millisecond range). The main transmitter for fast EPSPs is acetylcholine acting postsynaptically on nicotinic receptors. However, there is evidence indicating that some fast EPSPs might be mediated by serotonin, ATP or glutamate [11, 19]. Parasympathetic input is exclusively mediated through cholinergic fast EPSPs, indicating that parasympathetic efferents activate enteric neurons through the release of acetylcholine [34]. Excitation and inhibition of muscle activity after vagal stimulation are therefore mediated by vagal activation of enteric excitatory and inhibitory muscle motor neurons.

Putative mediators of slow EPSPs, which last for several seconds or minutes, are: acetylcholine (muscarinic receptors), substance P (NK-1 and/or NK-3 receptors), serotonin (5-HT_{1P} receptors), glutamate (NMDA receptors), GABA, calcitonin gene-related peptide and vasoactive intestinal peptide (VIP) (see [41]). Slow EPSP-like responses may be evoked by numerous other substances, many of which increase intracellular cAMP levels [41]. There are regional differences in the occurrence of slow EPSPs, which are readily inducible in enteric neurons in the small intestine but in less than 50 % of gastric neurons [32]. The excitatory effect of GABA on enteric neurons is noteworthy because the inhibitory effects of many anesthetics on neurons of the central nervous system are mediated through GABA receptors.

Substances involved in slow IPSPs (inhibitory postsynaptic potentials) are: noradrenaline (α_2 receptors), somatostatin, adenosine, ATP, galanin and opioids (see [41]). As for the slow EPSPs, slow IPSPs are mainly recorded in enteric neurons from the small and large intestine, but are very rare in myenteric neurons of the stomach.

Among the substances involved in presynaptic inhibition are noradrenaline (α_2-receptors), adenosine and neuropeptide Y (see [41]). Presynaptic inhibition may occur at fast and slow synapses and is one important mechanism of selective inhibition of particular synapses. Thus, it has been reported that noradrenaline mainly inhibits cholinergic excitatory neurons [32]. This appears to be the primary action of the sympathetic nervous system, which upon activation and release of noradrenaline inhibits enteric neurons and thereby leads to inhibition of motility.

Functional Circuitry in the ENS

The enormous diversity of synaptic transmission is one of the obstacles in unraveling enteric circuits. Although significant advances in our understanding of enteric circuits has been made over the last 20 years it is still not totally clear today what the circumstances are in which the transmission process is activated.

Even the early experiments by Magnus and by Bayliss and Starling suggested the existence of inhibitory and excitatory motor neurons. However, it was the adaptation of retrograde tracing techniques to the ENS that made direct demonstration of the projection polarities of enteric neurons and their respective transmitter coding possible [3]. This in turn made it possible to label enteric muscle motor neurons by applying a small DiI-crystal to the circular muscle, because the terminals of the motor neurons will take up the dye and transport the dye retrogradely to the cell body. As well as the peristaltic reflex referred to as the law of the intestine, there is also a comparable general rule concerning its neural correlate within the ENS: excitatory muscle motor neurons have ascending projections, whereas inhibitory muscle motor neurons have descending projections (Fig. 1). These projection preferences are found throughout the gut and are the hard-wired neuronal basis for the polarized motor components of the peristaltic reflex. The primary transmitters of the excitatory motor neurons are acetylcholine and substance P, whereas the transmitters of inhibitory neurons are nitric oxide, vasoactive intestinal peptide and ATP. The release of the transmitters is believed to be frequency dependent; that is to say that acetylcholine will be released initially, whereas release of substance P requires high-frequency action potential discharge at the terminals innervating the smooth muscle.

The Primary Afferent Neurons in the ENS

Since physiological stimuli elicit reflexes in an isolated intestinal segment, the existence and the pivotal role of enteric sensory neurons have been strongly advocated. Significant advances have been made recently in the identification of primary afferent neurons in the ENS (see [10]). The current concepts indicate that sensory neurons in the gut wall respond to different modalities. Chemo- and mechanosensitive neurons exist in the myenteric plexus. Primary afferent neurons in the submucous plexus code for mechanical distortion of the mucosa [16]. At least in the guinea-pig small and large intestine, it has been proposed that most, if not all, myenteric neurons with mucosal projections are primary afferent neurons [23, 35]. There is substantial evidence indicating that the terminals of primary afferent neurons in the myenteric plexus respond directly or indirectly to muscle tension, chemicals, pH or osmolarity within the lumen of the gut (see [2, 10, 18]). The indirect mode means that activation of enteric neurons depends on activation of other cells and the release of intermediary substances. Thus, the current concept suggests that the enterochromaffin cells act like "taste buds," which will sense changes in luminal content or detect mechanical distortion of the mucosa. Transmission of the information to the afferent neuron is then accomplished through the release of serotonin, which is one of the mediators released by enterochromaffin cells [16]. Mechanosensitivity of myenteric primary afferent neurons depends on the capability of the muscle to develop tension [18]. Thus, primary afferent neurons will not respond to stretching and will not initiate coordinated motor responses if the muscle is paralyzed. The importance of excitatory muscle response at the site of the distension stimulus was noted very early by Lüderitz [20], and for this reason the peristaltic reflex was originally referred to as the Bayliss-Starling-Lüderitz reflex. While this local excitation is crucial for the initiation of peristalsis, it is not clear whether this is a myogenic response (comparable to the myogenic tone of blood vessels) or a local excitation through enteric nerves. An increase in muscle tone as evidence of direct myogenic responses has been described in the stomach in response to filling [14].

At least one of the processes of the multipolar AH neurons (the intrinsic primary afferent neurons) projects to the mucosa. These terminals are believed to code for the stimuli that could originate in the lumen of the gut or within the submucosa/mucosa layer. Recently, evidence for a direct sensitivity of the cell body of multipolar AH neurons was obtained in colonic myenteric neurons, which respond directly to somal application of butyrate [26].

At least in the guinea-pig small and large intestine, putative primary afferents have characteristic electrophysiological and morphological properties. They belong to the class of AH neurons (named after their typical long-lasting afterhypolarization) and are multipolar [10, 26, 35]. Most of them synthesize acetylcholine and substance P, and they contain the calcium-binding protein calbindin. Although no putative afferent neurons in the intestine, or only a very few, receive fast synaptic input, all of them can be activated by slow EPSPs, which are very probably mediated by the release of substance P acting through NK-3 receptors [26]. This suggests that the primary afferent neurons in the intestine are synaptically coupled and act as "sensory circuits," although it is not known how many neurons might belong to such a circuit. This supports the concept of a self-reinforcing system or a feed-forward activation, which would allow recruitment of a large number of afferent neurons in response to a local mucosal stimulus and would lead to activation of other target neurons, such as interneurons and/or motor neurons (Fig. 1) [10, 41].

Calbindin immunoreactivity together with electrophysiological AH properties has been used as a marker for primary afferent neurons in the guinea-pig ENS. However, it has to be noted that calbindin might not be a useful marker in all regions of the gut and is certainly not a specific marker for enteric afferent neurons in other species [39].

The Circular Muscle Motor Neurons in the ENS

In the entire gut there are excitatory and inhibitory motor neurons to the circular muscle (Fig. 1). The excitatory motor neurons co-release acetylcholine and tachykinins in a frequency-dependent manner (very probably substance P and neurokinin A). While acetylcholine excites circular muscles through muscarinic receptors, both NK-1 and NK-2 receptors are involved in the excitatory effects of tachykinins [15]. The inhibitory circular muscle motor neurons are all noncholinergic and nonadrenergic and are referred to as NANC neurons. Most of them contain nitric oxide synthase and vasoactive intestinal peptide. Some of them contain neuropeptide Y, enkephalins, pituitary adenylate cyclase-activating polypeptide (PACAP) and alkaline phosphatase in various combinations in addition (see [7]). The colocalization of many transmitters in these inhibitory neurons is in agreement with the existence of multiple inhibitory transmission mechanisms to the muscle. ATP, nitric oxide, VIP and PACAP are all strong candidates for mediating inhibition of the circular muscle. Overall the ENS input to the smooth muscle is inhibitory and protects the gut from overexcitation. This inhibition is most obvious during phase I of the migrating motor complex, in which the gut remains silent. Whenever inhibition dominates and overpowers excitation coordinated gut behavior will cease, because excitatory responses are necessary for propulsion of luminal content. However, impairment of propulsion will also occur if excitation dominates, which in the worst case could lead to constriction of an intestinal segment and stenosis. Thus, the occurrence of inhibitory and excitatory responses coordinated in time and space is crucial for normal motility.

The projections of circular muscle motor neurons is in agreement with the muscle responses during the peristaltic reflex (Fig. 1). Ascending cholinergic neurons would release excitatory transmitters oral to the stimulus while descending nitrergic neurons release their inhibitory transmitters. This polarized projection has been demonstrated by retrograde tracing techniques in the small intestine and the stomach [3, 28–30]. Enteric motor neurons show region-specific characteristics, which might reflect their role in the regulation of different functions. One example is the striking dominance of ascending cholinergic motor neurons in the stomach and the different coding of circular muscle motor neurons in the stomach compared with the small intestine [7, 28–30].

Recently, it has been shown that muscle motor neurons can be differentially activated by 5-HT [22]. Thus, excitatory ascending enteric pathways consisting of cholinergic, substance P-ergic neurons were activated by 5-HT_3 receptors, whereas 5-HT_{1P} receptors were involved in activation of inhibitory descending pathways using nitrergic neurons. In agreement, contractile responses of the stomach were increased by a 5-HT_3 and decreased by a 5-HT_{1P} agonist [22]. A possible clinical relevance of this finding has been demonstrated in patients with functional dyspepsia [37]. In some of these patients impaired gastric accommodation can be restored by relaxing the fundus with the 5-HT_1 agonist sumatriptan.

The Longitudinal Muscle Motor Neurons in the ENS

In the small intestine most longitudinal muscle motor neurons appear to be cholinergic and excitatory [7]. In contrast, in the stomach a substantial number of longitudinal muscle motor neurons are nitrergic. There are also region-specific differences in the projections. While in the small intestine local short projections are predominant, clear-cut polarized projections are present in the stomach. The functional implication of this has not been resolved, but might be related to the importance of inhibitory tone during relaxation of the stomach in response to filling, which is in part mediated by enteric nerves [14].

The Secreto-motor Neurons in the ENS

Secreto-motor neurons in the small and large intestine are located in the submucosal plexus. In the stomach enteric neurons with projections to the mucosa are located in the myenteric plexus in the same ganglia as also contain muscle motor neurons. This is because submucosal ganglia are extremely sparse in the stomach.

In the guinea-pig small and large intestine there are distinct cholinergic and VIP-ergic submucosal neurons projecting to the mucosa [25, 36]. It should be emphasized that this clear-cut distinction is probably not present in other species. In humans, for example, a substantial number of submucosal neurons contain both the cholinergic marker choline acetyltransferase and VIP (authors' own, unpublished, results).

In the guinea-pig large intestine there is a projection preference of secreto-motor neurons [24, 25]. The descending projections are mainly VIP-ergic, whereas the ascending projections consist primarily of cholinergic neurons. Here the descending projections by far outnumber the ascending projections. As a consequence, activation of descending submucosal neurons induced a VIP-mediated increase in secretion in one study, whereas activation of ascending neurons induced an increase in secretion mediated by release of acetylcholine [25]. The same study further revealed a significant cross-potentiation of carbachol- and VIP-induced secretion as a possible functional role for the innervation of the mucosa by two populations releasing different secretagogues [25]. A polarized projection does not seem to exist in the submucous plexus of the small intestine [36].

As in the colon, polarized projections to the mucosa exist in the myenteric plexus of the stomach [28, 29, 31]. Here cholinergic ascending neurons outnumber nitrergic descending neurons. While the coding of neurons with projections to the mucosa is identical for the small and large intestine, significant differences in the coding exist for gastric enteric neurons with mucosal projections. Candidates for secreto-motor neurons in the stomach are ascending cholinergic neurons mainly colocalizing NPY and VIP and descending nitrergic neurons also colocalizing NPY and VIP.

Concluding Remarks

In summary, the ENS contains all crucial elements needed for autonomous regulation of various gut functions, such as motility and secretion. Results on neurochemical coding, transmission processes and projection preferences have advanced our knowledge on the functional circuitry in the ENS. One challenge in future research will be to relate these findings to pathophysiological states and to identify disorders in the ENS that may be associated with or the cause of gut-related diseases.

Acknowledgements. The authors wish to thank the Deutsche Forschungsgemeinschaft for continuous support since 1985.

References

1. Bayliss WM, Starling EH (1899) The movements and innervation of the small intestine. J Physiol (Lond) 24:99–143
2. Bertrand PP, Kunze WAA, Bornstein JC, Furness JB, Smith ML (1997) Analysis of the responses of the myenteric neuron in the small intestine to chemical stimulation of the mucosa. Am J Physiol 273:G1–G14
3. Brookes SJH, Costa M (1990) Identification of enteric motor neurones which innervate the circular muscle of the guinea pig small intestine. Neurosci Lett 11:227–230
4. Cooke HJ (1994) Neuroimmune signaling in regulation of intestinal ion transport. Am J Physiol 266:G167–G178
5. Cooke HJ, Reddix R (1994) Neural regulation of intestinal electrolyte transport. In: Johnson LR (ed) Physiology of the gastrointestinal tract. Raven Press, New York, pp 2083–2132
6. Cooke HJ, Sidhu M, Fox P, Wang YZ, Zimmermann EM (1997) Substance P as a mediator of colonic secretory reflexes. Am J Physiol 272:G238–G245
7. Costa M, Brookes SJH, Steele P, Gibbins I, Burcher E, Kandiah CJ (1996) Neurochemical classification of myenteric neurons in the guinea-pig ileum Neuroscience 75:949–967
8. Fasth S, Hulten L, Lundgren O, Nordgren S (1997) Vascular responses to mechanical stimulation of the mucosa of the cat colon. Acta Physiol Scand 101:98–104
9. Frieling T, Rupprecht C, Dobreva G, Schemann M (1997) Differential effects of inflammatory mediators on ion secretion in the guinea-pig colon. Comp Biochem Physiol [A] 118:341–343
10. Furness JB, Kunze WAA, Bertrand PP, Clerc N, Bornstein JC (1998) Intrinsic primary afferent neurons of the intestine. Prog Neurobiol 54:1–18
11. Galligan JJ, Bertrand PP (1994) ATP mediates fast synaptic potentials in enteric neurons. J Neurosci 14:7563–7571
12. Geishauser T, Reiche D, Schemann M (1998). In vitro motility disorders associated with abomasal displacement in dairy cows. Neurogastroenterol Mot 10:395–401
13. Goyal RK, Hirano I (1996) The enteric nervous system. N Engl J Med 334:1106–1115
14. Henning GW, Brookes SJH, Costa M (1997) Excitatory and inhibitory motor reflexes in the isolated guinea-pig stomach. J Physiol (Lond) 501:197–212
15. Holzer P, Holzer-Petsche U (1997) Tachykinins in the gut. I. Expression, release and motor function. Pharmacol Ther 73:173–217
16. Kirchgessner Y, Tamir H, Gershon MD (1992) Identification and stimulation by serotonin of intrinsic sensory neurons of the submucosal plexus of the guinea pig gut: activity-induced expression of Fos immunoreactivity. J Neurosci 12:235–248
17. Kirchgessner AL, Liu MT, Alcantara F (1997) Excitotoxicity in the enteric nervous system. J Neurosci 17:8804–8816
18. Kunze WAA, Furness JB, Bertrand PP, Bornstein JC (1998) Intracellular recording from myenteric neurons of the guinea-pig ileum that respond to stretch. J Physiol (Lond) 506:827–842
19. Liu MT, Rothstein JD, Gershon MD, Kirchgessner AL (1997) Glutamatergic enteric neurons. J Neurosci 17:4764–4784
20. Lüderitz C (1891) Das motorische Verhalten des Magens bei Reizung seiner äußeren Fläche. Arch Ges Physiol 49:158–174
21. Magnus R (1908) Die Bewegungen des Verdauungskanals. Ergeb Physiol 7:27–64
22. Michel K, Sann H, Schaaf, C, Schemann M (1997) Subpopulations of gastric myenteric neurons are differentially activated via distinct serotonin receptors: projection, neurochemical coding, and functional implications. J Neurosci 17:8009–8017
23. Neunlist M, Schemann M (1997) Projections and neurochemical coding of myenteric neurons innervating the mucosa of the guinea pig proximal colon. Cell Tissue Res 287:119–125
24. Neunlist M, Schemann M (1998) Polarised innervation pattern of the mucosa of the guinea pig distal colon. Neurosci Lett 246:161–164

25. Neunlist M, Frieling T, Rupprecht C, Schemann M (1998) Polarised enteric submucosal circuits involved in secretory responses of the guinea pig proximal colon. J Physiol (Lond) 506:539–550
26. Neunlist M, Dobreva G, Schemann M (1999) Characteristics of mucosally-projecting myenteric neurones in the guinea-pig proximal colon. J Physiol (Lond) (in press)
27. Nocerino A, Iafusco M, Guandalini S (1995) Cholera toxin-induced small intestinal secretion has a secretory effect on the colon of the rat. Gastroenterology 108:34–39
28. Pfannkuche H, Reiche D, Sann H, Schemann M (1998) Different subpopulations of cholinergic and nitrergic myenteric neurones project to mucosa and circular muscle of the guinea-pig gastric fundus. Cell Tissue Res 292:463–470
29. Pfannkuche H, Reiche D, Firzlaff U, Sann H, Schemann M (1998) Enkephalin-immunoreactive subpopulations in the myenteric plexus of the guinea-pig fundus project primarily to the muscle and not the mucosa. Cell Tissue Res 294:45–55
30. Reiche D, Schemann M (1998) Ascending choline acetyltranferase and descending nitric oxide synthase immunoreactive neurones of the myenteric plexus project to the mucosa of the guinea pig gastric corpus. Neurosci Lett 241:61–64
31. Reiche D, Schemann M (1999) The mucosa of the guinea-pig gastric corpus is innervated by myenteric neurones with specific neurochemical coding and projection preferences. J Comp Neurol (in press)
32. Reiche D, Pfannkuche H, Michel K, Schemann M (1998) Structural and functional organisation of the enteric nervous system in the stomach. Dtsch Tierarztl Wochenschr 105:461–465
33. Salzmann AL (1995) Nitric oxide in the gut. New Horiz 3:352–364
34. Schemann M, Grundy D(1992) Electrophysiological identification of vagally innervated enteric neurones in the guinea pig gastric corpus. Am J Physiol 263:G709-G718
35. Song ZM, Brookes SJ, Costa M (1991) All calbindin-immunoreactive myenteric neurons project to the mucosa of the guinea pig small intestine. Neurosci Lett 180:219–222
36. Song ZM, Brookes SJ, Steele P, Costa M (1992) Projections and pathways of submucous neurons to the mucosa of the guinea-pig small intestine. Cell Tissue Res 269:87–98
37. Tack J, Piessevaux H, Coulie B, Caenepeel P, Janssens J (1998) Role of impaired gastric accommodation to a meal in functional dyspepsia. Gastroenterology 115:1346–1352
38. Takahashi T, Nakamura K, Itoh H, Sima AAF, Owyang C (1997) Impaired expression of nitric oxide synthase in the gastric myenteric plexus of spontaneously diabetic rats. Gastroenterology 113:1525–1544
39. Timmermans JP, Adriaensen D, Cornelissen W, Scheuermann D (1997) Structural organisation and neuropeptide distribution in the mammalian enteric nervous system, with special attention to those components involved in mucosal reflexes. Comp Biochem Physiol 118:331–341
40. Vanner S, Surprenant A (1996) Neural reflexes controlling intestinal microcirculation. Am J Physiol 271:G223–G230
41. Wood JD (1994) Physiology of the enteric nervous system. In: Johnson LR (ed) Physiology of the gastrointestinal tract. Raven Press, New York, pp 423–482

INVITED ARTICLE

Pharmacotherapy of Gastrointestinal Motor Disorders

J. A. J. Schuurkes

Department of Gastrointestinal Pharmacology, Janssen Research Foundation, Turnhoutseweg 30, 2340 Beerse, Belgium

Abstract. Pharmacotherapy of motor disorders is complicated by the wide variety of drug targets and their interactions, the complex relationship between contractile patterns and propulsion, and regional and species differences. Drug classes for which clinical data are available include cholinergic agonists/antagonists, dopamine antagonists, calcium channel blockers and spasmolytics, serotonin 5-HT_4 agonists, cholecystokinin antagonists, motilin agonists, 5-HT_3 antagonists, opiate (ant)agonists, adrenergic alpha$_2$ agonists and laxatives. Recent studies have concentrated on new developments with 5-HT_1, 5-HT_4 and motilin agonists and CCK and substance P antagonists. The number of drug classes available for the treatment of gastrointestinal (GI) disorders is increasing rapidly. A proportion of these may provide more targeted treatment for the large number of GI disorders related to disturbed motility. An interesting new development is the search for compounds interfering with inhibitory (e.g., nitric oxide) or excitatory (e.g., substance P) transmitters of the enteric nervous system. These compounds will allow us to determine the role of novel transmitter substances in GI physiology and may lead to the definition of new targets for future drug screening. A recent development in the study of the pathophysiology of motility-related disorders is our appreciation of the role of the sensory nerves in either regulating local reflexes or transmitting information to the central nervous system (CNS). The endogenous substances involved in sensory transmission may become an important area for the motility-modulating effect of future drugs.

Introduction

Contractile patterns in the gastrointestinal (GI) tract are determined by the activity of smooth muscle cells. The regulation of this activity depends on a complex organization involving different smooth muscle cell layers, interstitial cells of Cajal and intramural nerves. It is also subject to modulation by a variety of messengers derived from the extrinsic nervous system and the circulation and from inflammatory reactions and immune responses (Fig. 1). Moreover, these messengers modulate the release or activity of each other.

Thus, the number of target receptors for endogenous or exogenous substances, either within the cell or on the cell surface, via which GI motility can be affected, is almost unlimited. It is therefore not surprising that a large number of compounds from different pharmacological and chemical classes affect GI motility when tested carefully in different areas of the GI tract. Unfortunately, many of the receptors on

M. K. Herbert et al. (Eds.), Problems of the Gastrointestinal Tract in Anesthesia...

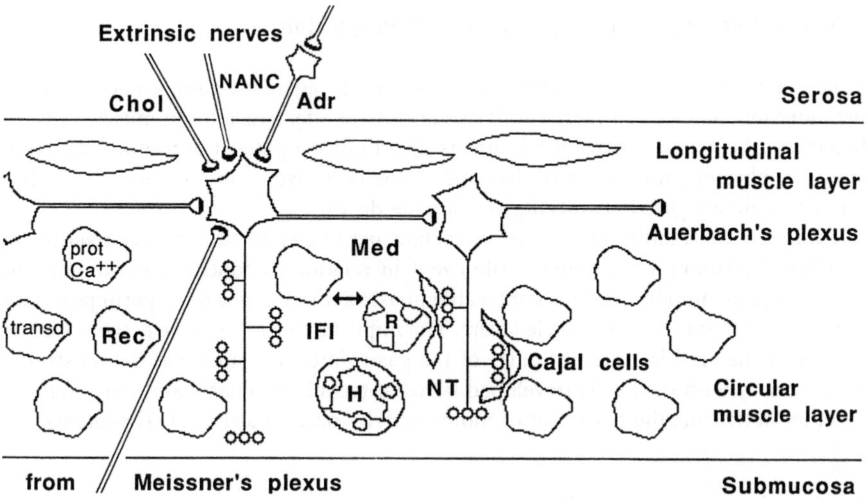

Fig. 1. Possible sites of drug action on the gastrointestinal muscularis. Receptors (*Rec, R*) on the smooth muscle cell surface or inside the cell interact with messengers present in the interstitial fluid (*IFL*) derived from other smooth muscle cells, interstitial cells of Cajal, the enteric nervous system (neurotransmitters, *NT*) or bloodstream (hormones, *H*), or released during inflammatory reactions or immune responses (mediators, *Med*). The action of these messengers is not limited to the smooth muscle cells. They may also interfere with each other – e.g., hormonal modulation of neurotransmitter release. Reproduced, with permission, from Schuurkes (1991)

which these compounds act also occur outside the muscularis, leading to nonspecific responses or unwanted side effects.

This review will not discuss the pharmacological effects of all classes of compounds available to the pharmacologist, but will focus on those classes that can be used to affect motility in a specific manner and that have yielded results indicating that the agents may be relevant to clinical practice.

Contractile Force Alone Does Not Determine the Net Effect on Propulsion

Decreased Contractile Activity ≠ Decreased Propulsion

Anticholinergics, spasmolytics, calcium channel blockers, alpha$_2$ agonists and opiate agonists all inhibit contractile activity, as has been demonstrated in guinea pig ileum during electrical stimulation. However, when these compounds are tested for their effects on propulsion of fecal pellets in the descending colon of the guinea pig, only anticholinergics, alpha$_2$ agonists and opiate μ agonists, such as loperamide, inhibit propulsion. Mixed μ and κ agonists, such as trimebutine, have no effect, whereas the spasmolytic papaverine and the calcium channel blocker verapamil accelerate propulsion. Thus, propulsion can be improved not only by enhancing the force of a propulsive contraction but also by reducing the force of a segmentary, local contraction or by decreasing tone, thereby reducing resistance to flow.

Increased Contractile Activity ≠ Enhanced Propulsion

This can be easily demonstrated with cholinergic agonists. Compounds such as bethanechol enhance contractile activity via a direct effect on smooth muscle cells. In bypassing the neural control mechanisms they induce a pattern of motility different from the physiological patterns observed in the digestive or interdigestive state but do not accelerate gastric emptying at tolerable doses.

Although contractile force is an important parameter in the characterization of motility, the timing of the contractile event in relation to contractions in adjacent areas is equally important. This contractile phasic activity is always superimposed on the basal tonic state of the muscle layers. The importance of this tonic activity for the storage of material in different parts of the gastrointestinal tract was demonstrated only recently with the newly developed barostat technique. Phasic and tonic activity together determine the net result of motor activity on propulsion of GI contents.

Regional and Species Differences

The GI tract consists of a series of compartments with different functions, separated by sphincters. The effects of agonists or antagonists can be region specific. The pharmacology of the sphincter regions deserves special attention, because they have a distinct receptor population and may have functional responses opposing those found in adjacent regions. For example, the colon is known to relax after the administration of noradrenaline, whereas noradrenaline induces a contraction in the internal anal sphincter. The explanation for these paradoxes most often lies in an interaction with different receptors or a difference in the location of these receptors (e.g., smooth muscle cells vs nerve cells).

Species differences can be limited to quantitative differences, but in some cases – for example, with motilin agonists – they are qualitative. Motilin contracts strips from rabbit duodenum in a dose-dependent manner. However, motilin has no effect on duodenal strips from the guinea pig, rat or dog.

Drug Class

Cholinergic Agonists/Antagonists

Acetylcholine is the main driving force of GI motility. Cholinergic agonists such as bethanechol have been shown to enhance tone in the lower esophageal sphincter and may thus prevent gastroesophageal reflux. Unfortunately, these compounds enhance acid secretion at the doses needed to increase pressure in the sphincter and are therefore of no use in clinical practice. Similarly, bethanechol can accelerate gastric emptying in human volunteers, but only at doses inducing cholinergic side effects. When tolerable doses are administered, bethanechol does not enhance gastric emptying in patients in whom it is delayed (McCallum et al. 1983).

Anticholinergic compounds such as scopolamine can be effectively used to reduce contractile activity, e.g. in patients with irritable bowel syndrome (IBS). New muscarinic-3 developments in this area are aimed at selecting receptor subtype-specific antagonists (e.g., muscarinic$_3$ receptor antagonists) in order to avoid some of the side effects of anticholinergic treatment. The recent finding that atropine reduces the number of transient relaxations of the lower esophageal sphincter suggests a role for these subtype-specific antagonists in the treatment of reflux (Mittal et al. 1997)

Adrenergic Agonists/Antagonists

While adrenergic agonists/antagonists (De Ponti et al. 1996) have well-known therapeutic value in the treatment of cardiovascular and respiratory disease, these agents cannot be regarded as established therapeutic tools in the treatment of motility disorders. Although the beta$_3$-adrenergic agonist SR 58611 A has been shown to reduce colonic motility in conscious dogs, the occurrence of tachycardia limits its usefulness as a therapeutic agent. The clinical use of the alpha$_2$ agonists clonidine and lidamidine is limited to patients with opiate-refractory diarrhea.

Dopamine Antagonists

Dopamine antagonists are effective in the prevention of nausea and vomiting via their effect on D_2 receptors in the chemoreceptor trigger zone, at the floor of the fourth ventricle. They also affect GI motility. Dopamine is an effective inhibitor of esophageal peristalsis, gastric peristalsis and antroduodenal coordination; it also lowers esophageal sphincter and gastric tone. Dopamine antagonists such as domperidone, metoclopramide and clebopride act on D_2 receptors and can prevent the inhibitory effects of dopamine on upper gut motility. Dopamine antagonists given alone accelerated gastric emptying in a dog model for delayed gastric emptying. In diabetic patients with dyspepsia (Koch et al. 1989) they reduce symptoms, accelerate gastric emptying and normalize the rhythm of the gastric pacesetter potential. Their effects are limited to the upper gut.

Domperidone is a specific dopamine antagonist that acts on peripheral dopamine receptors. Domperidone does not pass the blood–brain barrier and therefore cannot reach the dopamine receptors in the striatum that are responsible for the effects of neuroleptic compounds such as haloperidol. In contrast, metoclopramide can to some extent reach central dopamine receptors, explaining some of its side effects, such as drowsiness and dystonia. Moreover, metoclopramide is not selective; it also acts on 5-HT_3 and 5-HT_4 receptors.

Calcium Channel Blockers and Spasmolytics

The influx of calcium into the smooth muscle cells is a prerequisite for contraction. This influx can be inhibited specifically by calcium channel blockers (De Ponti et al. 1993), such as nifedipine, diltiazem or verapamil, or by drugs that act on the cell membrane, such as papaverine and mebeverine. Mebeverine has weak anticholinergic properties and is used mainly to treat spasms of the lower gut, whereas specific calcium channel blockers can be used in esophageal disorders, such as diffuse spasms and achalasia.

Opiate Agonists

The nerves of the enteric nervous system express opiate receptors. In general the interaction of an opiate agonist with these receptors will reduce the activity in a nerve fiber.

The μ opiate-receptor agonist loperamide, which does not reach the CNS, inhibits propulsive motility, intestinal secretion and relaxation of the internal anal sphincter, thus explaining its antidiarrheal properties.

An alternative way to achieve an antidiarrheal effect via opiate receptors is the use of enkephalinase inhibitors. Enkephalinases are responsible for the breakdown of endogenous opiates. This approach, however, requires the presence of endogenous opiates before these compounds can be effective in diarrhea. The preserved endogenous opiates may interact with a variety of opiate receptors. Furthermore, compounds such as acetorphan are peptidase inhibitors and do not selectively inhibit enkephalinase activity. Thus, the use of peripheral μ-opiate agonists seems to be a more specific way to obtain an antidiarrheal effect.

The combined μ- and κ-opiate-receptor agonists trimebutine and fedotozine can induce phase III activity in the small intestine. Although these compounds have only a moderate effect on motility, they may be of use in inhibiting afferent nerve activity in patients with a sensitized gut, as in dyspepsia or IBS.

Laxatives

A number of laxatives can lead indirectly to changes in small or large intestinal motility. Within this group, no compounds are available that specifically improve colonic transit by affecting motility.

This class of compounds is heterogeneous. Apart from bulk-forming and osmotic laxatives, it also contains drugs that interfere with the mucosa and lead to the release of secretogogues, such as prostaglandins. This explains why some of the effects of the surfactants, such as castor oil and dioctyl sodium sulfosuccinate, the anthraquinones, such as senna, cascara and danthron, and the diphenylmethane derivatives, such as bisacodyl and phenolphthalein, can be inhibited by pretreatment with indomethacin.

Side effects are limited, but chronic use of irritant laxatives may lead to substantial loss of electrolytes and mucosal damage, including damage to the enteric nerves. Whether abnormalities in the neuronal networks are the cause or consequence of the use of these laxatives remains to be determined.

Serotonin 5-HT_3 Antagonists

5-HT_3 antagonists such as tropisetron, ondansetron and granisetron are effective inhibitors of emetic episodes induced by chemotherapy or irradiation. Their effects on motility are limited to reduction of gastric contractile amplitude and inhibition of the occurrence of phase III of the migratory motor complex (MMC) in the stomach. They are not indicated for the treatment of upper gut motility disorders, but may reduce diarrhea and the symptoms of diarrhea-predominant IBS via an effect on 5-HT_3 receptors on afferent sensory nerves. A mild constipating action has been reported (Talley et al. 1990), which may be caused either by an inhibition of motility or by reduced intestinal secretion.

Serotonin 5-HT_4 Agonists

Substituted benzamides (Briejer et al. 1996) such as cisapride, clebopride and metoclopramide facilitate cholinergic neurotransmission in the guinea-pig ileum in vitro. This facilitatory action on the cholinergic driving system of GI motility is believed to explain the effects of these compounds in patients and healthy volunteers. 5-HT_4 receptors located in the enteric nervous system and on smooth muscle cells account for the effects of the benzamides on GI motility. Cisapride is the only selective compound available for clinical application; the other available substituted benzamides, clebopride and metoclopramide, combine 5-HT_4-agonistic properties amongst others with D_2-antagonistic effects. Other 5-HT_4 receptor agonists, e.g. mosapride (Ruth et al. 1998), are presently being tested in clinical practice for their effects on upper gut motility.

Cisapride (Wiseman and Faulds 1994) enhances esophageal peristalsis and increases lower esophageal sphincter tone and gastric emptying, and it is therefore used in patients with reflux symptoms and esophagitis. Cisapride does not bypass the neuronal mechanisms that control motility, but acts to facilitate them by inducing a physiological motor pattern and improving propulsion throughout the GI tract. It enhances contractile force and frequency in the stomach, improves antropyloroduodenal coordination and reduces the number of isolated pyloric contractions (Fig. 2). As a result it accelerates gastric emptying, with this effect more pronounced when gastric emptying is delayed. Therefore, 5-HT_4 agonists such as cisapride are indicated not only in gastroesophageal reflux but also in the treatment of dyspepsia and gastroparesis. Similar mechanisms are responsible for its accelerating effect on transit through the small intestine and proximal colon. Side effects are limited to transient formation of loose stools in a small number of patients.

This latter effect prompted the search for compounds with a more pronounced effect on large bowel motility. Prucalopride (Briejer and Schuurkes 1998; Briejer et al. 1998) and SDZ HTF 919 (Nguyen et al. 1997) are now in clinical testing. Prucalopride induces giant migrating contractions in the dog colon. It stimulates proximal and inhibits distal colonic motility. These effects are mediated via an action on 5-HT_4 receptors, as the latter can be antagonized by a 5-HT_4 receptor antagonist. These compounds hold promise as the first representatives of a new class of prokinetic compounds termed enterokinetics, which are aimed at alleviating constipation by acting directly to enhance propulsive motility (Emmanuel et al. 1998).

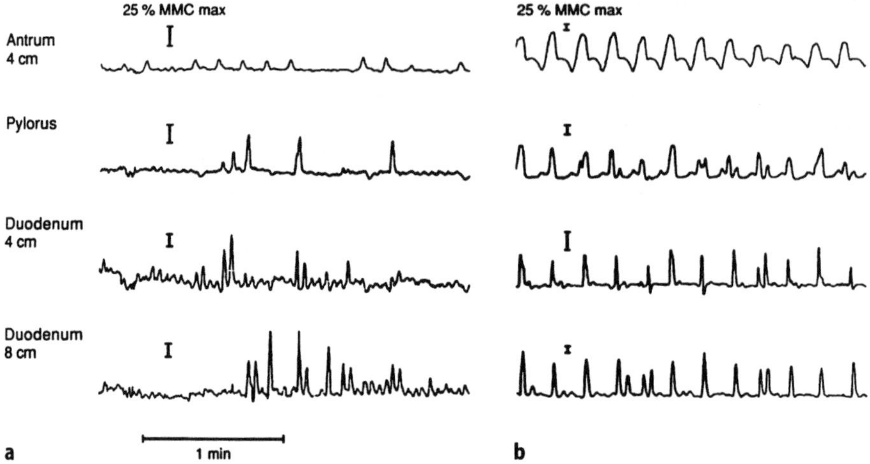

Fig. 2a, b. Cisapride (1.25 mg/kg p.o.) stimulates antropyloroduodenal motility and induces a coordinated motor pattern in the digestive state in a conscious dog (beagle 7017, exp. 729). **a** 30 min after the administration of a small (5 g/kg) test meal containing milk powder, rice, meat and water. **b** 90 min after the administration of cisapride. Cisapride was administered 2 h after the test meal. Since duodenal contractions after cisapride occur at the time of pyloric closure, they favor aboral transport of chyme without inducing duodeno-gastric reflux. Reproduced, with permission, from Schuurkes (1990b)

Selective 5-HT_4 antagonists are now also available. Their value in reducing the motility-stimulating effects of endogenous serotonin is currently under study.

Cholecystokinin Antagonists

Cholecystokinin (CCK) is a GI hormone acting via CCK-A receptors in the digestive state to improve gallbladder contraction, pancreatic secretion and sphincter of Oddi activity. It also enhances gastric secretion via CCK-B receptors. Since the administration of CCK delays gastric emptying, CCK-A antagonists such as devazepide and loxiglumide have been tested for their effects on gastric emptying. In dogs, devazepide inhibits the delayed gastric emptying induced by CCK but not that induced by intralipid. However, in healthy volunteers, the CCK-A antagonist loxiglumide was shown to reduce the inhibitory effects of intraduodenal lipids on gastric motility. It also reduced the occurrence of meal-like fullness and nausea and increased the pressures at which sensations were reported (Feinle et al. 1996). This may indicate a role for CCK-A antagonists in the treatment of fatty meal-induced symptoms, such as those seen in functional dyspepsia.

Recently, devazepide and loxiglumide were also shown to reduce the occurrence of transient lower esophageal sphincter relaxations induced by gastric distension in conscious dogs and healthy volunteers (Boulant et al. 1997). This suggests a possible role for CCK-A antagonists in the treatment of gastroesophageal reflux disease (GORD).

Whether CCK-A-antagonists may be helpful in biliary duct/sphincter of Oddi dyskinesia remains to be determined. The effects of CCK in enhancing large bowel motility are more pronounced in patients with IBS than in non-IBS patients. This has prompted the use of CCK-A antagonists in constipation-predominant IBS.

Motilin Agonists

Motilin is a GI hormone that selectively initiates a migrating motor complex (MMC) in the fasted state. Its plasma levels fluctuate with the occurrence of natural MMCs. Endogenous motilin plays an important role in the initiation of a natural MMC, especially in the stomach. The strong contractions during phase III of the MMC are responsible for emptying of indigestible solids from the stomach into the duodenum. Motilin acts on motilin receptors located in the stomach and duodenum but not in the colon, explaining its selective effect on the upper gut.

Erythromycin (Peeters 1993) has an effect similar to that of motilin and acts on motilin receptors. Although erythromycin has no effect on canine gastric strips in vitro, it accelerates gastric emptying in conscious dogs by inducing forceful gastric contractions. These strong contractions prevent the normal sieving function of the antropyloroduodenal region. The physiological relevance of this observation remains to be determined. In patients with severe gastroparesis, such as that seen in diabetic neuropathy, motilin and erythromycin are both effective in accelerating gastric emptying. More studies are needed to quantify the effects of these compounds on symptom improvement. The role of motilin agonists in GORD appears limited by the small and inconsistent effects of these agents on lower esophageal sphincter pressure.

A second generation of motilin agonists is now being tested. These compounds are erythromycin derivatives [e.g., ABT-229 (Verhagen et al. 1997), EM-574 (Choi et al. 1998)] devoid of antibacterial activity. They effectively accelerate gastric emptying in healthy volunteers. Their role in the reduction of symptoms associated with upper GI tract motility disorders remains to be established.

Future Developments

Nitric Oxide

The discovery of nitric oxide (NO) as an important neurotransmitter, together with vasoactive intestinal peptide (VIP) and adenosine triphosphate (ATP), will stimulate researchers to find ways of modulating this important part of the GI nervous system (Stark and Szurszewski 1992). For example, vagally induced relaxation of the stomach, of major importance for the accommodation of food, is largely dependent on the release of NO.

Compounds such as nitroprusside and nitroglycerin, which are NO donors, relax GI smooth muscle cells by releasing NO and are therefore used in esophageal disorders such as achalasia and diffuse spasms. Recent data suggest a role for NO donors in the treatment of functional dyspepsia. Total symptom score was reduced after glyceryl trinitrate, most probably by its facilitatory action on gastric accommodation (Gilja et al. 1997). The role of NO is not, however, limited to the upper gut. Balloon-evoked relaxations of the internal anal sphincter can be prevented by the administration of L-nitro-arginine, an inhibitor of nitric oxide synthase.

Tachykinins

Substance P and neurokinins A and B belong to a family of neuropeptides referred to as tachykinins owing to their ability to induce rapid contractions of smooth muscle. These peptides interact with at least three different receptors, NK_1, NK_2 and NK_3. A series of antagonists have been used experimentally to study the role of the tachykinins. Although data suggest a possible role for the tachykinins in pain transduction and in contracting smooth muscle, attention has been focused on the role of NK_1-antagonists as antiemetic compounds. In various animal species these antagonists have been shown to be effective against a wide range of emetic stimuli. However, their relevance in the treatment of emesis has not yet been proven (Andrews et al. 1998).

Sensory Function

Another important area for future research is the sensitized gut. Balloon inflation of the stomach of human volunteers allows us to determine the perception threshold. Some compounds, such as fedotozine, a combined κ- and μ-opiate agonist, have been shown to enhance this threshold value. Whether this effect is caused by inhibition of central perception or sensory input to the brain, by a change in compliance of the stomach or by a combination of these mechanisms remains to be elucidated. Thus the gut may be 'sensitive' or even 'sensitized' to repeated exposure to stimuli – e.g., food constituents. Serotonin and CCK are candidates as mediators for these effects. Other mediators derived from the immune system or from inflammatory processes may play an important part in the 'sensitized' gut. Therefore, it might be possible to reduce GI symptoms by interfering with sensory pathways, without affecting GI motility itself.

Local intraluminal sensory pathways play an important part in the regulation of the motor response of the GI wall to intraluminal contents. Sensory nerves in the wall of the intestine initiate and control peristaltic activity by releasing calcitonin gene-related peptide (CGRP), which acts to excite inhibitory (anal) and excitatory (oral) nerves. Recent studies indicate that these nerves are endowed with 5-HT_4 receptors (Grider et al. 1996, 1998). Thus a 5-HT_4 receptor agonist can facilitate the action of the nerves and improve propulsive motility. This finding might explain the prokinetic effects of 5-HT_4 agonists.

Serotonin 5-HT_1 Receptors

The observation that the 5-HT_{1d} agonist sumatriptan delayed gastric emptying of liquids in humans (Houghton et al. 1992) prompted the question as to whether this was caused via an effect on the gastric fundus. In a study of healthy volunteers, sumatriptan was found to reduce gastric tone. This effect indicates a possible role for sumatriptan or sumatriptan-like compounds in conditions in which gastric tone is enhanced. In dyspeptic patients, for instance, duodenal distension leads to a lower degree of gastric relaxation than in healthy volunteers. Sumatriptan was recently shown to relax the fundus in dyspeptic patients and, moreover, to enhance the threshold for discomfort (Coulie 1996). Whether this will lead to a reduction in dyspeptic symptoms remains a subject for further study.

Conclusions

Increased or decreased contractile activity does not necessarily lead to enhanced or decreased propulsion.

The myenteric plexus, with its multiple transmitters and receptors, is a major target for compounds aimed at modifying GI motility.

Although a variety of agents affect GI motility, only a few classes specifically interfere with contractile processes and their neuronal control mechanisms. These are:

- Upper GI tract: D_2 antagonists, 5-HT_4 agonists or motilin agonists can be used to enhance, and calcium channel blockers, nitric oxide donors to reduce, motor activity.
- Lower GI tract: 5-HT_4 agonists can be used to enhance, and CCK antagonists, 5–HT_3 antagonists, opiate agonists and spasmolytics to reduce, motor activity.

Pharmacological stimulation or inhibition of nitric oxide synthase, neurokinin receptors or 5-HT_1 receptors, or interference with afferent nerves or mechanisms of sensitization, may lead to promising new therapeutic tools.

Acknowledgements. The author is indebted to Dr. Alexander Gray for editing the manuscript and to Mrs. Diane Verkuringen for preparation of the manuscript.

References

Andrews PLR, Naylor RJ, Joss RA (1998) Neuropharmacology of emesis and its relevance to anti-emetic therapy. Support Care Cancer 6:197–203

Boulant J, Mathieu S, D'Amato M, Abergel A, Dapoigny M, Bommelaer G (1997) Cholecystokinin in transient lower oesophageal sphincter relaxation due to gastric distension in humans. Gut 40:575–581

Briejer MR, Akkermans LMA, Schuurkes JAJ (1996) Gastrointestinal prokinetic benzamides: the pharmacology underlying stimulation of motility. Pharmacol Rev 47:631–651

Briejer MR, Bosmans J-P, Van Daele P, Schuurkes JAJ (1999) The in vitro pharmacological profile of prucalopride (R093877), a novel enterokinetic compound. (Submitted for publication)

Briejer MR, Schuurkes JAJ (1999) Effects of the enterokinetic prucalopride (R093877) on colonic motility in fasted dogs. (Submitted for publication)

Choi M-G, Camilleri M, Burton DD, Johnson S, Edmonds A (1998) Dose-related effects of *N*-demethyl-*N*-isopropyl-8,9-anhydroerythromycin A 6,9-hemiacetal on gastric emptying of solids in healthy human volunteers. J Pharmacol Exp Ther 285:37–40

Coulie B (1996) Role of 5-hydroxytryptamine-1 receptors in the regulation of gastrointestinal motility (Acta Biomedica thesis). Leuven University Press, Leuven

De Ponti F, Giaroni C, Cosentino M, Lecchini S, Frigo G (1993) Calcium-channel blockers and gastrointestinal motility: basic and clinical aspects. Pharmacol Ther 60:121–148

De Ponti F, Giaroni C, Cosentino M, Lecchini S, Frigo G (1996) Adrenergic mechanisms in the control of gastrointestinal motility: From basic science to clinical applications. Pharmacol Ther 69:59–78

Emmanuel AV, Kamm MA, Roy AJ, Antonelli K (1998) Effect of a novel prokinetic drug, R093877, on gastrointestinal transit in healthy volunteers. Gut 42:511–516

Feinle C, D'Amato M, Read NW (1996) Cholecystokinin-A receptors modulate gastric sensory and motor responses to gastric distention and duodenal lipid. Gastroenterology 110:1379–1385

Gilja OH, Hausken T, Bang CJ, Berstad A (1997) Effect of glyceryl trinitrate on gastric accommodation and symptoms in functional dyspepsia. Dig Dis Sci 42:2124–2131

Grider JR, Foxx-Orenstein AE, Jin J-G (1998) 5-Hydroxytryptamine$_4$ receptor agonists initiate the peristaltic reflex in human, rat, and guinea pig intestine. Gastroenterology 115:370–380
Grider JR, Kuemmerle JF, Jin JG (1996) 5-HT released by mucosal stimuli initiates peristalsis by activating 5-HT$_4$/5-HT$_{1p}$ receptors on sensory CGRP neurons. Am J Physiol 270:G778-G782
Houghton LA, Fowler P, Keene ON, Read NW (1992) Effect of sumatriptan, a new selective 5HT$_1$-like agonist, on liquid gastric emptying in man. Aliment Pharmacol Ther 6:685–691
Koch KL, Stern RM, Stewart WR, Vasey MW (1989) Gastric emptying and gastric myoelectrical activity in patients with diabetic gastroparesis: effect of long-term domperidone treatment. Am J Gastroenterol 84:1069–1075
McCallum RW, Fink SM, Lerner E, Berkowitz DM (1983) Effects of metoclopramide and bethanechol on delayed gastric emptying present in gastroesophageal reflux patients. Gastroenterology 84:1573–1577
Mittal RK, Chiareli C, Liu J, Holloway RH, Dixon W Jr (1997) Atropine inhibits gastric distension and pharyngeal receptor mediated lower oesophageal sphincter relaxation. Gut 41:285–290
Nguyen A, Camilleri M, Kost LJ, Metzger A, Sarr MG, Hanson RB, Fett SL, Zinsmeister AMR (1998) SDZ HTF 919 stimulates canine colonic motility and transit in vivo. J Pharmacol Exp Ther 280:1270–1276
Peeters TL (1993) Erythromycin and other macrolides as prokinetic agents. Gastroenterology 103:1886–1899
Ruth M, Hamelin B, Röhss K, Lundell L (1998) The effect of mosapride, a novel prokinetic, on acid reflux variables in patients with gastro-oesophageal reflux disease. Aliment Pharmacol Ther 12:35–40
Schuurkes J (1991a) Pharmacotherapy of gastrointestinal transit. In: Kamm MA, Lennard-Jones JE (eds) Gastrointestinal transit: pathophysiology and pharmacology. Wrightson Biomedical, Petersfield, pp 171–178]
Schuurkes J (1990b) Effect of cisapride on gastric motility. Z Gastroenterol 28 [Suppl 1]:27–30
Stark ME, Szurszewski JH (1992) Role of nitric oxide in gastrointestinal and hepatic function and disease. Gastroenterology 103:1928–1949
Talley NJ, Phillips SF, Haddad A, Miller LJ, Twomey C, Zinsmeister AR, MacCarty RL, Ciociola A (1990) GR38032F (ondansetron) a selective 5-HT$_3$ receptor antagonist, slows colonic transit in healthy man. Dig Dis Sci 35:477–480
Verhagen MAMT, Samson M, Maes B, Geypens BJ, Ghoos YF, Smout AJPM (1997) Effects of a new motilide, ABT-229, on gastric emptying and postprandial antroduodenal motility in healthy volunteers. Aliment Pharmacol Ther 11:1077–1086
Wiseman LR, Faulds D (1994) Cisapide: an updated review of its pharmacology and therapeutic efficacy as a prokinetic agent in gastrointestinal motility disorders. Drugs 47:116–152

Suggested Further Reading on Pharmacology of Gastrointestinal Motility

Allescher HD (1991) Medikamentöse Beeinflussung der gastro-intestinalen Motilität und Sekretion. Z Gastroenterol 29 [Suppl 3]:27–30
Burks TF (1987) Actions of drugs on gastrointestinal motility. In: Johnson LR (ed) Physiology of the GI tract, 2nd edn, chap 23. Raven Press, New York, pp 723–743
Daniel EE, Collins SM, Fox J-AET, Huizinga JD (1989) Pharmacology of drugs acting on gastrointestinal motility. In: Schultz SG, Wood JD, Rauner BB (eds) Handbook of physiology, sect 6: The gastrointestinal system, chap 19. American Physiological Society, Bethesda, pp 715–757
Daniel EE, Collins SM, Fox J-AET, Huizinga JD (1989) Pharmacology of neuroendocrine peptides. In: Schultz SG, Wood JD, Rauner BB (eds) Handbook of physiology, sect 6: The gastrointestinal system, chap 20. American Physiological Society, Bethesda, Maryland, pp 759–816
Dunn CDR (1991) Gastrointestinal disease management. II. Motility disorders and their management. Scrip PJB Publications, Richmond
Galmiche J-P, Bruley Des Varannes S, Le Bodic L (1991) Les médicaments prokinétiques en gastroentérologie. Gastroenterol Clin Biol 15:T7–T10
Wienbeck M, Barnert J (1990) Prinzipien der Pharmacotherapie. Z Gastroenterol 28 [Suppl 1]:22–26

Effect of Interleukin-1β on Cholinergic Contractions in the Gastrointestinal Tract of the Rat

T. G. Moreels · J. G. De Man · B. Y. De Winter · A. G. Herman
P. A. Pelckmans

Division of Gastroenterology and Pharmacology, University of Antwerp (UIA), 2610 Wilrijk, Belgium

Introduction

Tumor necrosis factor alpha (TNFα), interleukin 1 beta (IL1β) and interleukin 6 (IL6) are key inflammatory cytokines mediating the acute-phase response (Dinarello 1991). Studies in patients and in animal models have shown that the concentrations of these cytokines increase both systemically and in the peritoneal fluid during and after major surgical trauma (Baigrie et al. 1992; Tsukada et al. 1993). They are considered to be responsible for the induction of the general manifestations of the acute-phase response like fever, tachycardia, loss of appetite, elevated prostaglandin and acute-phase protein levels. Recently, experimental studies have emerged a role for these inflammatory cytokines in the modulation of the enteric neuromuscular function (Collins 1996). Both neuronal and smooth muscle cells of the gastrointestinal tract seem to be targets of these cytokines.

Major surgical trauma is followed by postoperative ileus. Ileus is defined as an inhibition of the propulsive intestinal motility, a failure of transport along the alimentary tract. Although the pathogenesis of postoperative ileus is still debated, recent evidence has revealed that postoperative ileus can result from the activation of a neuronal reflex pathway, leading to an hyperactivity of the adrenergic and enteric inhibitory non-adrenergic non-cholinergic neurones (De Winter et al. 1997, 1998).

Therefore, it is possible that during the perioperative period the enteric neuromuscular function is altered due to the release of inflammatory cytokines, leading to gastrointestinal motility disorders like postoperative ileus. In this pharmacological study we examined the effect of human recombinant IL1β (hrIL1β) on cholinergic contractions of different parts of the gastrointestinal tract in the rat.

Materials and Methods

Male Wistar rats (250–350 g) were fasted for 24 h with free access to drinking water. The animals were anesthetized in vaporized diethylether and sacrificed by bleeding. The ileum and the stomach were rapidly removed and placed in ice-cold Krebs-Ringer solution (118.3 mM NaCl, 4.7 mM KCl, 1.2 mM $MgSO_4$, 1.2 mM KH_2PO_4, 2.5 mM $CaCl_2$, 25 mM $NaHCO_3$, 0.026 mM CaEDTA and 11.1 mM glucose). Ileal longitudinal muscle – myenteric plexus (LM-MP) preparations were prepared following the method of Paton and Zar (1968). After removal of the mucosa, four equal longitudinal muscle strips were prepared from the gastric fundus. The LM-MP preparations

M. K. Herbert et al. (Eds.), Problems of the Gastrointestinal Tract in Anesthesia...

and the muscle strips were mounted in organ baths (5 ml) filled with Krebs-Ringer solution maintained at 37 °C and aerated with a mixture of 5 % CO_2 and 95 % O_2. The LM-MP preparation or the muscle strip was connected to a strain gauge transducer (Statham UC2) for continuous recording of isometric tension. The strips were brought at their optimal point of length–tension relationship using 0.1 μM carbachol, by a method modified from that of Pelckmans et al. (1989) and then allowed to equilibrate for at least 60 min before experimentation. During the equilibration period the preparations were washed every ten minutes with fresh Krebs-Ringer solution.

In a preliminary series of experiments, we investigated the well known effect of hrIL1β (R&D Systems, Abingdon, UK) on acetylcholine (ACh)-induced contractions of the ileal LM-MP preparation to validate our own study. The LM-MP preparations were incubated with hrIL1β (10 ng/ml) for 60 min. Subsequently the strips were washed and the effect of incubation with the cytokine was studied on a cumulative dose response curve to ACh (1 nM–100 μM). In rat ileal LM-MP preparations hrIL1β has been shown to inhibit the contractile response to ACh (Aubé et al. 1996).

In a first series of experiments the effect of increasing concentrations of hrIL1β was investigated over different time periods on electrically induced contractions of longitudinal muscle strips of the rat gastric fundus. The strips were incubated with different concentrations of hrIL1β (0.1–10 ng/ml) and during the incubation period contractions were induced by electrical field stimulation (EFS, 2 Hz, 1 ms pulse duration, 10 s pulse trains) every 15 min, for a total incubation time of 60 min. In control conditions the strips were incubated with the vehicle of the hrIL1β solution.

In a second series of experiments, the effect of hrIL1β (10 ng/ml–60 min) was investigated on cholinergic contractions, induced by EFS (0.25–8 Hz, 1 ms pulse duration, 10 s pulse trains) and by cumulative doses of exogenously administered acetylcholine (ACh, 1<nM to 10 μM). The specificity of the effect of hrIL1β in the gastric fundus was studied by means of the human recombinant interleukin-1 receptor antagonist (hrIL1RA, 200 ng/ml, R&D Systems, Abingdon, UK). The hrIL1RA was administered 15 minutes prior to the hrIL1β incubation period.

The contractions were expressed as the percentage of a 120 mM KCl-induced contraction in the ileum and as a 50 mM KCl-induced contraction in the gastric fundus at the end of each experiment after incubation with the neurotoxin tetrodotoxin (TTX, 3 μM). Finally the muscle strips were blotted dry and weighted. Contractions induced by KCl were expressed as mN/mg tissue mass. Values are shown as mean ± SEM for the number of rats indicated. For statistical analysis, Student's *t* test for paired values and one-way analysis of variance followed by Dunnett's test or the Student-Newman-Keuls test were used where appropriate. *P* values of less than 0.05 were considered to be significant.

This study was approved by the Ethics Committee of the University of Antwerp, according to the Helsinki Declaration (1975).

Results

Effect of hrIL1β on ACh-induced Contractions in the Ileal LM-MPs

ACh induced concentration-dependent contractions in ileal LM-MPs with an EC_{50} of approximately 1 μM. After incubation with hrIL1β (10 ng/ml – 60 min) the response to ACh was significantly decreased (for 1 μM ACh : 66.0 ± 4.3 % in controls to 49.6 ± 4.9 % after hrIL1β, *n* = 7). These results are in accordance with those obtained by Aubé et al. (1996). HrIL1β did not change the reference contraction to 120 mM KCl, since the ratio of the KCl-induced contraction to the weight of the LM-MP preparation was similar with (2.1 ± 0.1 mN/mg tissue mass) or without (2.0 ± 0.2 mN/mg tissue mass) incubation with hrIL1β (*n* = 7). Since we were able to reproduce previously reported results, we could assume that the hrIL1β was functionally active.

Time and Dose Response of hrIL1β on EFS-induced Contractions in the Gastric Fundus

EFS with a frequency of 2 Hz induced a contraction of 56.9 ± 5.5 % in control conditions. This contraction was of cholinergic origin since it was completely blocked by TTX (3 μM) or by the non-selective muscarine receptor antagonist atropine (1 μM) (data not shown). Incubation of the muscle strips with increasing doses of hrIL1β (0.1–10 ng/ml) induced time- and dose-dependent increments of the response to EFS (Fig. 1). Only the dose of 10 ng/ml resulted in a statistically significant increase: from 55.8 ± 5.1 % in controls to 72.5 ± 2.3 % after 15 min of incubation with 10 ng/ml hrIL1β, and from 57.3 ± 5.1 % in controls to 78.7 ± 3.1 % after 60 min of incubation with 10 ng/ml hrIL1β (*n* = 8). Incubation with hrIL1β for 60 min did not change the reference contraction to 50 mM KCl, since the ratio of the KCl-induced contraction to

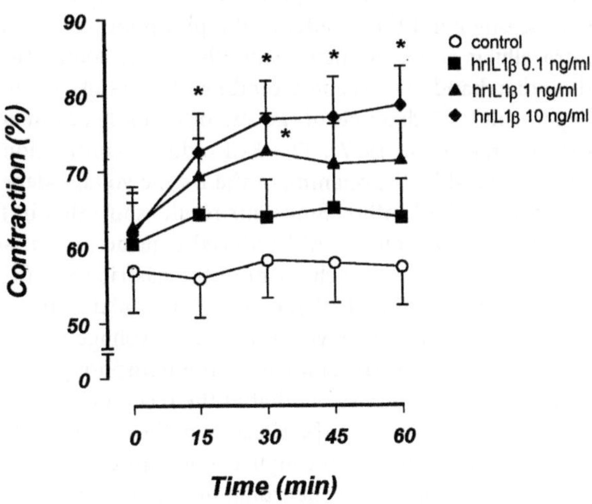

Fig. 1. Time- and dose-dependent effect of human recombinant interleukin-1β (hrIL1β) on cholinergic contractions induced by electrical field stimulation (EFS, 2 Hz, 1 ms pulse duration, 10 s pulse trains) in longitudinal muscle strips of the rat gastric fundus. Results are expressed as percentages of a 50 mM KCl-induced contraction and shown as mean ± SEM for *n* = 8. *$P<0.05$, significantly different from control, one-way ANOVA followed by Dunnett's test

the weight of the muscle strip (in mN/mg tissue mass) was similar in controls and for all concentrations of hrIL1β: 5.1 ± 0.3 in controls, 5.90 ± 0.6 after 0.1 ng/ml hrIL1β, 5.6 ± 0.4 after 1 ng/ml hrIL1β and 5.3 ± 0.3 after 10 ng/ml hrIL1β ($n = 8$).

Effect of hrIL1β and hrIL1RA on EFS- and ACh-induced Contractions in the Gastric Fundus

In control conditions, EFS (0.25–8 Hz, 1 ms pulse duration, 10 s pulse trains) and ACh (1 nM to 10 μM) induced frequency- and dose-dependent contractions in longitudinal muscle strips of the gastric fundus with an EF_{50} of approximately 2 Hz and an EC_{50} of approximately 0.1 μM. After incubation with hrIL1β (10 ng/ml – 60 min) the response to both EFS and ACh was significantly increased (for 2 Hz: from 36.6 ± 11.7 % in controls to 74.9 ± 4.7 % after hrIL1β; for 0.1 μM ACh: from 75.7 ± 5.4 % in controls to 110.4 ± 4.4 % after hrIL1β, $n = 5$). Pretreatment of the muscle strips with hrIL1RA (200 ng/ml) completely blocked the effect of hrIL1β on EFS- and ACh-induced cholinergic contractions (for 2 Hz : 46.0 ± 7.7 % after hrIL1RA plus hrIL1β; for 0.1 μM ACh: 71.7 ± 5.9 % after hrIL1RA plus hrIL1β, $n = 5$). These results indicate that the effect of hrIL1β in the gastric fundus was specifically mediated through IL1 receptors.

Discussion

This study reconfirms that hrIL1β decreases cholinergic contractions in ileal LM-MPs of the rat and it demonstrates that cholinergic contractions of longitudinal smooth muscle strips of the rat gastric fundus are increased by hrIL1β. The effect of hrIL1β in the gastric fundus was specific, since it was completely blocked by hrIL1RA. However, the KCl-induced contractions were not altered by incubation with hrIL1β.

The ACh-induced contraction of gastrointestinal smooth muscle cells is mediated through muscarinic M_3 receptors which are coupled to a G-protein (Eglen et al. 1996). On the one hand this results in the phospholipase C-mediated release of Ca^{2+} from intracellular stores, inducing smooth muscle contraction (Horowitz et al. 1996). On the other hand, M_3 receptor binding also results in the opening of L-type voltage-dependent Ca^{2+} channels of the smooth muscle cell membrane, inducing an influx of Ca^{2+} (Karaki et al. 1997). The KCl-induced contraction is a non-receptor-mediated event induced by the opening of the L-type voltage-dependent Ca^{2+} channels and the induction of Ca^{2+} influx. Since our results show that in the rat gastric fundus hrIL1β had no influence on the KCl-induced contractions, it seems that the non-receptor-mediated contractile mechanism of the gastric smooth muscle cells is unaffected by hrIL1β. Therefore, hrIL1β incubation modulated the cholinergic contractions at a level different from the level of the L-type voltage-dependent Ca^{2+} channels. It is possible that at the postreceptor level the phospholipase C-mediated release of Ca^{2+} is increased. It is also possible that at the receptor level the sensitivity of the M_3 receptors is increased by hrIL1β. These hypotheses can be tested by means of other contractile agonists that act through a G protein-coupled receptor. Since hrIL1β has been shown to alter the enteric neuronal function (Collins 1996), it is also possible that the cholinergic contractions are modulated at the prejunctional level. This hypothesis can be tested by means of a neurotoxin.

In conclusion, these results indicate that hrIL1β modulates cholinergic neurotransmission differently in the ileum and the gastric fundus of the rat, without altering KCl-induced contractions. The mechanism of action of hrIL1β in the gastric fundus is mediated through IL1 receptors and needs further investigation. Taken together, these results might shed a new light on the underlying pathophysiological mechanisms of disturbed motility patterns in the perioperative period.

References

Aubé AC, Blottière HM, Scarpignato C, Cherbut C, Rozé C, Galmiche JP (1996) Inhibition of acetylcholine induced intestinal motility by interleukin 1β in the rat. Gut 39:470–474

Baigrie RJ, Lamont PM, Kwiatkowski D, Dallman MJ, Morris PJ (1992) Systemic cytokine response after major surgery. Br J Surg 79: 757–760.

Collins SM (1996) The immunomodulation of enteric neuromuscular function: implications for motility and inflammatory disorders. Gastroenterology 111:1683–1699

De Winter BY, Boeckxstaens GE, De Man JG, Moreels TG, Herman AG, Pelckmans PA (1997) Effect of adrenergic and nitrergic blockade on experimental ileus in rats. Br J Pharmacol 120:464–468.

De Winter BY, Robberecht P, Boeckxstaens GE, De Man JG, Moreels TG, Herman AG, Pelckmans PA (1998) Role of VIP1/PACAP receptors in postoperative ileus in rats. Br J Pharmacol 124:1181–1186

Dinarello CA (1991) Interleukin-1 and interleukin-1 antagonism. Blood 77:1627–1652

Eglen RM, Hegde SS, Watson N (1996) Muscarinic receptor subtypes and smooth muscle function. Pharmacol Rev 48:531–565

Horowitz A, Menice CB, Laporte R, Morgan KG (1996) Mechanisms of smooth muscle contraction. Physiol Rev 76:967–1003

Karaki H, Ozaki H, Hori M, Mitsui-Saito M, Amano KI, Harada KI, Miyamoto S, Nakazawa H, Won KJ, Sato K (1997) Calcium movements, distribution, and functions in smooth muscle. Pharmacol Rev 49:157–230

Paton WDM, Zar MA (1968) The origin of acetylcholine released from guinea-pig intestine and longitudinal muscle strips. J Physiol (Lond) 194:13–33

Pelckmans PA, Boeckxstaens GE, Van Maercke YM, Herman AG, Verbeuren TJ (1989) Acetylcholine is an indirect inhibitory transmitter in the canine ileocolonic junction. Eur J Pharmacol 170:235–242

Tsukada K, Katoh H, Shiojima M, Suzuki T, Takenoshita S, Nagamachi Y (1993) Concentrations of cytokines in peritoneal fluid after abdominal surgery. Eur J Surg 159:475–479

INVITED ARTICLE

Impairment of Intestinal Motility in the Critically Ill Patient. Clinical Implications and Contribution of Drugs and Mediators

M. K. Herbert

Dept. of Anesthesiology, University of Würzburg, Josef-Schneider-Strasse 2,
97080 Würzburg, Germany

Introduction

Impaired gastrointestinal motility is increasingly recognized as a major problem in critically ill patients in intensive care units. Impaired motility is observed to vary in frequency and degree under different conditions and in individual patients at different times, ranging between complete inhibition and slowing down of gastrointestinal transit. The disturbance of motility can occur in all parts of the gastrointestinal tract, and a stasis of clinical relevance is mostly observed in the stomach, the small intestine, and the colon. Although the reasons for the disturbance of a regular transit of ingested food are heterogeneous and manifold in the different parts of the gastrointestinal tract, all lead to the same consequence: nutrition via the enteral route is hampered or impossible or continuation of enteral nutrition bears the risk of complications.

Regulation of Gastrointestinal Motility

As described in detail in the first chapter of this book, a variety of extrinsic neural, intrinsic enteric, and humoral mechanisms regulate intestinal motility. A number of special features of the motor system of the gastrointestinal tract, i.e. smooth muscles, the enteric nervous system, and both excitatory and inhibitory (e.g. nitric oxide, NO) enteric transmitters enable peristaltic reflexes to occur and thus to mix and propel the ingested food through the gastrointestinal tract from the oral to the aboral end. Intestinal motility is regulated by the specific anatomical arrangement of smooth muscle layers and neural plexuses, the pacemaker sites within the stomach and intestine, the spontaneous electrical rhythmicity of the gastrointestinal muscle and the functional integration of the enteric nervous system with the central nervous systems. Propulsive peristalsis is the result of a coordinated and balanced action of descending inhibitory and ascending excitatory motor neurons of the enteric nervous system (Furness and Costa 1987; Waterman and Costa 1994; Waterman et al. 1994a, b). The motility pattern of the gastrointestinal tract also depends on the presence of an adequate stimulus, i.e. ingested food, so that a specific postprandial and interdigestive motility pattern can be distinguished. Normally, the interdigestive motility, which has the function of cleaning the bowel and preventing bacterial overgrowth, switches from interdigestive to postprandial propulsive motility when food is ingested and passes through the lumen of the intestine. During fasting, the flow of intestinal content

M. K. Herbert et al. (Eds.), Problems of the
Gastrointestinal Tract in Anesthesia...

varies according to the specific phases of the interdigestive cycle. It is most pronounced at the time of phase 3 of the migrating motor complex (MMC), but is not insignificant even during motor quiescence of phase 1.

Consequences of and Problems Arising from Impaired Gastrointestinal Motility. Benefit of Enteral Nutrition

Besides specific internal and neurological diseases that compromise propulsive intestinal motility, intra-abdominal surgery, drugs used in anesthesia and in the postoperative period, and pharmacological and nonpharmacological therapeutic strategies applied in intensive care medicine can all contribute to the inhibition of gastrointestinal motility.

In the perioperative period and in intensive care medicine a number of factors inducing and promoting stasis of the gastrointestinal transit are unavoidable and necessary, for example to make an operation possible or to improve the life-threatening condition that has brought the patient to the intensive care unit. On the other hand, there are various consequences and complications of the absence of intestinal motility or failure of gastric emptying. These secondary complications may initiate a vicious circle of promoting intestinal stasis and subsequently inducing a variety of disturbances, and thus perpetuate the initial imbalance, which in the worst possible case can culminate in multiple organ failure.

The diagnosis of impaired gastric emptying or absence of intestinal transit is mainly based on clinical signs or on physical examination of the patient, but these signs are often contradictory in interpretation and, especially, with regard to their clinical relevance. Whereas impaired gastric emptying can be deduced reliably from gastric content aspiration volumes of more than 300 ml via a nasogastric tube, the differentiation between a totally abolished or partially reduced transpyloric passage is more difficult or even impossible. Taking into consideration that the volume of gastric secretions is usually about 2000 ml per day, the respective aspiration volume obtained with a nasogastric tube only indirectly indicates the degree of inhibition of transpyloric transit. In recent years efforts have been made in cutaneous electrogastrography, a technique for monitoring electrical activity of presumably gastric pacemaker circuits from cutaneous surface electrodes on the abdominal wall (Desvarannes et al. 1991; Chen and McCallum 1993; Chen et al. 1994; Liang and Chen 1997). Although there is evidence for abnormal gastric slow waves in patients with delayed gastric emptying (Chen et al. 1994), forthcoming research will reveal the real impact of cutaneous registration of gastric myoelectrical activity as a correlate of impaired gastric motility. An inhibition of intestinal or colonic transit of digested matter is judged from the absence of defecation, which again is a rather rough and indirect clinical parameter with a broad range of frequencies of stool under physiological conditions from one or two per day to approximately one per 4 or 5 days.

The clinically often used parameter of audible bowel sounds on auscultation is a poor or unreliable correlate of propulsive peristalsis in the intestine. Thus, it is controversial whether the audible bowel sounds originate from the colon, small intestine, upper gastrointestinal tract, or whether they are elicited by propulsive peristaltic waves, segmental spastic contractions of an intestinal lumen partially filled with gas and liquids or are caused, for example, by the activity front of phase 3 of interdigestive migrating motor activity. Only a few investigators have assessed bowel motility sonographically (Pape et al. 1994).

Why Is It so Important to Have a Normal Gastrointestinal Motility?

According to a more traditional opinion, traumatized patients or those who have undergone major surgery are usually fed by the parenteral route in absence of gastrointestinal motility until the production of the first flatus or stool. A primarily parenteral nutrition seems reasonable for a limited time interval after extensive intraperitoneal resections, for example. Research carried out in recent years, however, has shown that enteral nutrition via the normal gastrointestinal route is superior to parenteral alimentation in several respects (Heyland et al. 1993). First, the overall clinical outcome of critically ill patients is statistically improved with enteral versus parenteral nutrition (Kudsk et al. 1992; Kompan et al. 1999). As shown by laboratory (Kudsk et al. 1981, 1983) and prospective clinical trials (Moore and Jones 1986; Moore et al. 1989), morbidity and mortality after trauma are reduced when nutrients are provided through the gastrointestinal rather than intravenous route.

Multiple organ failure remains the main cause of death following severe injury in patients in intensive care (Landow and Andersen 1994). Loss of the gut barrier function and the subsequent increased bacterial and endotoxin translocation play an important part in the pathogenesis of multiple organ failure (Schlag et al. 1991; Landow and Andersen 1994; Moore and Moore 1995).There is direct and indirect evidence for an increased intestinal permeability (Harris et al. 1992) and translocation of bacteria in humans after shock or injury, in burn patients (Brathwaite et al. 1993; Deitch 1990; Kompan et al. 1999; Langkamp-Henken et al. 1994; LeVoyer et al. 1992; Pape et al. 1994; Roumen et al. 1993; Rush et al. 1988) and in patients undergoing heart or major abdominal surgery (Carr et al. 1996; Sinclair et al. 1995). In addition, in multiply injured and shocked patients, intestinal ischemia and reperfusion injury precipitate mucosal injury (Landow and Andersen 1994; Pape et al. 1994; Rush et al. 1988; Roumen et al. 1993). Increased intestinal permeability has been found early after a trauma, such as burn injury (Deitch 1990; Gianotti et al. 1994; LeVoyer et al. 1992) or blunt or penetrating abdominal trauma (Langkamp-Henken et al. 1995). Loss of intestinal mucosal barrier function is seen also after starvation and parenteral nutrition without any preceding trauma, a condition that improves on institution of enteral nutrition (Carr et al. 1996; Hadfield et al. 1995; Pape et al. 1994; Van der Hulst et al. 1998). Randomized trials confirmed the benefit of enteral versus parenteral feeding (Kudsk et al. 1992). These advantages of enteral food supply can be further improved by an early start of nutritional support within 24 hours or less after trauma or an operation (Beier-Holgersen and Boesby 1996; Chiarelli et al. 1990; Grahm et al. 1989; Mochizuki et al. 1984; Moore and Jones 1986; Sagar et al. 1979; Sullivan et al. 1998).

Besides the scepticism of many clinicians about providing alimentation via the enteral route in the early postoperative period, gastric intolerance was the most frequent reason why attempts at instituting early enteral nutrition failed (Adam and Batson 1997). Impaired gastric emptying led to discrepancies between the delivered and prescribed volume of feed. A study in five intensive care units in the United Kingdom established that on average only 76 % of the quantity of feed prescribed was delivered to the patients. High gastric residual volumes or aspirates after a period of rest following feeding were used as a marker of gastric intolerance (Adam and Batson 1997). In general, residual volumes of 50–150 ml have been recommended as cut-off points for discontinuation of enteral delivery (Cataldi-Betcher et al. 1983; Koruda et al 1987; McClave et al. 1992). An alternative approach, to circumvent impaired gastric emptying, is to administer feed via a nasojejunal tube or percutaneous endoscopic gastrojejunostomy (Gottfried and Plumser 1984; Gray et al. 1989). This feeding into the small bowel was preferred over gastric feeding in the early period. However, the incidence of intolerance to early jejunal feeding ranges from 13 % to 37 % (Adams et al. 1986; Cerra et al. 1988; Jones et al. 1989; Moore and Jones 1986).

Drugs and Mediators Contributing to the Inhibition of Gastrointestinal Motility

Pharmacological substances used for induction of anesthesia or for analgosedation of critically ill patients in the intensive care unit are thought to inhibit gastrointestinal motility. In recent years research on inhibition of gastrointestinal motility has focused mostly on inhibition of gastric emptying and on pharmacological approaches to improve gastric transit. Although the jejunum and ileum represents the longest route in the passage of digested matter, little is known about drug-induced inhibition of small intestinal motility.

Inhibition of Gastric Emptying

The multitude of reasons that account for impaired or delayed gastric emptying have been reviewed in detail (Minami and McCallum 1984). This chapter will not discuss the pharmacological effects of all substances that impair gastric emptying, but will focus on the action of opioids used in anesthesia and intensive care medicine and on recent findings which might be or may become of clinical relevance.

A well-established effect of opioids is inhibition of gastric emptying. This effect has been demonstrated with agents such as morphine, diamorphine, pethidine (meperidine), sufentanil and buprenorphine in a variety of clinical settings, e.g. anesthetic premedication, pain relief in labor (Milligan et al. 1988; Nimmo et al. 1975; Todd and Nimmo 1983) and in healthy volunteers (Adelhoj et al. 1985). Opioid peptides and their receptors are found throughout the gastrointestinal system, with particularly high concentrations in the gastric antrum and proximal duodenum (Bagnol et al. 1997; Polak and Bloom 1979). The mechanism of inhibition of gastric emptying by exogenous and endogenous opioids is still controversial, and although central and peripheral mechanisms may be involved, their relative contribution remains uncertain (Manara and Bianchetti 1985). A central mechanism has been postulated, because intracerebroventricular injection of morphine in the rat inhibits gastrointestinal propulsion (Porecca et al. 1983). Other findings obtained in rodents (Manara et al. 1986), which have been confirmed in humans, show that opioids inhibit gastric emptying by a peripheral mechanism. Using methylnaltrexone, a highly ionized quaternary derivative of naltrexone which does not penetrate the blood–brain barrier, morphine-induced gastric delay was reversed in healthy volunteers (Murphy et al. 1997). This finding provides a new therapeutic strategy for the reversal of opioid-induced inhibition of the motility in the stomach and small intestine without affecting opioid-induced analgesia (Yuan et al. 1995, 1996).

Inhibition of the Intestinal Peristaltic Reflex

Intestinal peristalsis was studied in vitro with an experimental setup using a constant intraluminal perfusion system (Holzer et al. 1997). Extrapolation of the data to the clinical situation must be considered with caution, because of possible species differences and differences between in vivo and in vitro conditions. Ileal segments of adult guinea-pigs were mounted in organ baths that contained oxygenated Tyrode solution. Prewarmed Tyrode solution was infused into the intestinal lumen at a constant infusion rate, and the fluid passing the gut lumen was directed into a vertical outlet tubing 4 cm (reflecting a pressure of 400 Pa) above the fluid level of the organ bath. This arrangement caused gradual filling of the intestine. When the intraluminal pressure reached a threshold, an aborally moving wave of circular muscle contraction, measured as a spike-like increase in intraluminal pressure, propelled the intraluminal fluid to leave the system and thus caused emptying of the segment. The pressure threshold for eliciting peristaltic waves was used to quantify the effects of drugs on peristaltic activity (Holzer et al. 1997). Inhibition of peristalsis was reflected by an increase of the pressure threshold and abolition of peristalsis manifested itself in a lack of peristaltic activity in spite of an intraluminal pressure of 400 Pa. After an equilibration period of 30 min and registration of normal peristalsis the segments were exposed to a drug. Using this experimental setup the effects of narcotics, sedatives, opioids and propulsive substances on intestinal motility were investigated.

Propofol and etomidate are routinely used narcotics for the induction of anesthesia and propofol for the sedation of patients in intensive care units. Both substances affect the intestinal motility in vitro in a concentration-dependent manner by increasing the pressure threshold to elicit a peristaltic contraction and by inhibition of the peristaltic reflex (Markus et al. 1998). Since comparable doses of both drugs are used in clinical routine in humans, it seems rather likely that both drugs also affect the propulsive motility in the human intestine. Midazolam, a short-acting benzodiazepine, increases the pressure threshold at a bath concentration of 10 μM and abolishes the reflex at 100 μM (Wenderoth et al. 1998). Opioids, which are used as potent analgesics, have the major side effect of constipation when used for any length of time. In the experiments evaluating the acute effect of opioids on the peristaltic reflex, selective ligands for μ-receptors [(D-Ala^2,*N*-Me-Phe^4, glycerol^5)-enkephalin, DAMGO], κ-receptors (*U50,488*), and δ_1-receptors ((D -Pen^2, *p*-chloro-phe^4, D -Pen^5)-enkephalin, DPDPE) were administered to the ileal segments. All three types of opioid ligands inhibited propulsive peristalsis in a concentration-dependent manner in the nanomolar range. A similar inhibition was observed with the clinically used derivatives fentanyl and the short-acting remifentanil (Arzet et al. 1998a). The inhibitory action of fentanyl, remifentanil and the selective receptor ligands was prevented or reversed by the opioid antagonist naloxone. Interestingly, by use of selective receptor antagonists it has been shown that the inhibitory effect of the δ-opioid ligand DPDPE, which occurs at rather high concentrations only (Herbert et al. 1997), is presumably mediated by μ-opioid receptors (Arzet et al. 1998b). Whether the lack of a δ-receptor-mediated effect of DPDPE is species dependent or due to the absence of δ-opioid receptors in the guinea-pig ileum remains open. Ketamine, another drug with potent analgesic properties, provides a good alternative to opioids under clinical conditions. The experiments concerning their effect on ileal motility revealed that racemic as well as the *S*(+) enantiomer of ketamine inhibited the intestinal reflex in a concentration-dependent manner, but about 1,000-fold concentrations of ketamine were required compared with fentanyl to completely abolish intestinal motility (Herbert et al. 1998a). The results of these in vitro experiments are in line with clinical data of a moderate inhibitory effect of ketamine on gastrointestinal motility in patients (Freye and Knüfermann 1994).

Nitric oxide (NO) is an inhibitory transmitter in the enteric nervous system (Sanders and Ward 1992; Smits and Lefebvre 1996; Suzuki et al. 1994). The application of a NO donor, sodium nitroprusside, extraserosally to the organ bath mimics the inhibitory effect of the intrinsic transmitter in the guinea-pig ileum (Holzer et al. 1997). Various mediators, e.g. lipopolysaccharides, cytokines and inflammatory mediators, that are released during pathological conditions such as sepsis, exert their action via the release or synthesis of NO. Thus NO liberated from macrophages and other cells might be a candidate mediator that contributes to the inhibition of intestinal motility in critically ill patients. Enhanced formation of NO by the inducible isoform of NO synthase in septic shock has been confirmed by measurement of highly elevated plasma levels of nitrite and/or nitrate, the main stable end products of NO (Doughty et al. 1998; Evans et al. 1993; Wong et al. 1995; Tagan et al. 1998). NO accounts for many sequelae observed in these patients, such as decreased cardiac contractility, vasodilatation and vascular hyporesponsiveness to vasoconstrictors, sepsis-induced liver dysfunction and lung injury, and finally, multiple organ failure (Julou-Schaeffer et al. 1990; Ochoa et al. 1991; Evans et al. 1993; Petros et al. 1994; Keller et al. 1995; Schulz et al. 1995; Thiemermann et al. 1995; Cobb and Danner 1996). It seems reasonable to speculate that NO, released from macrophages during sepsis syndrome, might interfere with or augment the inhibitory effect of drugs used in intensive care medicine, e.g. sedatives and opioid analgesics. This hypothesis has been confirmed in recent experiments using midazolam in a concentration of 10 μM, which never caused complete inhibition of intestinal motility in vitro when tested alone. After preincubation of the ileal segments in 10 μM sodium nitroprusside, a concentration which usually enhanced the pressure threshold to evoke a peristaltic wave, but failed to induce complete inhibition of the peristaltic reflex in the guinea-pig ileum, 10 μM midazolam abolished intestinal peristalsis in about 50 % of the segments tested (Herbert et al. 1998c).

Drugs with Prokinetic Actions

As outlined above, many drugs used in clinical routine affect gastrointestinal motility. While it is important to know the potential inhibitory effect of these drugs, it is even more essential to counteract this inhibition of gastrointestinal motility with prokinetic agents. A primary goal in states of intestinal dysmotility is to resolve the ileus and restore normal peristalsis.

Cerulein, metoclopramide, neostigmine, and cisapride are routinely used to stimulate gastrointestinal motility under intensive care conditions. However, especially in critically ill patients suffering from sepsis syndrome these agents often fail to exert a propulsive effect. In postoperative ileus cisapride has inconsistent effects. Some studies show either an earlier return of bowel sounds (Boghaert et al. 1987) and/or passage of flatus or stool (Pescatori 1987; Verlinden et al 1987; Tollesson et al. 1991), whereas others do not (Von Ritter et al. 1987; Clevers et al. 1988; Hallerbäck et al. 1991). In accordance with this modest beneficial effect on small bowel motor activity after intra-abdominal surgery (Benson et al. 1994), cisapride's major prokinetic effect seems to be acceleration of gastric emptying (Van Rooy et al. 1988). Cerulein has been proven to be the most effective stimulatory agent on peristalsis in the guinea-pig ileal reflex in vitro tested so far. Cerulein (0.1–100 nM) brought about a concentration-dependent reduction of the pressure threshold to elicit a peristaltic wave and increased the frequency of contractions. With 100 nM cerulein the frequency of contractions was more than doubled over the entire observation period (Herbert et al. 1998c). Metoclopramide has either no effect or an inhibitory effect on peristalsis in the small intestine in vitro (Kuhn et al. 1998). Metoclopramide at concentrations of 1–10 μM did not affect the pressure threshold or the frequency of contractions. After administration of 30 μM metoclopramide the peristalsis parameters remained unchanged in 5 of 10 segments, whereas in the other 5 segments the contractions were completely abolished (Kuhn et al. 1998). The mechanism of this inhibition, which was observed in all segments after 100 μM metoclopramide, is unknown and needs further investigation. These preliminary experiments, however, suggest that metoclopramide is not a suitable drug to improve intestinal dysmotility, since propulsive peristalsis is disturbed or abolished by high doses of metoclopramide. The rationale for the use of neostigmine in the treatment of intestinal atonia is inhibition of the cleavage of endogenous acetycholine with a resulting accumulation of this excitatory enteric transmitter. Experiments with the guinea-pig ileum show a steep concentration-response relationship for the stimulant effect of neostigmine in vitro (Petnehazy et al. 1998). Concentrations of neostigmine that were effective in lowering the pressure threshold and enhancing the frequency of peristaltic contraction also caused intermittent bursts of stationary contractions with no propulsive quality, which lasted 2–3 min (Petnehazy et al. 1998). Thus, neostigmine also does not seem to be a suitable drug for the treatment of intestinal dysmotility.

Conclusions

Propulsive peristalsis of the gastrointestinal tract is complexly regulated by an interplay of the enteric nervous system and smooth muscle via enteric transmitters. Over the past two decades several experimental and clinical studies have provided convincing evidence of the benefit of early enteral versus parenteral nutrition in intensive care medicine. Since propulsive peristalsis is often a prerequisite for enteral alimentation, the start of enteral food supply is hampered by the inhibition of gastrointestinal motility through a number of factors, e.g., endogenous mediators, drugs, and therapeutic strategies. As tested so far in vivo and in vitro, nearly all pharmacological substances used in anesthesia and intensive care impair gastric emptying and/or intestinal motility in a dose-dependent manner. Drugs with a prokinetic action exert only a limited effect on gastrointestinal stasis under intensive care conditions or on disturbed motility compromised by pharmacological drugs.

References

Adam S, Batson S (1997) A study of problems associated with delivery of enteral feed in critically ill patients in five ICUs in the UK. Intensive Care Med 23: 261–266

Adams MB, Seabrook GR, Quebbeman EA, Condon RE (1986) Jejunostomy: a rarely indicated procedure. Arch Surg 121: 236–238

Adams S, Dellinger EP, Wertz MJ, Orekovich MR, Simonowitz D, Johansen K (1986) Enteral versus parenteral nutrition support following laparotomy for trauma: a randomized prospective trial. J Trauma 26: 882–890

Adelhoj B, Petring OU, Ibsen M, Brynnum J, Poulsen HE (1985) Buprenorphine delays drug absorption and gastric emptying in man. Acta Anaesthesiol Scand 29: 599–601

Arzet H, Herbert MK, Markus CK, Holzer P, Roewer N (1998a) The inhibitory effect of the δ-opioid ligand DPDPE on intestinal peristalsis in the guinea-pig ileum *in vitro* is mediated by μ-receptors. Anasthesiol Intensivmed Notfallmed Schmerzther 33: 605

Arzet H, Herbert MK, Markus CK, Holzer P, Roewer N (1998b) Fentanyl and remifentanil inhibit intestinal peristalsis in the guinea-pig *in vitro*. Anasthesiol Intensivmed Notfallmed Schmerzther 33: 605

Bagnol D, Mansour A, Akil H, Watson SJ (1997) Cellular localization and distribution of cloned mu and kappa opioid receptors in rat gastrointestinal tract. Neuroscience 81: 579–591

Beier-Holgerson R, Boesby S (1996) Influence of postoperative early nutrition on postsurgical infections. Gut 39: 833–835

Benson MJ, Roberts JP, Wingate DL, Rogers J, Deeks JJ, Castillo FD, Williams NS (1994) Small bowel motility following major intra-abdominal surgery: the effects of opiates and rectal cisapride. Gastroenterology 106: 924–936

Boghaert A, Haesaert G, Mourisse P, Verlinden M (1987) Placebo-controlled trial in postoperative ileus. Acta Anaesth Belg 38: 195–197

Brathwaite CE, Ross SE, Nagele R, Mure AJ, O'Malley KF, Garcia-Perez FA (1993) Bacterial translocation occurs in humans after traumatic injury: evidence using immunofluorescence. J trauma 34: 586–590

Carr CS, Ling KDE, Boulos P, Singer M (1996) Randomised trial of safety and efficacy of immediate postoperative enteral feeding in patients undergoing gastrointestinal resection. BMJ 312: 869–871

Cataldi-Betcher EL, Seltzer MH, Slocum BA, Jones KW (1983) Complications occurring during enteral nutrition support. A prospective study. JPEN J Parenter Enteral Nutr 7: 546–552

Cerra FB, McPherson JP, Konstantinides FN, Konstantinides KM, Teasley KM (1988) Early nutrition does not prevent multiple organ failure syndrome (MOFS) after sepsis. Surgery 104: 727–733

Chen J, McCallum RW (1993) Clinical applications of electrogastrogram. Am J Gastroenterol 88: 1324–1336

Chen J, Schirmer BD, McCallum RW (1994) Serosal and cutaneous recordings of gastric myoelectrical activity in patients with gastroparesis. Am J Physiol 266: G90-G98

Chiarelli, Enzi G, Casadei, Bagio B, Valerio A, Mazzoleni F (1990) Very early nutrition supplementation in burned patients. Am J Clin Nutr 51: 1035–1039

Clevers GJ, Smout AJPM, Akkermans LMA, Wittepol P (1988) Restoration of gastrointestinal transit and colonic motility after major abdominal surgery; effects of cisapride. Surg Res Commun 4: 205–213

Cobb JP, Danner RL (1996) Nitric oxide and septic shock. JAMA 275: 1192–1196

Deitch EA (1990) Intestinal permeability is increased in burn patients shortly after injury. Surgery 107: 411–416

Desvarannes SM, Mizrahi, Dubois A (1991) Relation between postprandial gastric emptying and cutaneous electrogastrogram in primates. Am J Physiol 261: G248-G255

Doughty L, Carcillo JA, Kaplan S, Janosky J (1998) Plasma nitrite and nitrate concentrations and multiple organ failure in pediatric sepsis. Crit Care Med 26: 157–162

Evans T, Carpenter A, Kinderman H, Cohen J (1993) Evidence of increased nitric oxide production in patients with sepsis syndrome. Circ Shock 41: 77–81

Freye E, Knüfermann V (1994) No inhibition of intestinal motility following ketamine-midazolam anesthesia. A comparison of anesthesia with enflurane and fentanyl/midazolam. Anasthesist 43: 87–91

Furness JB, Costa M (1987) The enteric nervous system. Churchill Livingstone, Edinburgh

Gianotti L, Alexander JW, Nelson JL, Fukushima R, Pyles T, Chalk CL (1994) Role of early enteral feeding and acute starvation on postburn bacterial translocation and host defense: Prospective, randomized trial. Crit Care Med 22: 265–272

Gottfried EM, Plumser AB (1984) Endoscopic gastrojejunostomy: A technique to establish small bowel feeding without laparotomy: Gastrointest Endosc 30: 355–357

Grahm TW, Zadrozny DB, Harrington T (1989) The benefits of early jejunal hyperalimentation in the head-injured patient. Neurosurgery 25: 729–735

Gray RR, St Louis EL, Grosman H (1989) Modified catheter for percutaneous gastrojejunostomy. Radiology 173: 275–278

Hadfield RJ, Sinclair DG, Houldsworth PE, Evans TW (1995) Effects of enteral and parenteral nutrition in gut mucosal permeability in the critically ill. Am J Respir Crit Care Med 152: 1545–1548

Hallerbäck B, Bergman B, Bong H, Ekström P, Glise H, Lundgren K, Risberg O (1991) Cisapride in the treatment of postoperative ileus. Aliment Pharmacol Ther 5: 503–511

Harris CE, Griffith RD, Freestone N, Billington D, Altherton ST, Macmillan RR (1992) Intestinal permeability in the critically ill. Intensive Care Med 18: 38–41

Herbert MK, Arzet H, Holzer P, Roewer N (1997) Selective ligands for δ-opioid receptors have less inhibitory effect on intestinal peristalsis than μ- or κ-agonists in the guinea-pig ileum(abstract). Anesthesiology 87 [Suppl. 3A]: A646

Herbert MK, Kuhn H, Roewer N (1998a) Effect of racemic and S(+)-ketamine on the peristaltic reflex in guinea-pig ileum *in vitro*. Comparison to fentanyl. Anästhesiol. Intensivmed. Notfallmed. Schmerzther. 33, 613–614

Herbert MK, Kuhn H, Holzer P, Roewer N (1998b) Properistaltic effect of caerulein in guinea-pig ileum *in vitro*. Anästhesiol. Intensivmed. Notfallmed. Schmerzther. 33, 615

Herbert MK, Wenderoth H, Roewer N (1998c) Nitric oxide (NO) augments the inhibitory effect of midazolam on peristalsis in the guinea-pig ileum *in vitro*. Anästhesiol Intensivmed Notfallmed Schmerzther 33: 614-615

Heyland DK, Cook DJ, Guyatt GH (1993) Enteral nutrition in the critically ill patient: a critical review of the evidence. Intensive Care Med 19: 435–442

Holzer P, Lippe IT, Lotfi Tabrizi A, Lenard L Jr., Bartho L (1997) Dual excitatory and inhibitory effect of nitric oxide on peristalsis in the guinea pig intestine. J Pharmacol Exp Ther 280: 154–161

Jones TN, Moore FA, Moore EE, McCroskey BL (1989) Gastrointrestinal symptoms attributed to jejunostomy feeding after major abdominal trauma – a critical analysis. Crit Care Med 17: 1146–1150

Julou-Schaeffer G, Gray GA, Fleming I, Schott C, Parratt JR, Stoclet JC (1990) Loss of vascular responsiveness induced by endotoxin involves l-arginine pathways. Am J Physiol 259: H1038-H1043

Keller RS, Jones JJ, Kim KF, Myers PR, Adams HR, Parker JL, Rubin LJ (1995) Endotoxin-induced myocardial dysfunction: Is there a role for nitric oxide? Shock 4: 338–344

Kompan L, Kremzar B, Gadzijev, Prosek M (1999) Effects of early enteral nutrition on intestinal permeability and the development of multiple organ failure after multiple injury. Intensive Care Med 25: 157–161

Koruda MJ, Guenter P, Rombeau JL (1987) Enteral nutrition in the critically ill. Crit Care Clin 3: 133–153

Kudsk KA, Carpenter G, Petersen SR, Sheldon GF (1981) Effective enteral and parenteral feeding in malnourished rats with hemoglobin-*E. coli* adjuvant peritonitis. J Surg Res 31: 105–110

Kudsk KA, Stone JM, Carpenter G, Sheldon GF (1983) Enteral an parenteral feeding influences mortality after hemoglobin-*E. coli* peritonitis in rats. J Trauma 23: 605–609

Kudsk KA, Croce MA, Fabian TC, Minard G, Tolley EA, Poret A, Kuhl MR, Brown RO (1992) Enteral versus parenteral feeding. Effects on septic morbidity after blunt and penetrating abdominal trauma. Ann Surg 5: 503–511

Kuhn H, Herbert MK, Holzer P, Roewer N (1998) Metoclopramide has either no or an inhibitory effect on peristalsis in small intestine *in vitro*. Anasthesiol Intensivmed Notfallmed Schmerzther 33: 615

Landow L, Andersen LW (1994) Splanchnic ischemia and its role in multiple organ failure. Acta Anaesthesiol Scand 38: 626–639

Langkamp-Henken B, Donovan TB, Pate LM, Maull CD, Kudsk KA (1995) Increased intestinal permeability following blunt and penetrating trauma. Crit Care Med 23: 660–664

Le Voyer T, Cioffi WG, Pratt L, Shippee R, McManus WF, Mason AD Jr, Pruitt BA Jr (1992) Alterations in intestinal permeability after thermal injury. Arch Surg 127: 26–29

Liang J, Chen JDZ (1997) What can be measured from surface electrogastrography. Computer simulations. Dig Dis Sci 42: 1331–1343

Manara L, Bianchetti A (1985) The peripheral and central influences of opioids on gastrointestinal propulsion. Annu Rev Pharmacol Toxicol 25: 249–273

Manara L, Bianchi G, Ferretti P, Tavani A (1986) Inhibition of gastrointestinal transit by morphine results primarily from direct drug action on gut opioid sites. J Pharmacol Exp Ther 237: 945–949

Markus CK, Herbert MK, Arzet H, Holzer P, Roewer N (1998) Propofol and etomidate inhibit intestinal peristalsis in the guinea-pig ileum *in vitro*. Anasthesiol Intensivmed Notfallmed Schmerzther 33: 614

McClave S, Snider HL, Lowen DD, McLaughlin AJ, Greene LM, McCombs J, Rodgers L, Wright RA, Roy TM, Schumer MP, Pfeifer MA (1992) Use of residual volume as a marker for enteral feeding intolerance: prospective blinded comparison with physical examination and radiographic findings. JPEN J Parenter Enteral Nutr 16: 99–105

Milligan KR, Howe JP, McClean E, Dundee JW (1988) Postoperative gastric emptying in outpatient anesthesia: the effect of opioid supplementation. J Clin Anesth 1: 9–11

Minami H, McCallum RW (1984) The physiology and pathophysiology of gastric emptying in humans. Gastroenterology 86: 1592–1610

Mochizuki H, Trocki R, Dominioni L, Brackett KA, Joffe SN, Alexander JW (1984) Mechanism of prevention of postburn hypermetabolism and catabolism by early enteral feeding. Ann Surg 200: 297–310

Moore FA, Jones TN (1986) Benefits of immediate jejunostomy feeding after abdominal trauma: a prospective randomized study. J Trauma 26: 874–881

Moore FA, Moore EE (1995) Evolving concepts in the pathogenesis of postinjury multiple organ failure. Surg Clin North Am 75: 257–277

Moore FA, Moore EE, Jones TN, McCroskey BL, Petersson VM (1989) TEN vs. TPN following major abdominal trauma: reduced septic morbidity. J Trauma 29: 916–923

Murphy DB, Sutton JA, Prescott LF, Murphy MB (1997) Opioid-induced delay in gastric emptying. Anesthesiology 87: 765–770

Nimmo WS, Wilson J, Prescott LF (1975) Narcotic analgesics and delayed gastric emptying during labour. Lancet I: 890–893

Ochoa JB, Udekwu AO, Billiar TR, Curran RD, Cerra FB, Simmens RL, Peitzman AB (1991) Nitrogen oxide levels in patients after trauma and during sepsis. Ann Surg 214: 621–626

Pape HC, Dwengler A, Regel G, Auf'M'Kolck, Gollub F, Wisner D, Sturm JAQ, Tscherne H (1994) Increased gut permeability after multiple trauma. Br J Surg 81: 850–852

Pescatori M (1987) Effect of cisapride on clinical parameters on postoperative ileus. Prog Med 43 [Suppl 1]: 111–114

Petnehazy T, Scheidl S, Holzer P, Hammer HF (1998) Evaluation of the effect of neostigmine on peristalsis in the guinea pig ileum. Anasthesiol Intensivmed Notfallmed Schmerzther 33: 611–612

Petros A, Lamb G, Leone A, Moncada S, Bennett D, Vallance P (1994) Effects of nitric oxide synthase inhibitors in humans with septic shock. Cardiovasc Res 28: 34–39

Polak JM, Bloom SR (1979) Neuropeptides of the gut: a newly discovered control mechanism. World J Surg 3: 393–399

Porreca F, Cowan A, Raffa RB, Tallarida RJ (1983) Ketazocines and morphine: effects on gastrointestinal transit after central and peripheral injection. Life Sci 32: 1785–1790

Roumen RMH, Hendriks T, Wevers AR, Gorris JA (1993) Intestinal permeability after severe trauma and hemorrhagic shock is increased without relation to septic complications. Arch Surg 128: 453–457

Rush BF, Sori AJ, Murphy TF, Smith S, Flanagan JJ, Machiedo GW (1988) Endotoxemia and bacteremia during hemorrhagic shock. The link between trauma and sepsis? Ann Surg 207: 549–554

Sagar S, Harland P, Shields R (1979) Early postoperative feeding with elemental diet. Br Med J I: 293–295

Sanders KM, Ward SM (1992) Nitric oxide as a mediator of nonadrenergic noncholinergic neurotransmission. Am J Physiol 262: G379-G392

Schlag G, Redl H, Halstrom S (1991) The cell in shock: the origin of multiple organ failure. Resuscitation 21: 127–180

Schulz R, Panas DL, Catena R, Moncada S, Olley PM, Lopaschuk GD (1995) The role of nitric oxide in cardiac depression induced by interleukin-1ß and tumor necrosis factor-alpha. Br J Pharmacol 114: 27–34

Sinclair DG, Haslam PL, Houldsworth PE, Pepper JR, Evans TW (1995) The effect of cardiopulmonary bypass upon intestinal and pulmonary endothelial permeability. Chest 108: 718–724

Smits GJM, Lefebvre RA (1996) ATP and nitric oxide: inhibitory NANC neurotransmitters in the longitudinal muscle-myenteric plexus preparation of the rat ileum. Br J Pharmacol 118: 695–703

Sullivan DH, Nelson CL, Bopp MM, Puskarich-May CL, Wall RC (1998) Nightly enteral nutrition support of elderly hip fracture patients. A phase I trial. J Am Coll Nutr 17: 155–161

Suzuki N, Mizuno K, Gomi Y (1994) Role of nitric oxide in the peristalsis in the isolated guinea-pig ileum. Eur J Pharmacol 251: 221–227
Tagan D, Eckert P, Markert M, Feihl F, Schaller MD (1998) Blood nitrate levels in septic and cardiogenic shock. Clin Intensive Care 9: 71–76
Thiemermann C, Ruetten H, Wu CC, Vane JR (1995) The multiple organ dysfunction syndrome caused by endotoxin in the rat: attenuation of liver dysfunction by inhibitors of nitric oxide synthase. Br J Pharmacol 116: 2845–2851
Todd JG, Nimmo WS (1983) Effect of premedication on drug absorption and gastric emptying. Br J Anaesth 55: 1189–1193
Tollesson PO, Cassuto J, Rimbäck G, Faxen A, Bergman L, Mattson E (1991) Treatment of postoperative ileus with cisapride. Scand J Gastroenterol 26: 477–482
Van der Hulst RRWJ, Von Meyenfeldt MF, van Kreel BK, Thunnissen FBJM, Brummer RJM, Arends JW, Soeters PB (1998) Gut permeability, intestinal morphology, and nutritional depletion. Nutrition 14: 1–6
Van Rooy F, Creve U, Verlinden M, Hubens A (1988) Effect of cisapride on post-cholecystectomy upper gastrointestinal transit time. Int J Clin Pharmacol Ther Toxicol 26: 265–268
Verlinden M, Michielis G, Boghaert A, deCoster M, Dehertogs P (1987) Treatment of postoperative gastrointestinal atony. Br J Surg 74: 614–617
Von Ritter C, Hunter S, Hinder RA (1987) Cisapride does not reduce postoperative paralytic ileus. S Afr J Surg 25: 19–21
Waterman SA, Costa M (1994) The role of inhibitory motor neurons in peristalsis in the isolated guinea-pig small intestine. J Physiol 477: 459–468
Waterman SA, Costa M, Tonini M (1994a) Accommodation mediated by enteric inhibitory reflexes in the isolated guinea-pig small intestine. J Physiol 474: 539–546
Waterman SA, Tonini M, Costa M (1994b) The role of ascending excitatory and descending inhibitory pathways in the peristalsis in isolated guinea-pig small intestine. J Physiol 481: 223–232
Wenderoth H, Herbert MK, Roewer N (1998) The benzodiazepine midazolam inhibits the peristaltic reflex in guinea-pig ileum *in vitro*. Anasthesiol Intensivmed Notfallmed Schmerzther 33: 614
Wong HR, Carcillo JA, Burckart G, Shah N, Janovsky JE (1995) Increased serum nitrite and nitrate concentrations in children with sepsis syndrome. Crit Care Med 23: 835–842
Yuan C, Foss JF, Moss J (1995) Effects of methylnaltrexone on morphine-induced inhibition of contraction in isolated guinea-pig ileum and human intestine. Eur J Pharmacol 276: 107–111
Yuan CS, Foss JF, O'Connor M, Toledano A, Roizen MF, Moss J (1996) Methylnaltrexone prevents morphine induced delay in oral-cecal transit times without affecting analgesia. A double blind randomised placebo-controlled trial. Clin Pharmacol Ther 59: 469–475

INVITED ARTICLE

Potential of Motilides in the Treatment of Hypomotility Syndromes

T. L. Peeters

Center for Gastroenterological Research, Department of Pathophysiology, Katholieke Universiteit Leuven, 3000 Leuven, Belgium

Historical Perspective

The 22-amino-acid polypeptide motilin was discovered as a result of the study of the relationship between changes in duodenal pH and gastric motility (Brown et al. 1966, 1972). As soon as the synthesis of the peptide was achieved, it was logical for the effect on gastric emptying to be explored. However, the results were contradictory: acceleration, lack of effect and retardation were all reported, and given that the peptide was expensive and the methodology for measuring gastric emptying tedious, the topic was abandoned. Because intestinal pH changes also affect pressure in the lower esophageal sphincter (LES), attention was then directed to the effect of motilin on the LES, and the induction of a rise in basal LES pressure was soon demonstrated. Then the study of the physiology of motilin took a new direction with the discovery of the relation between plasma motilin levels and phase 3 of the migrating motor complex (MMC) in dogs (Itoh et al. 1978), just a few years after the MMC had been described in this species. This relation was soon confirmed in humans, and the finding that in dogs and in humans exogenous motilin induced phase 3 activity suggested that motilin's physiological role was the regulation of interdigestive motor activity. Despite numerous studies this hypothesis remains controversial.

In 1984 Itoh observed that erythromycin mimicked the effect of motilin and also induced phase 3 activity (Itoh et al. 1984). Soon erythromycin derivatives were developed with enhanced motility effects and decreased antibiotic potency (Omura et al. 1987; Itoh and Omura 1987). They were given the name motilides, and Takeda (Osaka, Japan) showed some interest in developing EM-523, a derivative synthesized by Dr. S. Omura at the Kitasato Institute in Tokyo, into a new drug. Because erythromycin induced a motilin release in the dog, Itoh et al. (1984) suggested that it acted through motilin. However, because erythromycin displaces receptor-bound motilin (Kondo et al. 1988; Peeters et al. 1989) and has the same regional and species specificity in vitro (Peeters et al. 1989), it appeared to act as a motilin agonist. The definitive proof for this hypothesis came with the development of the first motilin antagonists (Peeters et al. 1994; Depoortere et al. 1995).

Meanwhile, it was felt in our own group that with erythromycin as a (cheap) alternative for motilin, it would be easy to clarify the effect on gastric emptying. Assuming that a motilin agonist would accelerate gastric emptying, the effect of intravenous erythromycin was evaluated in patients with diabetic gastroparesis, and it was found that emptying of solids and lipids was markedly accelerated (Janssens et al. 1990). Presentation of these data at the meeting of the American Gastroenterological Associ-

M. K. Herbert et al. (Eds.), Problems of the Gastrointestinal Tract in Anesthesia...

ation in Washington in 1989 largely stimulated interest in this area, and the effect of erythromycin on gastrointestinal motility has since been explored in more detail by several groups (see below). The study indicated that motilides could find application in the treatment of gastroparesis and, in view of the known effects of motilin on the gastrointestinal system, also in other hypomotility syndromes. These considerations prompted several other drug companies to develop motilides and led to a reappraisal of the effects of motilin. In a way history was reversed, as it became of interest to show that motilin mimicked erythromycin. The effects of motilin on gastric (Schmid et al. 1991; Peeters et al. 1992a) and gallbladder emptying (Luiking et al. 1998), for example, received renewed attention.

Motilides

Itoh and Omura (1987) proposed using the name motilides for all macrolides with (a) a direct contractile effect in vitro on rabbit duodenal segments; and (b) the capacity to induce, in vivo, phase 3 activity in dogs. In view of their interaction with the motilin receptor they may now be redefined as macrolides acting as motilin agonists (Peeters et al. 1989).

Macrolides are lipophilic molecules composed of a lactone ring containing between 12 and 16 members (excluding nitrogen), to which one or two aminosugars or sugars are attached. They include a number of naturally occurring substances produced by actinomycetes, and semisynthetic derivatives of these products. Several natural macrolides are well-known antibiotics, such as erythromycin, streptomycin, aureomycin, oleandomycin and spiramycin. Semisynthetic antibiotics include roxithromycin, clarithromycin and azithromycin. All motilides now developed as candidate drugs are semisynthetic derivatives.

Structure–activity studies and considerations of stability and bioavailability, and probably also of patent rights, have led to the development of several candidate drugs. The first structure–activity studies were based on in vivo observations. They showed that 14-membered, but not 16-membered, macrolides induced MMCs in dogs (Itoh et al. 1985); that introduction of an enol configuration into the macrolide ring enhances the amplitude of antral contractile waves (Omura et al. 1987); and that contractile potency may be increased by changing the substituents of the 3'-amino function (Sunazuka et al. 1989; Tsuzuki et al. 1989). Later it was shown that the affinity for the motilin receptor of the rabbit antrum correlates with in vitro potency on the rabbit duodenum (Depoortere et al. 1989) and also with in vivo potency in the dog (Peeters 1993). The motilin receptor has therefore been proposed as a model for the development of motilides (Peeters and Depoortere 1994). This proposition is borne out by the fact that during the development of some compounds binding studies were used as a guideline. It will also be noted that macrolides with low affinity for the motilin receptor have less gastrointestinal side-effects and that motilides with a high affinity for the motilin receptor have low antibacterial activity.

The first compound with potent motility effects that was envisaged as candidate drug was EM-523 (Fig. 1). Probably because it has low bioavailability, it has been succeeded by EM-574 (also from Takeda, Osaka, Japan). In both compounds the macrolide ring is modified and contains an enol structure, a feature also found in all other

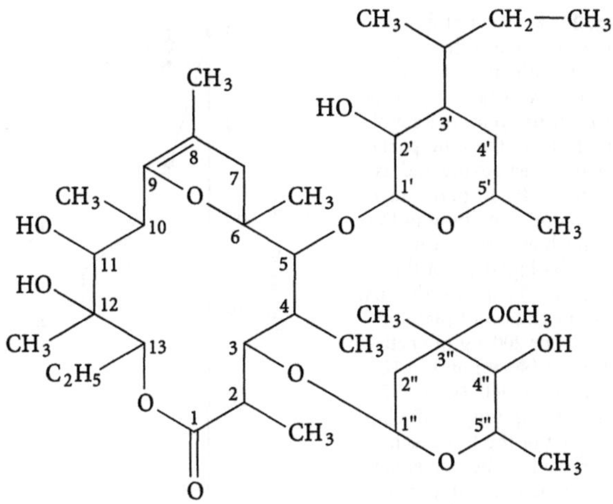

Fig. 1. Structure of EM-523, the first motilide developed as a candidate drug. In this compound an enol configuration has been introduced into the macrolide ring, and a methyl on the amino-N of the desosamine sugar has been replaced by ethyl. The full name of this compound is de(*N*-methyl)-*N*-ethyl-8,9-anhydroerythromycin A 6,9-hemiacetal. In EM-574 the ethyl is replaced by an isopropyl

motilides, because it is probably the most important feature enhancing potency. In EM-523 one of the methyl groups on the 3'-amino group is replaced by an ethyl, in EM-574 by an isopropyl. The enol moiety may easily lead to the formation of spiroketals which have low potency (Lartey et al. 1995). This can be prevented by blocking the hydroxyl on carbon-12, as is the case in ABT-229 (Abbott, Chicago, Ill.) and GM-611 (Chugai, Gotemba, Japan). Another approach is the shortening of the lacton-ring, as in KC-11458 (Kali Chemie, Hanover, Germany) and LY-274301 (Lilly Laboratories, Indianapolis, Ind.). EM-574, ABT-229, KC-11458 and GM-611 are presently undergoing clinical trials.

As yet few and limited data are available on these compounds, but the fact that erythromycin and motilin presumably have the same motility effects has been most useful in the exploration of their potential.

Therapeutic Potential of Motilides

Gastroparesis

The original report by Janssens et al. (1990) that erythromycin markedly accelerates gastric emptying in patients with diabetic gastroparesis (Fig. 2) has been confirmed by several groups. Erythromycin has also been successfully used in other conditions accompanied by gastroparesis, such as postvagotomy, systemic sclerosis, cancer therapy and anorexia nervosa, and reports continue to appear (Peeters 1993). Recently a meta-analysis compared the effect of cisapride, domperidone, metoclopramide and erythromycin and concluded that erythromycin was most effective in improving gastric emptying and metoclopramide, most effective in improving symptoms (Sturm et al. 1997).

Improvement of symptoms is indeed an important issue, and it is not always related to improvement of emptying. In so-called functional dyspepsia, for example, gastroparesis is probably related to the symptoms only in a subpopulation of patients.

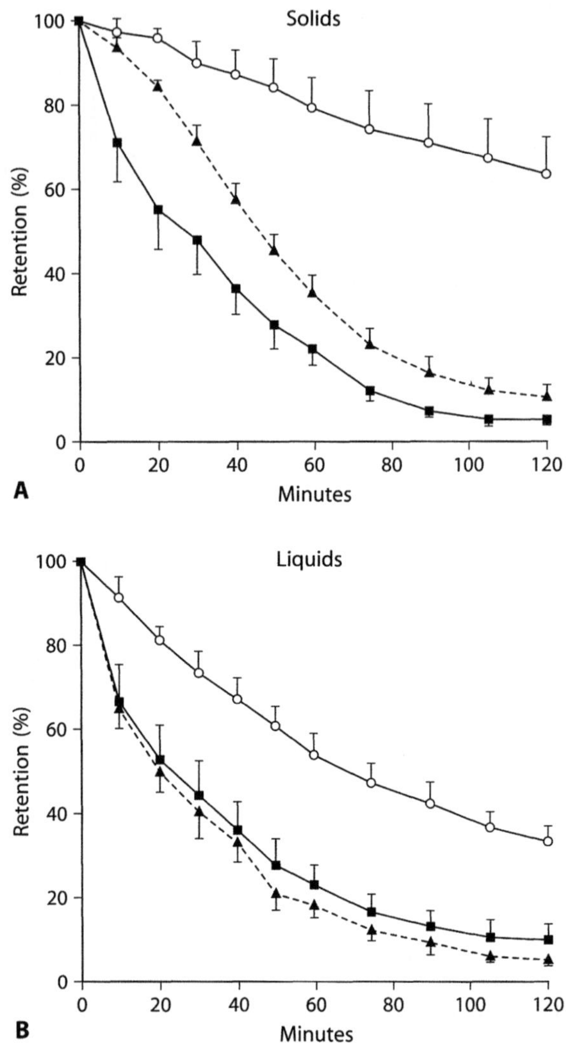

Fig. 2A, B . Rate of gastric emptying in healthy subjects and in patients with diabetic gastroparesis taking placebo or erythromycin. **A** Rate of emptying of the solid part of the test meal, expressed as the mean (±SE) percentage of isotope remaining in the stomach at various times after the ingestion of the meal, in 10 patients after i.v. administration of placebo (◇–◇) or 200 mg of erythromycin (◆–◆) and in 10 healthy subjects (◇–◇). **B** Rate of emptying of the liquid part of the test meal, expressed as the percentage of isotope remaining in 10 patients after the administration of placebo (○–○) or erythromycin (●–●) and in 10 healthy subjects (○–○). From Janssens et al. (1990), reprinted with permission

While in diabetics with gastroparesis the motilide EM523L improves insulin requirements (Ishii et al. 1997), and erythromycin improves dyspeptic symptoms (Samson et al. 1997), it may therefore well be that only a limited number of patients with functional dyspepsia benefit from an increase in their gastric emptying rate. Moreover, it is now known that the motor patterns responsible for the effect of erythromycin on gastric emptying include the induction of powerful peristaltic contractions in the antrum (Sarna et al. 1991), improvement of antroduodenal coordination, induction of phase 3-like patterns superimposed on the fed motility pattern (Annese et al. 1992), inhibition of pyloric pressure waves (Fraser et al. 1992), and enhancement of fundic tone (Des Varannes et al. 1995). It is certainly possible that in some dyspeptic patients the last effect may increase symptoms rather than reduce them, because impairment of fundic relaxation may also be related to dyspeptic symptoms. Another possible drawback may be that the induction of phase-3 like patterns is the reason why erythromycin abolishes the lag phase (Lin et al. 1994), and that the emptying rates of solids and liquids are the same (Janssens et al. 1990). This suggests that erythromycin accelerates gastric emptying at the expense of grinding and sieving. Indeed, in dogs erythromycin causes rapid gastric emptying of untriturated solids (Lin et al. 1994).

In volunteers in whom gastric emptying was retarded by motion sickness (induced by sitting in a rotating chair) erythromycin had no effect. This suggests that erythromycin is unable to reverse an inhibition that is most likely due to central mechanisms (Stewart et al. 1994).

Reflux Disease

Erythromycin increases LES pressure in man (Chaussade et al. 1994; Pennathur et al. 1993, 1994). In the cat the motilide LY-274301 increases basal LES pressure in a dose-dependent manner and increases the LES pressure lowered by instillation of HCl in the distal esophagus or by isoproterenol (Greenwood et al. 1994). However, these studies disclosed very limited effects on the esophageal body. The possibility that erythromycin induces the esophageal component of the MMC has received little attention; certainly the erythromycin analogue EM-523 had this effect in dog and in man (Itoh et al. 1991).

The effect on sphincter pressure and the gastrokinetic effect should reduce postprandial reflux, and this has indeed been found in two studies (Pehl et al. 1994; Pfeiffer et al. 1991). However, currently transient lower esophageal sphincter relaxations (TLESR) are recognized as the most common factor leading to reflux disease, and apparently erythromycin has no effect on their frequency (Sifrim, personal communication). This may explain why in patients with reflux disease erythromycin had no beneficial effect (Champion et al. 1994; Harrison et al. 1991).

Chronic Idiopathic Pseudo-obstruction

In chronic idiopathic pseudo-obstruction several reports indicate favorable effects obtained with erythromycin, but the data relate to only small numbers of patients or to case studies (Minami et al. 1996). Erythromycin is able to induce phase 3 activity in these patients, although the effect seems to depend upon the nature of the underlying disorder. Thus, in children without spontaneous phase 3 (Di Lorenzo et al. 1994) and in children with an underlying myogenic disorder (Cucchiara et al. 1997) it was without effect.

In may be noted that in children with the presumptive diagnosis of chronic intestinal pseudo-obstruction, erythromycin facilitates the postpyloric passage of tubes during duodenal intubation for antroduodenal manometry. The authors assume that propagating antral contractions sweep the tube through the open pyloric channel into the duodenum (Di Lorenzo et al. 1990).

Ileus

Motilin could benefit patients with postoperative or paralytic ileus, and certainly if one accepts that the return of the migrating motor complex marks the end of the ileus condition. Moreover, plasma motilin levels are decreased pre- and perioperatively, and the elevation postoperatively correlates with the return of normal motility (Rennie et al. 1980).

Shortly after the discovery of motilin, an attempt was made to use the peptide in patients with postoperative ileus, but without success (Ruppin et al. 1976). More recently in a preliminary study favorable results were found in 20 out of 25 cancer patients with paralytic ileus (Meyer et al. 1991). In dogs motilin shortens the reappearance time of the phase III activity in the stomach after laparotomy (Yokoyama et al. 1995). However, motilin did not ameliorate intestinal dysmotility and stasis after intestinal autotransplantation in dogs during the early postoperative period (Nakada et al. 1995).

Preliminary studies with motilides did also not lead to convincing data. In cholecystectomy patients erythromycin did not affect the appearance of flatus or bowel movements (Bonacini et al. 1993), although with EM-523 a dose-dependent decrease of the time before bowel sounds started was observed in a similar patient population (Hanyu et al. 1991).

Postoperative ileus is probably mostly caused by enhanced activity of inhibitory pathways. It may in fact correspond to a prolonged phase 1. It has long been known that during phase 1 the bowel is refractory to motilin. Thus, the dose of motilide or of motilin used, and the way it is administered (bolus or infusion), may be crucial.

Impaired Colonic Motility

In dogs intravenous erythromycin first induces a period of intense colonic motor activity, followed by a period of inhibition (Zara et al. 1985). Erythromycin also has a marked effect on the colon of the rabbit. In both species an effect of motilin has also been documented, and especially in the rabbit colon the density of motilin receptors is very high (Bickel and Belz 1988; Depoortere et al. 1991b).

In humans, however, the effect of motilin and erythromycin appears to be weak, limited to the fasted state and to the sigmoid region (Bradette et al. 1993). Perhaps this is because few motilin receptors are present (Van Assche et al. 1995).

In general the topic has received little attention, but it may deserve further exploration. Indeed one patient with reflex ileus and two with Ogilvie's syndrome have been successfully treated with erythromycin (Armstrong et al. 1991; Bonacini et al. 1991), while in a patient with pseudo-obstruction due to hereditary coproporphyria erythromycin had a marked effect when administered intravenously, although symptom improvement could not be maintained with oral therapy (Vassallo et al. 1992).

An increase in stool frequency after erythromycin has also been reported (Sharma et al. 1995).

Gallbladder

Erythromycin stimulates gallbladder contraction in normal volunteers, in postcholecystolithotomy patients, and in diabetics with autonomic neuropathy (Catnach et al. 1992, 1993; Fiorucci et al. 1992). The motilides EM-523 (Itoh et al. 1991) and KC-11458 (Eeckhout et al. 1994) are also effective. This seemed a surprising finding for a long time, as motilin was thought to have no effect. Recent studies, however, show gallbladder contraction after intravenous motilin (Luiking et al. 1998).

It has been suggested that motilides may find application in patients at risk of gallstone formation, such as those receiving parenteral nutrition, as a prophylactic to reduce recurrence, or to aid fragment clearance after extracorporeal shock-wave lithotripsy (Catnach et al. 1992).

Acute Applications (Intravenous Administration)

Intravenous erythromycin has been successfully used: (a) to empty the stomach before emergency surgery and in pregnant women undergoing cesarean delivery (Chaussade 1994); (b) to clear the stomach to facilitate endoscopy in patients with gastric stasis or with bezoar formation (Chaussade et al. 1992) and in patients with an obstructing blood clot in the cardia (Aubertin et al. 1995; Lawrence and McNally 1994); (c) to facilitate the postpyloric passage of tubes during duodenal intubation for antroduodenal manometry in children with the presumptive diagnosis of chronic intestinal pseudo-obstruction (Di Lorenzo et al. 1990); and (d) to facilitate the migration of an enteral feeding tube in volunteers (Keshavarzian and Isaac 1993) and in patients (Stern and Wolf 1994).

Mechanism of Action

Motilin's mechanism of action has not been fully elucidated. In vitro it induces contractions mediated via smooth muscle receptors in preparations from man, rabbit, cat and chicken. In vitro preparations from dog, rat and guinea pig, however, do not respond to motilin, although the dog has been the model of choice for the study of in vivo effects. In vivo, motilin's effect is neurally mediated, even in species in which a direct smooth muscle effect has been shown in vitro (man, rabbit). Motilin appears to stimulate the release of excitatory neurotransmitters via cholinergic, opioid and serotonergic pathways, but may also inhibit the release of inhibitory substances such as VIP and NO. A detailed review of these data is beyond the scope of this paper.

There is little doubt that in vitro motilides are able to interact with a motilin smooth muscle receptor. Motilin and motilides have the same species and regional specificity; share the same mechanism of action in vivo and in vitro; show cross-tachyphylaxis in vitro; and displace labeled motilin bound to rabbit antrum smooth muscle membranes (Peeters 1993). In the tissue bath, contractions of rabbit duodenal segments induced by motilides or motilin cannot be blocked by tetrodotoxin, atropine or hexamethonium, but are blocked by removal of calcium from the bath or calcium antagonists. The external calcium concentration affects motilin and erythromy-

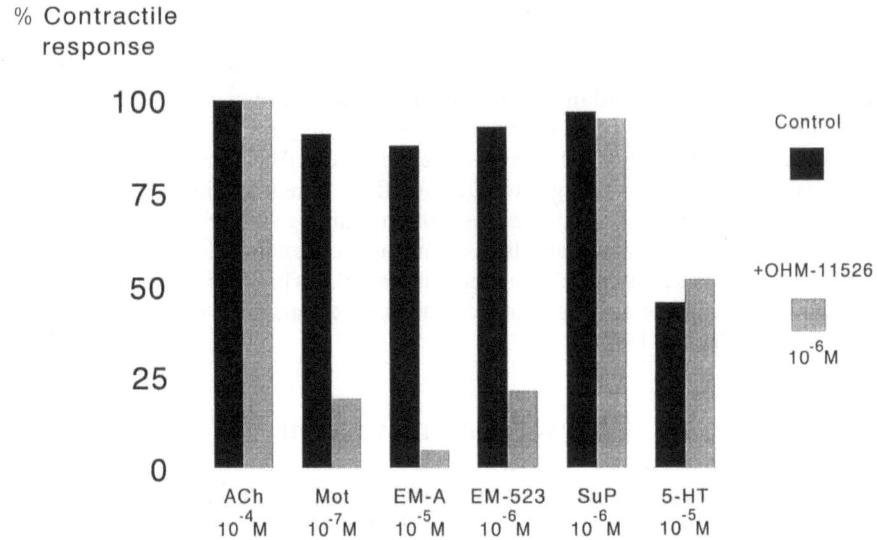

Fig. 3. Contractile response of rabbit duodenal segments to motilin (*Mot*, 10^{-7} M), erythromycin A (*EM-A*, 10^{-5} M), EM-523 (10^{-6} M), acetylcholine (*ACh*, 10^{-4} M), substance P (*SuP*, 10^{-6} M) and 5-hydroxytryptamine (*5-HT*, 10^{-5} M) under control conditions (response to 10^{-4} M acetylcholine is taken as 100%) and in the presence of 10^{-6} M of OHM-11526. Means of four experiments. From Depoortere et al. (1995), reprinted with permission

cin to the same extent (Peeters et al. 1991). Moreover, the transduction pathway of motilin and of motilides involves inositol phosphates (Depoortere and Peeters 1995). The definitive proof that all these observations are due to a direct interaction of motilides with the motilin receptor was obtained by the discovery of the first motilin antagonists which block motilide effects in vitro, as shown in Fig. 3 (Peeters et al. 1994; Depoortere et al. 1995).

In vivo, however, the effects of erythromycin are neurally mediated. The effect on the LES pressure is blocked by atropine (Chaussade et al. 1994), as is the effect on the stomach (Sarna et al. 1991) and on the gallbladder (Fiorucci et al. 1991). Serotoninergic pathways are also involved. Thus, 5-HT_3 antagonists prevent the initiation of antral phase 3 activity by EM-523 in dogs (Ohtawa et al. 1993) and by erythromycin in humans (Wilmer et al. 1993). Because the same is true for the in vivo effects of motilin, it seems likely that in vivo motilides, and motilin, act on a neuronal motilin receptor to increase the release of acetylcholine and perhaps other excitatory transmitters. This neuronal receptor is probably quite similar to the muscular one, because the potency of motilides to interact in vitro with the motilin receptor parallels not only the in vitro (Depoortere et al. 1989) but also the in vivo potency (Peeters 1993). The muscular motilin receptor has therefore been proposed as a model for the development of new motilides (Peeters and Depoortere 1994). Recently a central motilin receptor has been described in the rat cerebellum. This receptor, which is obviously not located on smooth muscle membranes, could be identical with the peripheral neural receptor, but further studies are needed (Depoortere and Peeters 1997).

The neural pathways are probably not located in the vagus, because erythromycin is still able to accelerate gastric emptying after vagotomy in humans and in dogs (Carlson et al. 1991). Because motilin and erythromycin are able to induce an MMC in an ex vivo rabbit intestinal preparation, an effect that is blocked by atropine, enteric cholinergic nerves appear to be involved (Marzio et al. 1994). Therefore one may assume that erythromycin acts on the myenteric plexus.

This hypothesis is supported by the findings that motilin and erythromycin act on the same subpopulation of myenteric neurons in the guinea pig antrum (Tack 1995) and that in the rabbit antrum motilin and ABT-229 enhance the response to electrical field stimulation (Van Assche et al. 1997, 1998). Apparently low concentrations stimulate the neural pathway, while higher concentrations may have a direct smooth muscle effect. This certainly corresponds with the observation in vivo that in the human antrum low concentrations of erythromycin induce phase 3 activity via an atropine-sensitive pathway, while higher concentrations induce antral contractile activity involving activation of a smooth muscle receptor (Coulie et al. 1998). The observation that in pseudo-obstruction the effect of erythromycin may depend upon the underlying disorder (see above) may also be understood in this perspective.

Motilin Analogues

As yet no compound has been reported with a higher affinity for the motilin receptor than motilin itself. It is not a surprise then that given via the intravenous route, motilin is more potent in stimulating gastrointestinal motor activity than the motilide EM-523. It is also more potent than accepted prokinetics, such as cisapride, metoclopramide and trimebutine (Inatomi et al. 1989). Therefore the peptide itself or peptide analogues may be considered as potential drugs, certainly if one takes into consideration that erythromycin has been shown to have its most pronounced effects when given intravenously.

A method has been developed by Kyowa Hakko Kyogo (Tokyo, Japan) to produce large amounts of the Leu^{13} analogue of porcine motilin by recombinant DNA technology (Miyashita et al. 1988). This compound is referred to as KW-5139, and the substitution of methionine by leucine in position 13 is aimed at stabilizing the product by preventing oxidation of the thiol group of methionine.

A similar approach was followed by Sanwa Kagaku Kenkyusho (Nagoya, Japan). In addition to the substitution of $methionine^{13}$ by leucine, their compound is extended at the C-terminal end with a homoserine lactone residue (Kurono 1990).

It has been shown that the biological activity of motilin resides in the N-terminal end and involves especially the residues 1, 4 and 7 (Peeters et al. 1989). An amidated 1–14 fragment has almost the same potency as the full-length peptide (Macielag et al. 1992). Based upon these observations an analogue was developed by Ohmeda (New Providence, N.J.), which received the code number OHM-11638 and corresponds to [*N*-trimethyl-$phenylalanine^{1}$, D-$arginine^{12}$, $leucine^{13}$, $lysine^{14}$] porcine motilin [1–14] amide. The modifications of residues 1 and 12 are aimed at protecting the compound against enzymatic degradation. This compound does accelerate gastric emptying in dogs (Macielag et al. 1995).

Conclusions and Perspectives

It is now well established that erythromycin has profound effects on gastrointestinal motility. Motilides may be useful in patients with gastroparesis and with a risk of gallstone formation. Given the limited number of therapeutic agents able to help patients with pseudo-obstruction, their potential in this condition certainly deserves attention. The usefulness in gastroesophageal reflux should not be discounted too quickly. Trials in gastritis, small intestinal bacterial overgrowth, postoperative ileus and constipation should be considered.

The most convincing data have been obtained after intravenous administration of erythromycin. The efficacy of oral therapy may be less, and the timing of the administration may be crucial. For example, in a patient with postvagotomy gastroparesis (Mozwecz et al. 1990) the drug was effective when taken 30 min, but not when taken 120 min prior to meals. Long-term treatment may pose another problem. As erythromycin is able to down-regulate the motilin receptor in the rabbit (Depoortere et al. 1991a), desensitization may develop.

Alternatives to the motilides for acute intravenous use are motilin or motilin analogues, but this remains to be explored.

Our laboratory maintains a hypertext review on motilides on the Internet, and this is soon to be expanded by the addition of a hypertext review on motilin. This information can be accessed via www.neurogastro.org, a site devoted to gastrointestinal motility.

Acknowledgements. The author's research is supported by grants from the Belgian National Science Foundation (NFWO grant no. G.3083.91) and the Belgian Ministry of Science (GOA 92/96–04 and IUAP P4/16).

References

Annese V, Janssens J, Vantrappen G, Tack J, Peeters TL, Willemse P, Vancutsem E (1992) Erythromycin accelerates gastric emptying by inducing antral contractions and improved gastroduodenal coordination. Gastroenterology 102:823–828

Armstrong D, Ballantyne G, Modlin I (1991) Erythromycin for reflex ileus in Ogilvie's syndrome (letter). Lancet 337:378

Aubertin JM, Levoir D, Becheur H, Bloch F, Petite JP (1995) Value of intravenous erythromycin before gastroscopy in the upper digestive hemorrhage (letter). Gastroenterol Clin Biol 19:645–646

Bickel M, Belz U (1988) Motilin and a synthetic enkephalin induce colonic motor complexes (CMC) in the conscious dog. Peptides 9:501–507

Bonacini M, Owen OS, Pritchard T (1991) Erythromycin as therapy for acute colonic pseudo-obstruction (Ogilvie's syndrome). J Clin Gastroenterol 13:475–487

Bonacini M, Quiason S, Reynolds M, Gaddis M, Pemberton B, Smith O (1993) Effect of intravenous erythromycin on postoperative ileus. Am J Gastroenterol 88:208–211

Bradette M, Poitras P, Boivin M (1993) Effect of motilin and erythromycin on the motor activity of the human colon. J Gastrointest Mot 5:247–251

Brown JC, Johnson LP, Magee DF (1966) Effect of duodenal alkalinization on gastric motility. Gastroenterology 50:333–339

Brown JC, Cook MA, Dryburgh JR (1972) Motilin, a gastric motor activity-stimulating polypeptide: final purification, amino acid composition, and C-terminal residues. Gastroenterology 62:401–404

Carlson RG, Hocking MP, Sninsky CA, Vogel SB (1991) Erythromycin acts through a cholinergic pathway to improve canine delayed gastric emptying following vagotomy and Roux-Y antrectomy. J Surg Res 50:494–498

Catnach SM, Fairclough PD, Trembath RC, Odonnell LJD, Mclean AM, Law PA, Wickham JEA (1992) Effect of oral erythromycin on gallbladder motility in normal subjects and subjects with gallstones. Gastroenterology 102:2071–2076

Catnach SM, Ballinger AB, Stevens M, Fairclough PD, Trembath RC, Drury PL, Watkins PJ (1993) Erythromycin induces supranormal gall bladder contraction in diabetic autonomic neuropathy. Gut 34:1123–1127

Champion G, Richter JE, Singh S, Schan C, Nellans H (1994) Effects of oral erythromycin on esophageal pH and pressure profiles in patients with gastroesophageal reflux disease. Dig Dis Sci 39:129–137

Chaussade S (1994) Does erythromycin have a therapeutic role in gastroenterology in 1994? Gastroenterol Clin Biol 18:917–919

Chaussade S, Michopoulos S, Sogni P, Guerre J, Couturier D (1994) Motilin agonist erythromycin increases human lower esophageal sphincter pressure by stimulation of cholinergic nerves. Dig Dis Sci 39:381–384

Chaussade S, Sogni P, Couturier D, Guerre J (1992) Intravenous erythromycin and gastric emptying. Gastrointest Endosc 38:733

Coulie B, Tack J, Peeters T, Janssens J (1998) Involvement of two different pathways in the motor effects of erythromycin on the gastric antrum in humans. Gut 43:395–400

Cucchiara S, Minella R, Scoppa A, Emiliano M, Calabrese F, Az-Zeqeh N, Rea B, Salvia G (1997) Antroduodenal motor effects of intravenous erythromycin in children with abnormalities of gastrointestinal motility. J Pediatr Gastroenterol Nutr 24:411–418

Depoortere I, Peeters TL (1995) Transduction mechanism of motilin and motilides in rabbit duodenal smooth muscle. Regul Peptides 55:227–235

Depoortere I, Peeters T (1997) Demonstration and characterization of motilin binding sites in the rabbit cerebellum. Am J Physiol G994-G999

Depoortere I, Peeters TL, Matthijs G, Cachet T, Hoogmartens J, Vantrappen G (1989) Structure-- activity relation of erythromycin related macrolides in inducing contractions and in displacing bound motilin in rabbit duodenum. J Gastrointest Mot 1:150–159

Depoortere I, Peeters TL, Vantrappen G (1991a) Effect of erythromycin and of octreotide on motilin receptor density in the rabbit. Regul Peptides 32:85–94

Depoortere I, Peeters TL, Vantrappen G (1991b) Motilin receptors of the rabbit colon. Peptides 12:89–94

Depoortere I, Macielag MJ, Galdes A, Peeters TL (1995) Antagonistic properties of [Phe^3,Leu^{13}]porcine motilin. Eur J Pharmacol 286:241–247

Des Varannes S, Parys V, Ropert A, Chayvialle J, Rozé C, Galmiche J (1995) Erythromycin enhances fasting and postprandial proximal gastric tone in humans. Gastroenterology 109:32–39

Di Lorenzo C, Lachman R, Hyman PE (1990) Intravenous erythromycin for postpyloric intubation. J Pediatr Gastroenterol Nutr 11:45–47

Di Lorenzo C, Flores AF, Tomomasa T, Hyman PE (1994) Effect of erythromycin on antroduodenal motility in children with chronic functional gastrointestinal symptoms. Dig Dis Sci 39:1399–404

Eeckhout C, Fioramonti J, Reling P, Hoeltje D, Buéno L (1994) Comparative effects of erythromycin and a new erythromycin derivative, KC 11458, on postprandial gallbladder emptying in dogs. Neurogastroenterol Mot 6:161

Fiorucci S, Bosso R, Morelli A (1992) Erythromycin stimulates gallbladder emptying and motilin release by atropine-sensitive pathways. Dig Dis Sci 37:1678–1684

Fraser R, Shearer T, Fuller J, Horowitz M, Dent J (1992) Intravenous erythromycin overcomes small intestinal feedback on antral, pyloric, and duodenal motility. Gastroenterology 103:114–119

Greenwood B, Dieckman D, Kirst HA, Gidda JS (1994) Effects of LY267108, an erythromycin analogue derivative, on lower esophageal sphincter function in the cat. Gastroenterology 106:624–628

Hanyu N, Aoki T, Itoh Z, Watanabe Y, Sugiyama M, Toyoda H, Ohmura S (1991) Effect of an erythromycin derivative, EM523L, on gastric motility in postoperative patients. Gastroenterology 100:A447

Harrison ME, Ruzkowski CJ, Young MF, Sanowski RA (1991) Erythromycin improves gastric emptying and esophageal motility without affecting gastroesophageal reflux. Gastroenterology 100:A80

Inatomi N, Satoh H, Maki Y, Hasimoto N, Itoh Z, Omura S (1989) An erythromycin derivative, EM-523, induces motilin-like gastrointestinal motility in dogs. J Pharmacol Exp Ther 251:707–712

Ishii M, Nakamura T, Kasai F, Baba T, Takebe K (1997) Erythromycin derivative improves gastric emptying and insulin requirement in diabetic patients with gastroparesis. Diabetes Care 20:1134–1137

Itoh Z, Omura S (1987) Motilide, a new family of macrolide compounds mimicking motilin. Dig Dis Sci 32:915

Itoh Z, Takeuchi S, Aizawa I, Mori K, Taminato T, Seino Y, Imura H, Yanaihara N (1978) Changes in plasma motilin concentration and gastrointestinal contractile activity in conscious dogs. Dig Dis Sci 23:929–935

Itoh Z, Nakaya M, Suzuki T, Arai H, Wakabayashi K (1984) Erythromycin mimics exogenous motilin in gastrointestinal contractile activity in the dog. Am J Physiol 247:G688-G694

Itoh Z, Suzuki T, Nakaya M, Inoue M, Arai H, Wakabayashi K (1985) Structure-activity relation among macrolide antibiotics in initiation of interdigestive migrating contractions in the canine gastrointestinal tract. Am J Physiol 248:G320-G325

Itoh Z, Mizumoto A, Hayashi N, Ohtawa M, Kawamura O, Kusano M, Sekiguchi T, Omura S (1991) Enhancement of contractile activity in man and dog lower esophageal sphincter (LES) by motilin agonist, EM523. Gastroenterology 100:A90

Janssens J, Peeters T, Vantrappen G, Tack J, Urbain J, De Roo M, Muls E, Bouillon R (1990) Improvement of gastric emptying in diabetic gastroparesis by erythromycin. Preliminary studies (see comments). N Engl J Med 322:1028–1031

Keshavarzian A, Isaac RM (1993) Erythromycin accelerates gastric emptying of indigestible solids and transpyloric migration of the tip of an enteral feeding tube in fasting and fed states. Am J Gastroenterol 88:193–197

Kondo K, Torii T, Omura S, Itoh Z (1988) Erythromycin and its derivatives with motilin-like biological activities inhibit the specific binding of 125-I-motilin to duodenal muscle. Biochem Biophys Res Commun 150:877–882

Kurono M (1990) Motilin-like polypeptide and the use thereof. European Patent Application 90100048.9

Lartey PA, Nellans HN, Faghih R, Petersen A, Edwards CM, Freiberg L, Quigley S, Marsh K, Klein LL, Plattner JJ (1995) Synthesis of 4"-deoxy motilides: identification of a potent and orally active prokinetic drug candidate. J Med Chem 38:1793–1798

Lawrence SP, McNally PR (1994) Intravenous erythromycin to clear the stomach of an obstructing blood clot (letter). Gastrointest Endosc 40:774–775

Lin HC, Sanders SL, Gu YG, Doty JE (1994) Erythromycin accelerates solid emptying at the expense of gastric sieving. Dig Dis Sci 39:124–128

Luiking YC, Peeters TL, Stolk MFJ, Nieuwenhuijs VB, Portincasa P, Depoortere I, van Berge Henegouwen GP, Akkermans L.M.A. (1998) Motilin induces gall bladder emptying and contractions in the fasted state in humans. Gut 42:830–835

Macielag MJ, Peeters TL, Konteatis ZD, Florance JR, Depoortere I, Lessor RA, Bare LA, Cheng YS, Galdes A (1992) Synthesis and in vitro evaluation of [Leu^{13}]porcine motilin fragments. Peptides 13:565–569

Macielag MJ, Gregory RL, Depoortere I, Florance J, Peeters TL, Ward J, KimDettelback J, Galdes A (1995) The motilin analog, OHM-11638, induces phase III-like contractions of the upper GUT and enhances gastric emptying in the conscious dog. Gastroenterology 108:A642

Marzio L, Grossi L, Martelli L, Falcucci M, Lapenna D (1994) Migrating motor complex recorded spontaneously and induced by motilin and erythromycin in an ex vivo rabbit intestinal preparation. Peptides 15:1067–1077

Meyer J, Sulkowski U, Preusser P (1991) Ergebnisse der Behandlung des paralytischen Ileus wegen diffuser intraabdomineller Metastasierung mit Motilin. Eine Pilotstudie an 25 Patienten. Med Klin 86:515–517

Minami T, Nishibayashi H, Shinomura Y, Matsuzawa Y (1996) Effects of erythromycin in chronic idiopathic intestinal pseudo-obstruction. J Gastroenterol 31:855–859

Miyashita E, Honda S, Saito A, Nishi T, Sekine S, Itoh S, Sato M (1988) High level production of a peptide hormone analogue [Leu^{13}] motilin in *E. coli*. Biotechnol Lett 10:763–768

Mozwecz H, Pavel D, Pitrak D, Orellana P, Schlesinger PK, Layden TJ (1990) Erythromycin stearate as prokinetic agent in postvagotomy gastroparesis. Dig Dis Sci 33:902–905

Nakada K, Ikoma A, Suzuki T, Reynolds JC, Campbell WL, Todo S, Starzl TE (1995) Amelioration of intestinal dysmotility and stasis by octreotide early after small-bowel autotransplantation in dogs. Am J Surg 169:294–299

Ohtawa M, Mizumoto A, Hayashi N, Yanagida K, Itoh Z, Omura S (1993) Mechanism of gastroprokinetic effect of EM523, an erythromycin derivative, in dogs. Gastroenterology 104:1320–1327

Omura S, Tsuzuki K, Sunazuka T, Marui S, Toyoda H, Inatomi N, Itoh Z (1987) Macrolides with gastrointestinal motor stimulating activity. J Med Chem 30:1941–1943

Peeters TL (1993) Erythromycin and other macrolides as prokinetic agents. Gastroenterology 105:1886–1899

Peeters TL, Depoortere I (1994) Motilin receptor: a model for development of prokinetics. Dig Dis Sci 39:76S-78S

Peeters TL, Matthijs G, Depoortere I, Cachet T, Hoogmartens J, Vantrappen G (1989) Erythromycin is a motilin receptor agonist. Am J Physiol 257:G470–G474

Peeters TL, Matthijs G, Vantrappen G (1991) The Ca-dependence of motilide induced contractions in rabbit duodenal muscle strips in vitro. Naunyn Schmiedebergs Arch Pharmacol 343:202–208

Peeters TL, Macielag MJ, Depoortere I, Konteatis ZD, Florance JR, Lessor RA, Galdes A (1992a) D-Amino acid and alanine scans of the bioactive portion of porcine motilin. Peptides 13:1103–1107
Peeters TL, Muls E, Janssens J, Urbain JL, Bex M, Van CE, Depoortere I, De RM, Vantrappen G, Bouillon R (1992b) Effect of motilin on gastric emptying in patients with diabetic gastroparesis. Gastroenterology 102:97–101
Peeters TL, Depoortere I, Macielag MJ, Dharanipragada R, Marvin MS, Florance JR, Galdes A (1994) The motilin antagonist Anq-11125 blocks motilide-induced contractions in vitro in the rabbit. Biochem Biophys Res Commun 98:411–416
Pehl C, Wendl B, Pfeiffer A, Schmidt T, Stellwag B, Kaess H (1994) Effect of erythromycin on postprandial reflux in patients with reflux disease. Gastroenterology 106:A158
Pennathur A, Cioppi M, Fayad JB, Little AG, Richter HM, Otterson MF, Maher JW (1993) Erythromycin, motilin, and the esophagus. Surgery 114:295–299
Pennathur A, Tran A, Cioppi M, Fayad J, Sieren GL, Little AG (1994) Erythromycin strengthens the defective lower esophageal sphincter in patients with gastroesophageal reflux disease. Am J Surg 167:169–173
Pfeiffer A, Wendl B, Pehl C, Kaess H (1991) Effect of erythromycin on gastroesophageal reflux. Gastroenterol Clin Biol 15:561–562
Rennie MJ, Christofides ND, Mitchenere P, Johnson AG, Bloom SR (1980) Motilin and human colonic activity. Gastroenterology 78:1243
Ruppin H, Domschke S, Domschke H, Wuensch E, Jaeger E, Demling L (1975) Effects of 13-Nle-motilin in man: inhibition of gastric evacuation and stimulation of pepsin secretion. Scand J Gastroenterol 10:199–202
Samson M, Jebbink RJ, Akkermans LM, Bravenboer B, van Berge Henegouwen GP, Smout AJ (1997) Effects of oral erythromycin on fasting and postprandial antroduodenal motility in patients with type I diabetes, measured with an ambulatory manometric technique. Diabetes Care 20:129–134
Sarna S, Soergel K, Koch T, Stone J, Wood C, Ryan R, Arndorfer R, Cavanaugh J, Nellans H, Lee M (1991) Gastrointestinal motor effects of erythromycin in humans. Gastroenterology 101:1488–1496
Schmid R, Schusdziarra V, Allescher HD, Bofilias I, Buttermann G, Classen M (1991) Effect of motilin on gastric emptying in patients with diabetic gastroparesis. Diabetes Care 14:65–68
Sharma SS, Bhargava N, Mathur SC (1995) Effect of oral erythromycin on colonic transit in patients with idiopathic constipation. A pilot study. Dig Dis Sci 40:2446–2449
Stern MA, Wolf DC (1994) Erythromycin as a prokinetic agent: a prospective, randomized, controlled study of efficacy in nasoenteric tube placement. Am J Gastroenterol 89:2011–2013
Stewart JJ, Wood MJ, Wood CD, Mims ME (1994) Effects of motion sickness and antimotion sickness drugs on gastric function. J Clin Pharmacol 34:635–643
Sturm A, Holtmann G, Goebell H (1997) Treatment of patients with gastroparesis: a meta-analysis of prokinetics. Gastroenterology 112:A833
Sunazuka T, Tsuzuki K, Marui S, Toyoda H, Omura S, Inatomi N, Itoh Z (1989) Motilides, macrolides with gastrointestinal motor stimulating activity. II. Quaternary N-substituted derivatives of 8,9-anhydroerythromycin A 6,9-dihydroerythromycin A 6,9-epoxide. Chem Pharm Bull (Tokyo) 10:2701–2709
Tack J (1995) Motilin and the enteric nervous system in the control of interdigestive and postprandial gastric motility. Acta Gastroenterol Belg 58:21
Tsuzuki K, Sunazuka T, Marui S, Toyoda H, Omura S, Inatomi N, Itoh Z (1989) Motilides, macrolides with gastrointestinal motor stimulating activity. I. *O*-Substituted and tertiary *N*-substituted derivatives of 8,9-anhydroerythromycin A 6,9-hemiacetal. Chem Pharm Bull (Tokyo) 10:2687–2700
Van Assche G, Thijs T, Depoortere I, Peeters TL (1995) Excitatory effect of motilin on the isolated human colon. Gastroenterology 108:A703
Van Assche I, Depoortere I, Thijs T, Peeters TL (1998) In the rabbit gastric antrum the neurogenic and myogenic effects of the motilide ABT-229 are mediated via motilin receptors. Neurogastroenterol Mot 10:106
Vassallo MJ, Camilleri M, Sullivan SN, Thomforde GM (1992) Effects of erythromycin on gut transit in pseudo-obstruction due to hereditary coproporphyria. J Clin Gastroenterol 14:255–259
Wilmer A, Tack J, Coremans G, Janssens J, Peeters T, Vantrappen G (1993) 5-Hydroxytryptamine-3 receptors are involved in the initiation of gastric phase-3 motor activity in humans. Gastroenterology 105:773–780
Yokoyama T, Kitazawa T, Takasaki K, Ishii A, Karasawa A (1995) Recovery of gastrointestinal motility from post-operative ileus in dogs: effects of Leu13-motilin (KW-5139) and prostaglandin F2 alpha. Neurogastroenterol Mot 7:199–210
Zara GP, Thompson HH, Pilot MA, Ritchie HD (1985) Effects of Erythromycin on gastrointestinal tract motility. J Antimicrob Ther 16:175–179

INVITED ARTICLE

The Pathogenesis of Postoperative Ileus in the Rat: Roles of Nitric Oxide, Vasoactive Intestinal Polypeptide and κ-Opioid Receptors

B. Y. De Winter[1] · J. G. De Man[1] · T. G. Moreels[1] · G. E. Boeckxstaens[1,2]
P. Robberecht[1,3] · A. G. Herman[1] · P. A. Pelckmans[1]

[1] Division of Gastroenterology and Pharmacology, University of Antwerp (UIA), 2610 Wilrijk, Belgium
[2] Division of Gastroenterology and Hepatology, Academic Medical Center (AMC), Amsterdam, The Netherlands
[3] Division of Biochemistry and Nutrition, Université Libre de Bruxelles (ULB), Brussels, Belgium

Introduction

Some excellent reviews are available on postoperative ileus (Livingston and Passaro 1990; Resnick et al. 1997a, b).

Postoperative ileus occurs to some degree after any abdominal operation, but it also occurs after extra-abdominal surgery. Ileus is defined as an inhibition of the propulsive intestinal motility, a failure of transport along the alimentary tract. Two different types of ileus can be distinguished: the mechanical ileus due to a structural inhibition, and the paralytic or adynamic ileus due to a functional inhibition of the propulsive intestinal motility. Postoperative ileus is the most common type of paralytic ileus (Dubois 1988). Clinically, postoperative ileus is characterized by abdominal distension, singultus, nausea, emesis, abdominal pain, constipation, and failure to pass gas. Clinical examination reveals a distended abdomen, tympanic percussion, and absence of bowel sounds. An X-ray of the abdomen is valuable: a step-ladder pattern occurs with air-fluid levels in the intestinal loops, presence of colonic gas, and colonic distension. The prognosis of postoperative ileus is usually good: in the majority of cases it resolves in 2–4 days (Dubois 1988; Kelley et al. 1993; Schröder and Möller 1987). Prolonged postoperative ileus occurs in 0.5–1.5 % of cases after abdominal surgery (Pichlmayr and Löhlein 1979).

However, the pathogenesis of postoperative ileus is still debated. Four major hypotheses concerning the pathogenesis of postoperative ileus have been put forward. The first hypothesis states that postoperative ileus is caused by hyperactivity of the inhibitory adrenergic neurons (Dubois 1988; Neely and Catchpole 1971). The adrenergic neurons inhibit gastrointestinal motility by decreasing the activity of the excitatory cholinergic neurons via activation of presynaptic α_2-receptors located on the cholinergic neurons. It is generally accepted that the inhibitory adrenergic neurons play an important part in the pathogenesis of postoperative ileus, but that other factors are also involved. Also, the numerous side-effects of adrenergic blockade limit their use in a clinical setting.

A second hypothesis incorporates the first and states that postoperative ileus results from the activation of a neural reflex pathway. The afferent limb of this pathway consists of capsaicin-sensitive sensory neurons, and the efferent limb consists of inhibitory adrenergic neurons. The importance of the afferent limb in the pathogene-

M. K. Herbert et al. (Eds.), Problems of the Gastrointestinal Tract in Anesthesia...

sis of postoperative ileus is demonstrated by several studies (Barquist et al. 1996; Holzer et al. 1986, 1992; Zittel et al. 1994).

The third hypothesis postulates a role for the enteric nervous system (ENS) (Dubois 1988; Livingston and Passaro 1990). The ENS can function independently of the central nervous system and consists of a network of small ganglia and connecting nerve fibers embedded in the gastrointestinal wall (Furness et al. 1992; Goyal and Hirano 1996). A population of the enteric neurons release neurotransmitters different from noradrenaline and acetylcholine; therefore, they are called nonadrenergic noncholinergic or NANC neurons. The NANC neurons release excitatory and inhibitory neurotransmitters and modulate gastrointestinal motility. The enteric inhibitory motor neurons release, among others, nitric oxide (NO), vasoactive intestinal polypeptide (VIP), pituitary adenylate cyclase-activating peptide (PACAP), and adenosine triphosphate (ATP) as neurotransmitters (Furness et al. 1992; Goyal and Hirano 1996). As these inhibitory NANC neurons are believed to provide the main inhibitory nerve supply to the gut, we hypothesized that postoperative ileus is caused by an hyperactivity of enteric inhibitory NANC neurons releasing inhibitory neurotransmitters such as NO and VIP.

A fourth hypothesis addresses the importance of hormones such as catecholamines and arginine vasopressin (AVP) (Dubois 1988; Livingston and Passaro 1990; Smith et al. 1977). During the stress response induced by surgery, several of these hormones are released. An increased release of catecholamines from the adrenal gland after surgery is demonstrated. Another hormone released during and after surgery is AVP.

At the moment, it is generally accepted that it is not one of these hypotheses, but the combination of these hypotheses that needs to be considered. The neural reflex pathway involved also needs further investigation. The nature of the afferent limb of the pathway, and the exact origin of the afferent limb, in the intestine and in other abdominal structures, needs to be studied. This could lead to new therapies reducing postoperative ileus by blocking the afferent and/or efferent limb of the reflex.

Role of Adrenergic Neurons and NO in the Pathogenesis of Postoperative Ileus (De Winter et al. 1997a)

Introduction

The activation of a neural reflex pathway plays an important part in the pathogenesis of postoperative ileus. In 1974, Furness and Costa described the existence of two types of intestinal adrenergic inhibitory reflexes: a low-threshold spinal reflex and a high-threshold peripheral reflex. Experimentally, postoperative ileus was markedly improved or prevented by chemical or pharmacological sympathectomy in several studies (Catchpole 1969; Dubois et al. 1973). However, after abdominal surgery adrenergic blockade did not always completely restore gastrointestinal motility (Heimbach and Crout 1971; Smith et al. 1977). Therefore, other mechanisms, such as an additional activation of inhibitory NANC nerves, which are believed to provide the main inhibitory supply to the gut (Burnstock and Costa 1973), may also have a role. Abrahamsson and Glise demonstrated the reflex activation of vagal nonadrenergic inhibitory fibers next to the stimulation of an adrenergic inhibitory reflex (Abrahamsson et al. 1979; Glise and Abrahamsson 1980). However, the exact nature of these vagal nonadrenergic inhibitory fibers remains unknown.

At present, NO is generally accepted as one of the main neurotransmitters of the inhibitory NANC nerves in different organ systems, including the gastrointestinal tract (Boeckxstaens and Pelckmans 1997; Rand and Li 1995; Stark and Szurszewski 1992). In the gastrointestinal tract NO plays an important role in several physiological reflex patterns, such as the receptive relaxation of the gastric fundus and the inhibitory component of the peristaltic reflex. Disturbances in NO biosynthesis have been implicated in numerous pathologic conditions such as achalasia, infantile pyloric hypertrophy and Hirschsprung's disease, and also in inflammatory conditions, such as ileitis, inflammatory bowel disease and sepsis (Goyal and Hirano 1996; Laszlo et al. 1995; Miller et al. 1993; Rand and Li 1995; Salzman 1995; Seago et al. 1995). Therefore, we investigated whether, in addition to the adrenergic pathway, an inhibitory nonadrenergic pathway is involved in postoperative ileus, and if so whether this pathway involves the activation of nitrergic nerves.

Development of a Rat Model

Male Wistar rats (150–250 g) were fasted for 48 h with free access to water. The rats were divided into three groups in a randomized way and underwent an operation under ether anesthesia. The first group underwent an abdominal skin incision (SI) after shaving and disinfection of the abdomen. The second group underwent a laparotomy (LAP) consisting of incision of the abdominal skin, abdominal muscle layers and peritoneum. The third group underwent a laparotomy followed by evisceration and manipulation (L+M) of the small intestine and cecum during 5 min. After the operations the rats were allowed to recover for 1 h. Then they received an intragastric injection of 0.1 ml Evans blue (50 mg in 1 ml 0.9 % sodium chloride) (Tanila et al. 1993) via a specially designed orogastric cannula introduced through the mouth. Twenty minutes later the rats were sacrificed under ether anesthesia and the intestinal transit was measured from the pylorus to the most distal point of migration of Evans blue and expressed in centimeters of migration, since the total length of the small intestine was not statistically different in the different groups.

In untreated rats (U) Evans blue migrated over a distance of 56.8 ± 4.1 cm ($n = 6$, Fig. 1). Neither ether anesthesia alone (E) nor skin incision (SI) had any effect on the gastrointestinal transit of Evans blue (Fig. 1). The transit after ether anesthesia was 61.5 ± 5.4 cm ($n = 5$), and the transit after the skin incision was 63.3 ± 2.3 cm ($n = 6$). However, laparotomy (LAP) significantly inhibited the intestinal transit to 29.1 ± 5.0 cm ($n = 7$, Fig. 1). Laparotomy associated with evisceration and manipulation of the small intestine and cecum (L+M) inhibited the transit even further, to 11.7 ± 1.8 cm ($n = 8$, Fig. 1). The transit after laparotomy and the transit after laparotomy plus manipulation were significantly different from the transit after the skin incision. The transit after laparotomy plus manipulation was also significantly different from the transit after laparotomy alone (Fig. 1).

By applying three different nociceptive stimuli, namely skin incision, laparotomy, and laparotomy plus manipulation of the small intestine and cecum, we achieved dif-

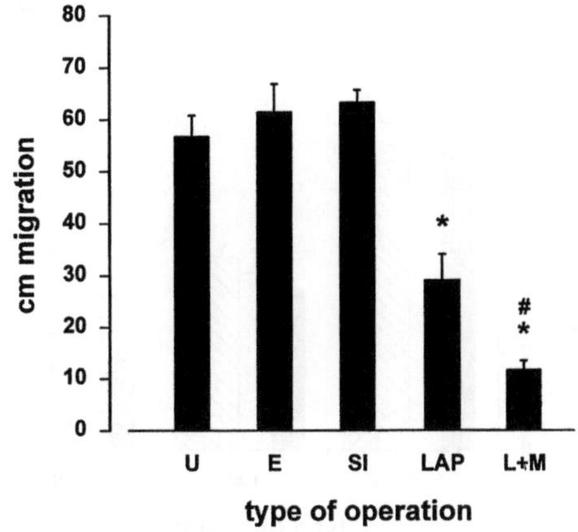

Fig. 1. Intestinal transit of Evans blue in untreated rats (*U*), in rats that underwent ether anesthesia (*E*) without abdominal operation and in rats that underwent a skin incision (*SI*), a laparotomy (LAP) or a laparotomy plus manipulation of the small intestine and cecum (*L+M*). Results are expressed as centimeters of migration of Evans blue and shown as mean ± SEM for ≥ 5. * $P \leq 0.05$, significantly different from the transit after SI; # $P \leq 0.05$, significantly different from the transit after LAP; one-way analysis of variance followed by the Bonferroni test

ferent degrees of inhibition of the intestinal transit. Ether anesthesia had no effect on the intestinal transit. Skin incision, resulting in the activation of somatic afferents, had no influence on the gastrointestinal transit and therefore served as control operation. Laparotomy, activating both somatic and visceral afferents, induced a significant inhibition of the gastrointestinal transit representative of postoperative ileus. This inhibition was more pronounced when the laparotomy was associated with mechanical stimulation of the gut, indicating that more intensive nociceptive stimulation results in an additional inhibition of the intestinal transit or a more pronounced ileus. Bueno et al. (1978) also demonstrated a different degree of disruption of the MMC pattern according to different stimuli. Therefore, we can conclude that the degree of nociceptive stimulation correlates with the degree of inhibition of the transit.

Result of Blockade of NO Synthase

Then we investigated the role of NO on the intestinal transit after the three operations. The rats were divided randomly into four groups. The first served as control group and received an intravenous (i. v.) injection of the vehicle in a tail vein 1 min before the operations. The second group received an i. v. injection of the NO synthase inhibitor L-nitroarginine 5 mg/kg in a tail vein. This dose of L-nitroarginine was previously shown to inhibit NO synthase in vivo in rats (Klabunde and Coston 1995; Wang et al. 1991). The third group was injected intravenously with the NO synthase substrate L-arginine 300 mg/kg. The dose of L-arginine was chosen in accordance with previous reports (Boughton-Smith et al. 1993; Laszlo et al. 1994). The fourth group received an i. v. injection of the combination of L-nitroarginine plus L-arginine. L-Nitroarginine, L-arginine and L-nitroarginine plus L-arginine had no effect on the transit after skin incision or laparotomy. The transit values were comparable to those obtained in control rats : 63.0 ± 3.7 cm after the skin incision and 32.4 ± 3.0 cm after the laparotomy (n = 9, Fig. 2). However, L-nitroarginine significantly enhanced the transit in rats that underwent a laparotomy plus manipulation of the small intestine and cecum, from 18.9 ± 1.7 cm (n = 9) in control rats to 34.1 ± 3.4 cm (n = 9) in

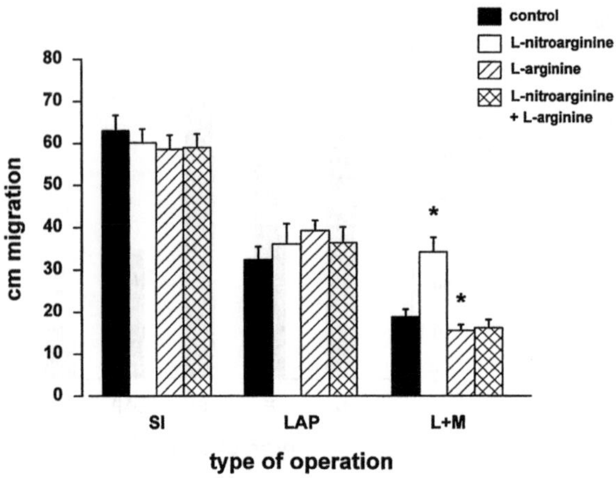

Fig. 2. Effect of skin incision (*SI*), laparotomy (*LAP*) or laparotomy plus manipulation of the small intestine and cecum (*L+M*) on the intestinal transit in control rats ($n = 9$) and in rats treated with L-nitroarginine (5 mg/kg, $n = 9$–11), with L-arginine (300 mg/kg, $n = 9$–10) or with the combination of L-nitroarginine plus L-arginine ($n = 9$). Results are expressed as centimeters of migration of Evans blue and shown as mean ± SEM. * $P \leq 0.05$, significant effect of the factors (L-nitroarginine, L-arginine) in rats that underwent L+M after two-way analysis of variance

L-nitroarginine-treated rats (Fig. 2). This effect of L-nitroarginine was prevented by concomitant administration of L-arginine (Fig. 2). L-Arginine alone caused a small, but significant, decrease in the transit after the laparotomy plus manipulation from 18.9 ± 1.7 cm in control rats to 15.6 ± 1.4 cm in L-arginine-treated rats ($n = 9$, Fig. 2).

After treatment with L-nitroarginine, the transit after laparotomy plus manipulation was no longer significantly different from the transit after laparotomy alone, indicating that L-nitroarginine was able to reverse the additional inhibition induced by mechanical stimulation of the gut.

In conclusion, treatment of the rats with L-nitroarginine, a NO biosynthesis inhibitor, did not affect the transit after the skin incision or the laparotomy. However, L-nitroarginine reversed the additional inhibition of the gastrointestinal transit induced by evisceration and manipulation, an effect prevented by concomitant administration of L-arginine, the substrate of NO synthase. Treatment with L-arginine alone had no effect on the transit after the skin incision or the laparotomy. However, L-arginine slightly, but significantly, increased the additional inhibitory effect of evisceration and manipulation. These findings support a role for an enhanced release of NO after mechanical stimulation of the gut.

Result of Adrenergic Neuron Blockade

To investigate the role of the adrenergic neurons, the rats were treated with reserpine, an adrenergic neuron-blocking drug. The rats were divided randomly into three groups. The first served as control group and received an intraperitoneal (i.p.) injection of the vehicle of reserpine 24 h before the operations. The second group received

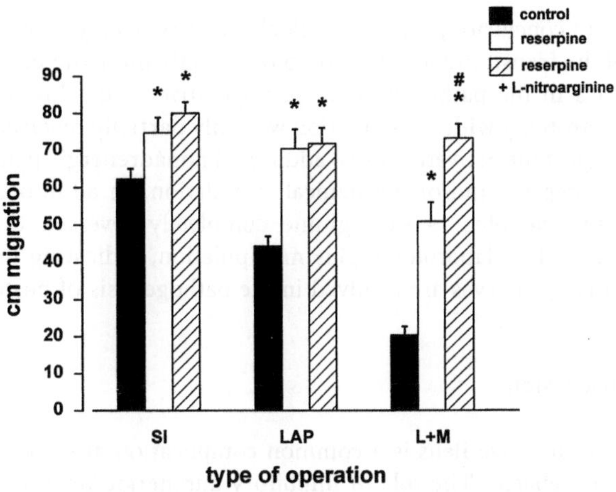

Fig. 3. Effect of skin incision (*SI*), laparotomy (*LAP*) or laparotomy plus manipulation of the small intestine and cecum (*L+M*) on the intestinal transit in control rats ($n = 9$–10) and in rats treated with reserpine (5 mg/kg, $n = 10$) or with the combination of reserpine and L-nitroarginine (5 mg/kg) ($n = 10$). Results are expressed as centimeters of migration of Evans blue and shown as mean ± SEM. * $P \leq 0.05$, significant difference from the transit in control rats with the same operation; # $P \leq 0.05$, significant difference from the transit in reserpine treated rats that underwent L+M; one-way analysis of variance followed by the Bonferroni test

an i.p. injection of reserpine 5 mg/kg (Boeckxstaens et al. 1991) 24 h before the operations. The third group received an i.p. injection of reserpine 5 mg/kg 24 h before the operations plus an i.v. injection of the NO synthase inhibitor L-nitroarginine, 5 mg/kg, in the tail vein 1 min before the operation.

Reserpine significantly increased the transit after the skin incision, from 62.2 ± 2.8 cm ($n = 9$) in control rats to 74.8 ± 4.1 cm ($n = 10$) in reserpine-treated rats (Fig. 3). The transit after the laparotomy was also significantly increased, from 44.3 ± 2.5 cm in control rats ($n = 9$) to 70.4 ± 5.3 cm in reserpine-treated rats ($n = 10$), abolishing the inhibitory effect on the transit induced by laparotomy alone (Fig. 3). After the laparotomy plus manipulation, the transit was also significantly enhanced by reserpine but not completely reversed, from 20.3 ± 2.3 cm in control rats to 50.8 ± 5.0 cm in reserpine-treated rats ($n = 10$, Fig. 3).

Treatment with reserpine plus L-nitroarginine had no additional effect on the transit after skin incision and laparotomy over that of reserpine alone ($n = 10$, Fig. 3). However, reserpine plus L-nitroarginine completely reversed the inhibition induced by laparotomy plus manipulation, from 20.3 ± 2.3 cm in control rats to 73.1 ± 3.8 cm in rats treated with reserpine plus L-nitroarginine ($n = 10$, Fig. 3).

In the rats treated with reserpine alone, the transit after laparotomy plus manipulation was significantly different from the transit after skin incision and after laparotomy alone. However, the difference between the transit after skin incision and the transit after laparotomy disappeared in the rats treated with reserpine alone. In the rats treated with reserpine plus L-nitroarginine the transit after skin incision, laparotomy and laparotomy plus manipulation were comparable, indicating a reversal of the inhibition induced by laparotomy with or without manipulation.

In conclusion, adrenergic blockade by reserpine completely reversed the inhibition of the transit induced by laparotomy, confirming the involvement of adrenergic pathways in the pathogenesis of postoperative ileus. However, the delayed transit after laparotomy with manipulation was only partially reversed by reserpine. These results suggest the activation of an additional nonadrenergic pathway following more intense nociceptive and/or mechanical stimulation. In addition, treatment of the rats with reserpine plus L-nitroarginine completely reversed the inhibition of the transit induced by laparotomy plus manipulation, indicating that both the adrenergic and nitrergic nerves are involved in the pathogenesis of postoperative ileus.

Discussion

Postoperative ileus is a common complication after surgery, and its pathogenesis is still debated. The role of inhibitory adrenergic neurons was investigated in our rat model of postoperative ileus by the use of reserpine, an adrenergic neuron-blocking drug. Reserpine completely reversed the inhibition induced by laparotomy alone, whereas the inhibition of the transit induced by laparotomy plus manipulation was only partially reversed, suggesting the activation of an additional nonadrenergic inhibitory mechanism by mechanical stimulation of the intestine.

Since NO is an inhibitory NANC neurotransmitter in the gastrointestinal tract (Boeckxstaens and Pelckmans 1997; Boeckxstaens et al. 1990; Bult et al. 1990), we investigated its putative role in the pathogenesis of postoperative ileus. L-Nitroarginine reversed the additional inhibition of the gastrointestinal transit induced by mechanical stimulation of the gut, an effect prevented by concomitant administration of L-arginine, the substrate of NO synthase. These findings support a role for an enhanced release of NO after mechanical stimulation of the gut. The combination of reserpine and NO synthase blockade completely reversed the inhibition of the transit induced by laparotomy plus manipulation.

The exact source of increased NO production after mechanical stimulation of the gut is not clear. Nitric oxide can be synthesized from L-arginine by three isoforms of NO synthase : two constitutive enzymes, namely the endothelial and the neuronal NO synthase, and an inducible enzyme. To identify the isoform of NO synthase involved, we investigated the effect of two selective inhibitors of the inducible NO synthase : *S*-methylisothiourea (Aranow et al. 1996; Southan et al. 1995; Szabo et al. 1994) and aminoguanidine (Wu et al. 1995, 1996). In our study, *S*-methylisothiourea and aminoguanidine had no effect on the intestinal transit after skin incision or after laparotomy, with or without manipulation, although these drugs were used in a concentration range shown to selectively inhibit the inducible isoform in vivo (Szabo et al. 1994; Wu et al. 1995). Therefore, the involvement of the inducible isoform of NO synthase is unlikely. The involvement of the endothelial isoform of NO synthase is difficult to exclude, since there are no selective inhibitors of this isoform. However, since L-nitroarginine and reserpine both have opposite effects on the blood pressure and since both have a beneficial effect on the transit after abdominal operations, it is not likely that the endothelial isoform of NO synthase is involved. Therefore, our results suggest that the enhanced release of NO is most probably produced by the constitutive neuronal rather than by the inducible NO synthase.

Role of VIP in the Pathogenesis of Postoperative Ileus
(De Winter et al. 1998)

Introduction

VIP (vasoactive intestinal polypeptide) and NO are both postulated as inhibitory neurotransmitters of the enteric nervous system (Boeckxstaens et al. 1991; Furness et al. 1992; Goyal and Hirano 1996; Goyal et al. 1980; Grider and Rivière 1990). Colocalization of VIP and NO was demonstrated in the enteric neurons of the guinea pig, opossum and rat gastrointestinal tract (Costa et al. 1992; Ekblad et al. 1994; Lynn et al. 1995). We have previously shown in our model of postoperative ileus that mechanical stimulation of the small intestine and cecum triggers a nonadrenergic pathway mediated by NO. Blockade of NO synthase by the arginine analogue L-nitroarginine completely reversed the additional inhibition of the transit induced by mechanical stimulation of the gut. On the other hand, several authors suggest an involvement of VIP in the pathophysiology of small bowel obstruction and postoperative ileus (Basson et al. 1989; Espat et al. 1995). Espat et al. reported an improvement in postoperative small bowel transit in the rat after treatment with a nonselective VIP receptor antagonist, VIP-ra (D-*p*-Cl-Phe^6, Leu^{17}) VIP (Espat et al. 1995).

The VIP receptors are a subclass of PACAP (pituitary adenylate cyclase activating polypeptide) type II receptors. The PACAP type II receptors are equally activated by PACAP and VIP. The PACAP type I receptors have greater affinity for PACAP than for VIP. The VIP receptors are now officially classified as VIP/PACAP receptors in the PACAP type II receptor class (Usdin et al. 1994). Recently the VIP_1/PACAP (VIP_1) and VIP_2/PACAP (VIP_2) receptors were cloned showing different distributions in the rat (Usdin et al. 1994). The VIP_2 receptor mRNA was most abundant in the stomach, whereas VIP_1 receptor mRNA was mostly present in the small intestine. Subsequently, VIP_1 and VIP_2 receptor agonists and antagonists were developed. Ac-His^1, D-Phe^2, K^{15}, R^{16}, VIP(3–7), GRF(8–27)-NH_2, a high-affinity selective antagonist of the VIP_1 receptor was synthesized and shown to be selective for the rat VIP_1 receptor in vitro (Gourlet et al. 1997a). This VIP_1 receptor antagonist was synthesized by analogy with the selective VIP_1 receptor agonist derived from growth hormone releasing factor (GRF) : K^{15}, R^{16}, VIP (1–7), GRF (8–27)-NH_2 (Gourlet et al. 1997b). RO 25-1553 was proven to be a highly selective VIP_2 receptor agonist in vitro (Gourlet et al. 1997c). Therefore, in the present study we investigated the effect of the selective VIP_1 receptor agonist and antagonist and VIP_2 receptor agonist in our rat model of postoperative ileus.

Result of Treatment with VIP_1/PACAP Receptor Agonists and Antagonists

We investigated the effect of the VIP_1 receptor agonist and the VIP_1 receptor antagonist on the intestinal transit after the three different operations. The rats were randomly divided into four groups. The first group served as control group and received an i.v. injection of the vehicle in the tail vein. Then the rats underwent a skin incision, laparotomy or laparotomy plus manipulation. The second group received an i.v.

injection of the VIP_1 receptor antagonist Ac-His[1], D-Phe[2], K[15], R[16], VIP(3–7), GRF(8–27)-NH_2 (5 μg/kg) 1 min before the operations (Gourlet et al. 1997a). The third group received an i.v. injection of a comparable dose of the VIP_1 receptor agonist K[15], R[16], VIP (1–7), GRF (8–27)-NH_2 (5 μg/kg) 1 min before the operations (Gourlet et al. 1997b). The fourth group was injected i.v. with the VIP_1 receptor antagonist immediately followed by an i.v. injection of the VIP_1 receptor agonist 1 min before the operations.

In control rats, treated with the vehicle, the transit after skin incision was 55.5 ± 3.2 cm. The laparotomy significantly delayed the transit to 43.1 ± 2.6 cm. This inhibition was more pronounced when the laparotomy was followed by a manipulation of the gut: the transit was 17.8 ± 1.8 cm (n = 9; Fig. 4).

Treatment of the rats with the VIP_1 receptor antagonist, the VIP_1 receptor agonist or the combination of the VIP_1 receptor antagonist and agonist had no effect on the transit after skin incision or laparotomy (n = 9; Fig. 4). However, the VIP_1 receptor antagonist significantly increased the transit after laparotomy plus manipulation from 17.8 ± 1.8 cm in control rats to 25.8 ± 2.3 cm in rats treated with the VIP_1 receptor antagonist (n = 9; Fig. 4). The VIP_1 receptor agonist, on the contrary, caused a small, but significant decrease in the transit after laparotomy plus manipulation from 17.8 ± 1.8 cm in control rats to 13.3 ± 2.1 cm in rats treated with the VIP_1 receptor agonist (n = 9; Fig. 4). The effect of the VIP_1 receptor antagonist and the effect of the VIP_1 receptor agonist were abolished when both treatments were combined: the transit after the laparotomy plus manipulation was 17.7 ± 2.5 cm (n = 9) and thus comparable to the transit after laparotomy plus manipulation in control rats (Fig. 4). However, even after the administration of the VIP_1 receptor antagonist, the transit after

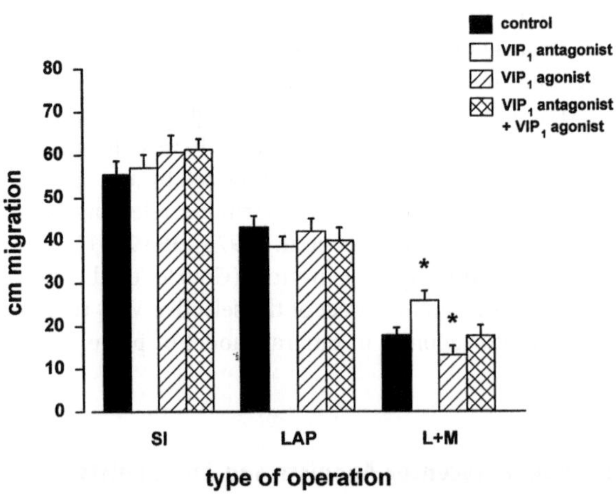

Fig. 4. Effect of skin incision (*SI*), laparotomy (*LAP*) or laparotomy plus manipulation of the small intestine and cecum (*L+M*) on the intestinal transit in control rats (n = 9) and in rats treated with the VIP_1 receptor antagonist (5 μg/kg, n = 9) or with the VIP_1 receptor agonist (5 μg/kg, n = 9) or with the combination of the VIP_1 receptor antagonist and the VIP_1 receptor agonist (n = 9). Results are expressed as centimeters of migration of Evans blue and shown as mean ± SEM. * $P \leq 0.05$, significant effect of the two factors (VIP_1 receptor antagonist, VIP_1 receptor agonist) after two-way analysis of variance

laparotomy plus manipulation was still significantly different from the transit after skin incision or laparotomy in all treatment groups, indicating that the VIP_1 receptor antagonist was not able to completely reverse the additional inhibition induced by mechanical stimulation of the gut.

In conclusion, the VIP_1 receptor agonist significantly enhanced the inhibition of the transit induced by mechanical stimulation of the gut. The VIP_1 receptor antagonist, in contrast, significantly improved the transit after the laparotomy plus manipulation. The effect of the VIP_1 receptor antagonist or agonist on the transit after the laparotomy plus manipulation disappeared when both treatments were combined. However, the VIP_2 receptor agonist was not able to alter the effect of the VIP_1 receptor antagonist on the transit after the laparotomy plus manipulation, and the VIP_2 receptor agonist also had no effect on the transit after the laparotomy plus manipulation on itself (De Winter et al. 1998), suggesting a specific effect on the VIP_1 receptor.

Discussion

We previously showed the involvement of NO in the additional inhibition of the transit induced by mechanical stimulation of the gut (De Winter et al. 1997a). In this chapter, we demonstrate an increased release of VIP, acting on VIP_1 receptors, after mechanical stimulation of the gut resulting in an inhibition of the gastrointestinal transit. This effect is specific for the VIP_1 receptor and is not altered by a VIP_2 receptor agonist. Previously, Espat et al. (1995) reported a beneficial effect of a nonselective VIP receptor antagonist on postoperative small bowel transit and a faster return of the migrating motor complex. However, the VIP_1 receptor antagonist was not able to reverse the additional inhibition of the transit induced by mechanical stimulation of the gut completely as did NO synthase blockade. The difference between the transit after laparotomy alone and the transit after laparotomy plus manipulation remained significant after treatment with the VIP_1 receptor antagonist. This may result from incomplete blockade of VIP receptors or from the involvement of another inhibitory neurotransmitter. Therefore, we can conclude that during mechanical stimulation of the gut VIP is also released, as well as NO, acting on VIP_1 receptors.

Role of Opioids in the Pathogenesis of Postoperative Ileus
(De Winter et al. 1997b)

Introduction

Opioids are widely used after abdominal surgery to control postoperative pain. Opioids can act on different receptors : three main receptor subtypes are known, namely μ-, κ- and δ-opioid receptors (Dhawan et al. 1996; Jaffe and Martin 1985). The most widely used opioid for analgesia is morphine, a preferential μ-opioid receptor agonist (Jaffe and Martin 1985; Livingston and Passaro 1990). In humans and rats, morphine was previously shown to delay gastric emptying, to inhibit small intestinal transit and to delay colonic transit, leading to its well-known complication of constipation. These effects of morphine are mediated by both central and peripheral pathways (Asai et al. 1997; Benson et al. 1994; Brown et al. 1988; Bueno et al. 1997; Galligan and Burks 1983; Kaufman et al. 1988; Manara et al. 1986; Thörn et al. 1996; Weisbrodt et al. 1980). However, morphine can increase intestinal and colonic electrical activity, but this increased activity did not result in effective propulsion, therefore the increased activity is defined as nonmigrating activity (Ferraz et al. 1995; Jaffe and Martin 1985; Livingston and Passaro 1990; Thörn et al. 1996). Opioids such as morphine are also known to prolong postoperative ileus (Ferraz et al. 1995; Livingston and Passaro 1990; Yukioka et al. 1987). Therefore, avoidance of opioids in the immediate postoperative period will lessen the postoperative ileus, but an alternative analgesic strategy is required to control the postoperative pain.

In contrast to morphine, fedotozine, a new peripheral κ-opioid receptor agonist, is able to reverse the inhibition of the gastrointestinal transit induced by peritoneal irritation in rats, suggesting a potential role in the treatment of ileus (Friese et al. 1997; Rivière et al. 1993, 1994). Peripheral κ-opioid receptor agonists also have analgesic properties (Bueno et al. 1997; Diop et al. 1994; Friese et al. 1997; Langlois et al. 1994). Friese et al. demonstrated a good correlation between the antinociceptive effect of κ-opioid receptor agonists and their potency to reverse ileus induced by peritoneal irritation (Friese et al. 1997). Sengupta et al. (1996) also suggested a role for peripheral κ- and not μ- or δ-opioid receptors in the modulation of visceral nociception. In the gastrointestinal tract both μ- and κ-opioid receptors are present on neurons in the myenteric and submucosal plexus and on the interstitial cells of Cajal (Fickel et al. 1997; Sengupta et al. 1996). Interstitial cells of Cajal are postulated to be pacemakers in the generation of the autorhythmicity of the gastrointestinal smooth muscles, conductors of excitable events, and mediators of the enteric neurotransmission (Sanders 1996). Therefore, the purpose of the present study was to investigate the role of μ- and κ-opioid receptors in experimental ileus induced by abdominal surgery. If κ-opioid receptor agonists are able to reverse ileus induced by abdominal surgery, they may represent an alternative to morphine for the treatment of postoperative pain.

Result of Treatment with a μ-Opioid Receptor Agonist

In a first series of experiments the effects of morphine, a preferential μ-opioid receptor agonist (Jaffe and Martin 1985), and naloxone, a nonselective opioid receptor antagonist (Jaffe and Martin 1985), were tested on the intestinal transit of Evans blue. The rats were randomly divided into four groups. The first group served as control group and received an intravenous (i.v.) injection of vehicle in a tail vein. Then the rats underwent a skin incision, laparotomy or laparotomy plus manipulation. The second group received an i.v. injection of morphine 1 mg/kg 1 min before the operations. This dose of morphine was previously shown to induce antinociception and to inhibit the small intestinal transit in the rat (Friese et al. 1997; Manara et al. 1986; Weisbrodt et al. 1980). The third group received an i.v. injection of naloxone 1 mg/kg 1 min before the operations. Naloxone is a nonselective opioid receptor antagonist blocking both μ- and κ-opioid receptors in this dose (Diop et al. 1994; Sengupta et al.

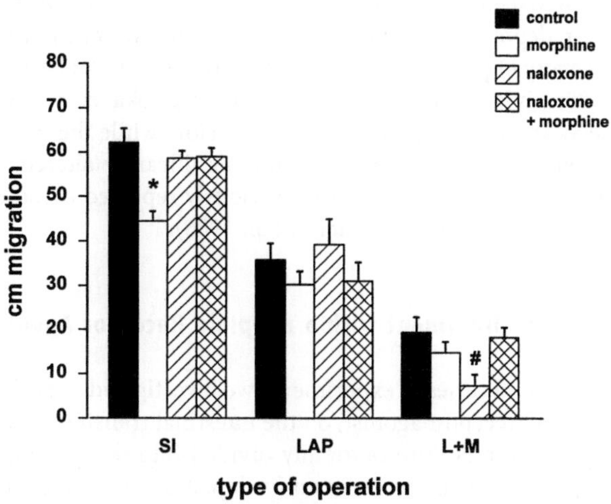

Fig. 5. Effect of skin incision (*SI*), laparotomy (*LAP*) or laparotomy plus manipulation of the small intestine and cecum (*L+M*) on the intestinal transit in control rats (*solid bars*, $n = 10$) and in rats treated with morphine (1 mg/kg, $n = 9–10$) or with naloxone (1 mg/kg, $n = 9–10$) or with naloxone plus morphine ($n = 9–10$). Results are expressed as centimeters of migration of Evans blue and shown as mean ± SEM. * $P \leq 0.05$, significant difference from the transit in rats that underwent SI; # $P \leq 0.05$ significant difference from the transit in control rats or rats treated with naloxone plus morphine after L+M; one-way analysis of variance followed by the Bonferroni test

1996). The fourth group was injected i.v. with naloxone 1 mg/kg, followed by an i.v. injection of morphine 1 mg/kg, 1 min before the operations.

Morphine significantly inhibited the transit after skin incision, from 62.2 ± 3.2 cm in control rats to 44.5 ± 2.2 cm in morphine-treated rats ($n = 10$) (Fig. 5). Although morphine tended to decrease the transit after laparotomy with or without manipulation compared with that in control rats, no statistical significance was reached (Fig. 5). Naloxone alone had no effect on the transit after skin incision or laparotomy compared with control rats ($n = 9–10$) (Fig. 5). However, the transit after laparotomy plus manipulation was significantly inhibited by naloxone from 19.3 ± 3.5 cm in control rats to 7.4 ± 2.5 cm in naloxone-treated rats ($n = 10$) (Fig. 5).

Consecutive injection of naloxone and morphine reversed the inhibitory effect of morphine on the transit after the skin incision from 44.5 ± 2.2 cm ($n = 10$) in morphine-treated rats to 59.0 ± 2.0 cm ($n = 9$) in rats treated with the combination of naloxone and morphine, comparable to the transit in control rats (Fig. 5). The combination of naloxone and morphine had no effect on the transit after the laparotomy (Fig. 5). However, naloxone plus morphine also reversed the inhibitory effect of naloxone on the transit after the laparotomy plus manipulation, from 7.4 ± 2.5 cm ($n = 10$) in rats treated with naloxone alone to 18.2 ± 2.2 cm ($n = 9$) in rats treated with the combination of naloxone and morphine. Also, this transit is comparable to the transit in control rats after laparotomy plus manipulation (Fig. 5).

The transit after skin incision was significantly different from the transit after laparotomy with or without manipulation in the different treatment groups. There was also a statistical significant difference between the transit after laparotomy and the transit after laparotomy plus manipulation in the different treatment groups.

Opioids such as morphine are widely used to control postoperative pain despite their depressant activity on the gastrointestinal motility leading to a delay in the recovery of postoperative ileus (Benson et al. 1994; Ferraz et al. 1995; Jaffe and Martin 1985; Livingston and Passaro 1990; Yukioka et al. 1987). Morphine significantly delayed the transit after the skin incision, while the transit after the laparotomy with or without manipulation was not significantly altered. The effect of morphine was reversed by naloxone as also previously reported by others (Brown et al. 1988; Galligan and Burks 1983; Manara et al. 1986).

Result of Treatment with a κ-Opioid Receptor Agonist

In a second series of experiments we investigated the effect of fedotozine, a peripheral κ-opioid receptor agonist, on the intestinal transit of Evans blue after the three operations. The rats were randomly divided into three groups. The first group served as control group and received an i.v. injection of vehicle. The second group was injected i.v. with fedotozine 5 mg/kg, 1 min before the operations. The dose of fedotozine was previously shown to induce antinociception and to reverse the inhibition of the gastrointestinal motility induced by peritoneal irritation in the rat (Diop et al. 1994; Rivière et al. 1993, 1994). The third group received an i.v. injection of naloxone 1 mg/kg followed by an i.v. injection of fedotozine 5 mg/kg 1 min before the operations.

Fedotozine had no effect on the transit after skin incision or laparotomy as compared with control rats (n = 9–10) (Fig. 6). However, fedotozine significantly enhanced the transit after the laparotomy plus manipulation from 20.4 ± 2.7 cm in

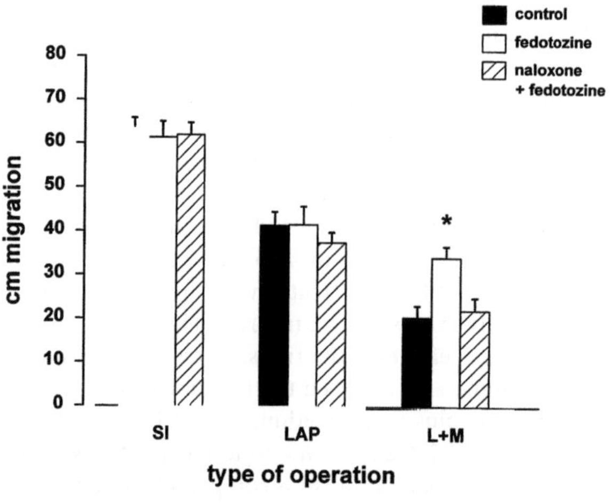

Fig. 6. Effect of skin incision (*SI*), laparotomy (*LAP*) or laparotomy plus manipulation of the small intestine and cecum (L+M) on the intestinal transit in control rats (n = 9) and in rats treated with fedotozine (5 mg/kg, n = 9–10) or with naloxone (1 mg/kg) plus fedotozine (n = 9–10). Results are expressed as centimeters of migration of Evans blue and shown as mean ± SEM. * $P \leq 0.05$, significant difference from the transit in rats that underwent L+M; one-way analysis of variance followed by the Bonferroni test

control rats to 34.1 ± 2.6 cm in fedotozine-treated rats (n = 9) (Fig. 6). Naloxone plus fedotozine had no effect on the transit after skin incision or laparotomy (n = 10) (Fig. 6). However, consecutive injection of naloxone and fedotozine reversed the effect of fedotozine alone on the transit after laparotomy plus manipulation from 34.1 ± 2.6 cm in fedotozine-treated rats to 22.0 ± 2.9 cm in rats treated with naloxone plus fedotozine (n = 9) (Fig. 6).

The difference between the transit after laparotomy and the transit after laparotomy plus manipulation was significant in the control rats and in the rats treated with naloxone plus fedotozine. However, after treatment of the rats with fedotozine alone, the transit after laparotomy plus manipulation was no longer significantly different from the transit after laparotomy alone, indicating that fedotozine reversed the additional inhibition of the transit induced by mechanical stimulation of the gut.

In the present study, we demonstrated that the opioid fedotozine, a peripheral κ-opioid receptor agonist, reversed the additional inhibition induced by mechanical stimulation of the gut. This effect of fedotozine was specific as it was reversed by naloxone. The concentration of naloxone we used was a non-receptor specific dose, antagonizing both μ- and κ-opioid receptors (Diop et al. 1994; Sengupta et al. 1996). Furthermore, fedotozine had no effect on the transit after skin incision and no effect on the delay in transit evoked by laparotomy showing that it was rather specific for mechanical stimulation of the gut. These results suggest that activation of peripheral κ-opioid receptors decreases the inhibitory reflex triggered by mechanical stimulation. Blockade of these peripheral κ-opioid receptors by naloxone indeed resulted in a further decrease in transit confirming this hypothesis. Endogenous opioids, localized within the gut wall, might attenuate the inhibition of the gastrointestinal transit induced by the manipulation, by activating the peripheral κ-opioid receptors. This positive effect of the peripheral κ-opioid receptors on the gastrointestinal transit is enhanced by exogenously administered κ-opioid receptor agonists like fedotozine.

Discussion

In this section, we have confirmed that morphine has an inhibitory effect on the gastrointestinal transit and that this effect is reversed by naloxone. We demonstrated that the transit after the laparotomy plus manipulation was enhanced by fedotozine while it was further inhibited by naloxone. These results support a role for peripheral κ-opioid receptors in the pathogenesis of postoperative ileus induced by abdominal surgery. Peripheral κ-opioid receptor agonists most probably act on the afferent limb of the inhibitory nervous reflex pathway induced by mechanical stimulation of the gut.

Interestingly, morphine and fedotozine had a differential effect on the transit after skin incision and after laparotomy plus manipulation, indicating a different mode of action. This different mode of action most probably results from the activation of different opioid receptors. Both μ- and κ-opioid receptors are expressed throughout the gastrointestinal tract, with a different distribution across the different regions (Fickel et al. 1997). Morphine is acting preferentially on μ-opioid receptors (Jaffe and Martin 1985), while fedotozine binds to peripheral κ-opioid receptors (Rivière et al. 1993). Therefore, these results suggest that only peripheral κ-opioid receptor agonists, and not μ-opioid receptor agonists, can decrease the inhibition of the transit induced by mechanical stimulation of the gut. They also accentuate the specificity of fedotozine as a κ-opioid receptor agonist. Since peripheral κ-opioid receptor agonists also possess antinociceptive activity, they might replace morphine in the treatment of postoperative pain, and at the same time have a beneficial effect on postoperative ileus.

General Discussion

Postoperative ileus is a common complication after abdominal surgery. It is generally accepted that postoperative ileus results from the activation of an inhibitory neural reflex pathway with the afferent limb consisting of capsaicin sensitive sensory neurons and the efferent limb consisting of adrenergic neurons. Hereby, we provide evidence that other additional mechanisms are involved such as the nitrergic and VIP-ergic innervation.

To explore the neural reflex pathways, we developed a rat model which enabled us to study postoperative ileus. Three different degrees of nociceptive stimulation, skin incision, laparotomy alone and laparotomy plus mechanical stimulation of the intestine, resulted in different degrees of inhibition of the gastrointestinal transit as measured by the migration of Evans blue. Using this model, we investigated different treatments to inhibit the reflex pathway at the afferent and/or efferent limb of the pathway.

To clarify the nature of the efferent limb, we first studied the involvement of the adrenergic innervation. Blockade of the adrenergic neurons with reserpine did not completely block the manipulation-induced decrease in the transit suggesting the involvement of an additional reflex pathway. Only the combined blockade of adrenergic neurons and nitric oxide synthase completely restored the transit after laparotomy plus mechanical stimulation of the gut. We also demonstrated that, next to nitric oxide, VIP is involved in the additional inhibition induced by mechanical stimulation of the gut via the activation of VIP_1 receptors. Therefore, we can conclude that both adrenergic and nonadrenergic pathways are involved; the nonadrenergic neurons release NO and VIP as neurotransmitters.

Opioids are widely used to control postoperative pain. Morphine, a preferential μ-opioid receptor agonist, is most widely used despite its depressant effect on the gastrointestinal transit. Recently, peripheral κ-opioid receptor agonists, like fedotozine, were developed. Fedotozine completely reversed the additional inhibition induced by mechanical stimulation of the intestine, probably by an effect on the afferent fibers arising from the intestine. Since peripheral κ-opioid receptor agonists have a beneficial effect on postoperative ileus and since they also possess antinociceptive activity, they may replace morphine in the postoperative period.

In conclusion, postoperative ileus results from the activation of neural reflex pathways. Treatment can be based on blockade of the afferent and/or efferent limb. The afferent limb can be inhibited by peripheral κ-opioid receptor agonists. The efferent limb can be completely blocked by the combination of adrenergic and nitrergic (or VIP-ergic) neuron blockade. Finally, a more intense activation of nociceptors results in a more severe ileus, therefore abdominal surgery should aim to minimize gut trauma as achieved by laparoscopic operations.

References

Abrahamsson H, Glise H, Glise K (1979) Reflex suppression of gastric motility during laparotomy and gastroduodenal nociceptive stimulation. Scand J Gastroenterol 14:101–106

Aranow JS, Zhuang J, Wang H, Larkin V, Smith M, Fink MP (1996) A selective inhibitor of inducible nitric oxide synthase prolongs survival in a rat model of bacterial peritonitis: comparison with two nonselective strategies. Shock 5:116–121

Asai T, Mapleson WW, Power I (1997) Differential effects of clonidine and dexmedetomidine on gastric emptying and gastrointestinal transit in the rat. Br J Anaesth 78:301–307

Barquist E, Bonaz B, Martinez V, Rivier J, Zinner MJ, Tache Y (1996) Neuronal pathways involved in abdominal surgery-induced gastric ileus in rats. Am J Physiol 270:R888-R894

Basson MD, Fielding LP, Bilchik AJ, Zucker KA, Ballantyne GH, Sussman J, Adrian TE, Modlin IM (1989) Does vasoactive intestinal polypeptide mediate the pathophysiology of bowel obstruction? Am J Surg 157:109–115

Benson MJ, Roberts JP, Wingate DL, Rogers J, Deeks JJ, Castillo FD, Williams NS (1994) Small bowel motility following major intra-abdominal surgery: the effects of opiates and rectal cisapride. Gastroenterology 106:924–936

Boeckxstaens GE, Pelckmans PA (1997) Nitric oxide and the non-adrenergic non-cholinergic neurotransmission. Comp Biochem Physiol 118:925–937

Boeckxstaens GE, Pelckmans PA, Bogers JJ, Bult H, De Man JG, Oosterbosch L, Herman AG, Van Maercke YM (1991) Release of nitric oxide upon stimulation of nonadrenergic noncholinergic nerves in the rat gastric fundus. J Pharmacol Exp Ther 256:441–447

Boeckxstaens GE, Pelckmans PA, Bult H, De Man JG, Herman AG, Van Maercke YM (1990) Non-adrenergic non-cholinergic relaxation mediated by nitric oxide in the canine ileocolonic junction. Eur J Pharmacol 190:239–246

Boughton-Smith NK, Evans SM, Laszlo F, Whittle BJ, Moncada S (1993) The induction of nitric oxide synthase and intestinal vascular permeability by endotoxin in the rat. Br J Pharmacol 110:1189–1195

Brown NJ, Coupar IM, Rumsey RD (1988) The effect of acute and chronic administration of morphine and morphine withdrawal on intestinal transit time in the rat. J Pharm Pharmacol 40:844–848

Bueno L, Ferre JP, Ruckebusch Y (1978) Effects of anesthesia and surgical procedures on intestinal myoelectric activity in rats. Am J Dig Dis 23:690–695

Bueno L, Fioramonti J, Delvaux M, Frexinos J (1997) Mediators and pharmacology of visceral sensitivity: from basic to clinical investigations. Gastroenterology 112:1714–1743

Bult H, Boeckxstaens GE, Pelckmans PA, Jordaens FH, Van Maercke YM, Herman AG (1990) Nitric oxide as an inhibitory non-adrenergic non-cholinergic neurotransmitter. Nature 345:346–347

Burnstock G, Costa M (1973) Inhibitory innervation of the gut. Gastroenterology 64:141–144

Catchpole BN (1969) Ileus: use of sympathetic blocking agents in its treatment. Surgery 66:811–820

Cochrane JPS, Forsling ML, Menzies Gow N, Le Quesne LP (1981) Arginine vasopressin release following surgical operations. Br J Surg 68:209–213

Costa M, Furness JB, Pompolo S, Brookes SJ, Bornstein JC, Bredt DS, Snyder SH (1992) Projections and chemical coding of neurons with immunoreactivity for nitric oxide synthase in the guinea-pig small intestine. Neurosci Lett 148:121–125

De Winter BY, Boeckxstaens GE, De Man JG, Moreels TG, Herman AG, Pelckmans PA (1997a) Effect of adrenergic and nitrergic blockade on experimental ileus in rats. Br J Pharmacol 120:464–468

De Winter BY, Boeckxstaens GE, De Man JG, Moreels TG, Herman AG, Pelckmans PA (1997b) Effect of μ- and κ-opioid receptors on postoperative ileus in rats. Eur J Pharmacol 339:63–67

De Winter BY, Robberecht P, Boeckxstaens GE, De Man JG, Moreels TG, Herman AG, Pelckmans PA (1998) Role of VIP1/PACAP receptors in postoperative ileus in rats. Br J Pharmacol 124:1181–1186

Dhawan BN, Cesselin F, Raghubir R, Reisine T, Bradley PB, Portoghese PS, Hamon M (1996) International union of pharmacology XII. Classification of opioid receptors. Pharmacol Rev 48:567–592

Diop L, Rivière PJ, Pascaud X, Junien JL (1994) Peripheral kappa-opioid receptors mediate the antinociceptive effect of fedotozine (correction of fetodozine) on the duodenal pain reflex in rat. Eur J Pharmacol 271:65–71

Dubois A (1988) Mechanical gastrointestinal obstruction and paralytic ileus. In: Kumar D, Gustavsson S (eds) An illustrated guide to gastrointestinal motility. Wiley, New York, pp 365–382

Dubois A, Weise VK, Kopin IJ (1973) Postoperative ileus in the rat: physiopathology, etiology and treatment. Ann Surg 178:781–786

Ekblad E, Mulder H, Uddman R, Sundler F (1994) NOS-containing neurons in the rat gut and coeliac ganglia. Neuropharmacology 33:1323–1331

Espat NJ, Cheng G, Kelley MC, Vogel SB, Sninsky CA, Hocking MP (1995) Vasoactive intestinal peptide and substance P receptor antagonists improve postoperative ileus. J Surg Res 58:719–723

Ferraz AA, Cowles VE, Condon RE, Carilli S, Ezberci F, Frantzides CT, Schulte WJ (1995) Nonopioid analgesics shorten the duration of postoperative ileus. Am Surg 61:1079–1083
Fickel J, Bagnol D, Watson SJ, Akil H (1997) Opioid receptor expression in the rat gastrointestinal tract: a quantitative study with comparison to the brain. Brain Res Mol Brain Res 46:1–8
Friese N, Chevalier E, Angel F, Pascaud X, Junien JL, Dahl SG, Rivière PJ (1997) Reversal by kappa-agonists of peritoneal irritation-induced ileus and visceral pain in rats. Life Sci 60:625–634
Furness JB, Bornstein JC, Murphy R, Pompolo S (1992) Roles of peptides in transmission in the enteric nervous system. Trends Neurosci 15:66–71
Furness JB, Costa M (1974) Adynamic ileus, its pathogenesis and treatment. Med Biol 52:82–89
Galligan JJ, Burks TF (1983) Centrally mediated inhibition of small intestinal transit and motility by morphine in the rat. J Pharmacol Exp Ther 226:356–361
Glise H, Abrahamsson H (1980) Reflex vagal inhibition of gastric motility by intestinal nociceptive stimulation in the cat. Scand J Gastroenterol 15:769–774
Gourlet P, De Neef P, Cnudde J, Waelbroeck M, Robberecht P (1997a) In vitro properties of a high affinity selective antagonist of the VIP1 receptor. Peptides 18:1555–1560
Gourlet P, Vandermeers A, Vertongen P, Rathe J, De Neef P, Cnudde J, Waelbroeck M, Robberecht P (1997b) Development of high affinity selective VIP1 receptor agonists. Peptides 18:1539–1545
Gourlet P, Vertongen P, Vandermeers A, Vandermeers-Piret MC, Rathe J, De Neef P, Waelbroeck M, Robberecht P (1997c) The long-acting vasoactive intestinal polypeptide agonist RO 25-1553 is highly selective of the VIP2 receptor subclass. Peptides 18:403–408
Goyal RK, Hirano I (1996) The enteric nervous system. N Engl J Med 334:1106–1115
Goyal RK, Rattan S, Said SI (1980) VIP as a possible neurotransmitter of non-cholinergic non- adrenergic inhibitory neurones. Nature 288:378–380
Grider JR, Rivier JR (1990) Vasoactive intestinal peptide (VIP) as transmitter of inhibitory motor neurons of the gut: evidence from the use of selective VIP antagonists and VIP antiserum. J Pharmacol Exp Ther 253:738–742
Heimbach DM, Crout JR (1971) Treatment of paralytic ileus with adrenergic neuronal blocking drugs. Surgery 69:582–587
Holzer P, Lippe IT, Amann R (1992) Participation of capsaicin-sensitive afferent neurons in gastric motor inhibition caused by laparotomy and intraperitoneal acid. Neuroscience 48:715–722
Holzer P, Lippe IT, Holzer-Petsche U (1986) Inhibition of gastrointestinal transit due to surgical trauma or peritoneal irritation is reduced in capsaicin-treated rats. Gastroenterology 91:360–363
Jaffe JH, Martin WR (1985) Opioid analgesics and antagonists. In: Goodman Gilman A, Goodman LS, Rall TW, Murad F (eds) Goodman and Gilman's The pharmacological basis of therapeutics. MacMillan, New York, pp 491–531
Kaufman PN, Krevsky B, Malmud LS, Maurer AH, Somers MB, Siegel JA, Fisher RS (1988) Role of opiate receptors in the regulation of colonic transit. Gastroenterology 94:1351–1356
Kelley MC, Hocking MP, Marchand SD, Sninsky CA (1993) Ketorolac prevents postoperative small intestinal ileus in rats. Am J Surg 165:107–111
Klabunde RE, Coston AF (1995) Nitric oxide synthase inhibition does not prevent cardiac depression in endotoxic shock. Shock 3:73–78
Langlois A, Diop L, Rivière PJ, Pascaud X, Junien JL (1994) Effect of fedotozine on the cardiovascular pain reflex induced by distension of the irritated colon in the anesthetized rat. Eur J Pharmacol 271:245–251
Laszlo F, Whittle BJ, Moncada S (1994) Time-dependent enhancement or inhibition of endotoxin-induced vascular injury in rat intestine by nitric oxide synthase inhibitors. Br J Pharmacol 111:1309–1315
Laszlo F, Whittle BJ, Evans SM, Moncada S (1995) Association of microvascular leakage with induction of nitric oxide synthase: effects of nitric oxide synthase inhibitors in various organs. Eur J Pharmacol 283:47–53
Livingston EH, Passaro EP (1990) Postoperative ileus. Dig Dis Sci 35:121–132
Lynn RB, Sankey SL, Chakder S, Rattan S (1995) Colocalization of NADPH-diaphorase staining and VIP immunoreactivity in neurons in opossum internal anal sphincter. Dig Dis Sci 40:781–791
Manara L, Bianchi G, Ferretti P, Tavani A (1986) Inhibition of gastrointestinal transit by morphine in rats results primarily from direct drug action on gut opioid sites. J Pharmacol Exp Ther 237:945–949
Mfller MJ, Chotinaruemol S, Sadowska-Krowicka H, Kakkis JL, Munshi UK, Zhang XJ, Clark DA.(1993) Nitric oxide: the Jekyll and Hyde of gut inflammation. Agents Actions 39:C180-C182
Neely & Catchpole (1971)
Pichlmayr R, Löhlein D (1979) Acute postsurgical syndromes. In: Blum AL, Siewert JR (eds) Clinics in gastroenterology. Saunders, Philadelphia, pp 249–269
Rand MJ, Li CG (1995) Nitric oxide as a neurotransmitter in peripheral nerves: nature of transmitter and mechanism of transmission. Annu Rev Physiol 57:659–682

Resnick J, Greenwald DA, Brandt LJ (1997a) Delayed gastric emptying and postoperative ileus after nongastric abdominal surgery. I. Am J Gastroenterol 92:751–762

Resnick J, Greenwald DA, Brandt LJ (1997b) Delayed gastric emptying and postoperative ileus after nongastric abdominal surgery. II. Am J Gastroenterol 92:934–940

Rivière PJ, Pascaud X, Chevalier E, Le Gallou B, Junien JL (1993) Fedotozine reverses ileus induced by surgery or peritonitis: action at peripheral kappa-opioid receptors. Gastroenterology 104:724–731

Rivière PJ, Pascaud X, Chevalier E, Junien JL (1994) Fedotozine reversal of peritoneal-irritation-induced ileus in rats: possible peripheral action on sensory afferents. J Pharmacol Exp Ther 270:846–850

Salzman AL (1995) Nitric oxide in the gut. New Horiz 3:33–45

Sanders KM (1996) A case for interstitial cells of Cajal as pacemakers and mediators of neurotransmission in the gastrointestinal tract. Gastroenterology 111: 492–515

Schröder H, Möller H (1987) Paralytic ileus-pathophysiology and clinical aspects. Zentralbl Chir 112:681–690

Seago ND, Thompson JH, Zhang X-J, Eloby-Childress S, Sadowska-Krowicka H, Rossi JL, Currie MG, Manning PT, Clark DA, Miller MJS (1995) Inducible nitric oxide synthase and guinea-pig ileitis induced by adjuvant. Mediators of Inflammation 4:19–24

Sengupta JN, Su X, Gebhart GF (1996) Kappa, but not mu or delta, opioids attenuate responses to distention of afferent fibers innervating the rat colon. Gastroenterology 111:968–980

Smith J, Kelly KA, Weinshilboum RM (1977) Pathophysiology of postoperative ileus. Arch Surg 112:203–209

Southan GJ, Szabo C, Thiemermann C (1995) Isothioureas: potent inhibitors of nitric oxide synthases with variable isoform selectivity. Br J Pharmacol 114:510–516

Stark ME, Szurszewski JH (1992) Role of nitric oxide in gastrointestinal and hepatic function and disease. Gastroenterology 103:1928–1949

Szabo C, Southan GJ, Thiemermann C (1994) Beneficial effects and improved survival in rodent models of septic shock with S-methylisothiourea sulfate, a potent and selective inhibitor of inducible nitric oxide synthase. Proc Natl Acad Sci USA 91:12472–12476

Tanila H, Kauppila T, Taira T (1993) Inhibition of intestinal motility and reversal of postlaparotomy ileus by selective alpha 2-adrenergic drugs in the rat. Gastroenterology 104:819–824

Thörn SE, Wattwil M, Lindberg G, Sawe J (1996) Systemic and central effects of morphine on gastroduodenal motility. Acta Anaesthesiol Scand 40:177–186

Usdin TB, Bonner TI, Mezey E (1994) Two receptors for vasoactive intestinal polypeptide with similar specificity and complementary distributions. Endocrinology 135:2662–2680

Wang Y-X, Zhou T, Pang CCY (1991) Pressor effects of L- and D-enantiomers of NG-nitro-arginine in conscious rats are antagonized by L- but not D-arginine. Eur J Pharmacol 200:77–81

Weisbrodt NW, Sussman SS, Stewart JJ, Burks TF (1980) Effect of morphine sulfate on intestinal transit and myoelectric activity of the small intestine of the rat. J Pharmacol Exp Ther 214:333–338

Wu CC, Chen SJ, Szabo C, Thiemermann C, Vane JR (1995) Aminoguanidine attenuates the delayed circulatory failure and improves survival in rodent models of endotoxic shock. Br J Pharmacol 114:1666–1672

Wu CC, Ruetten H, Thiemermann C (1996) Comparison of the effects of aminoguanidine and *N*-omega-nitro-L-arginine methyl ester on the multiple organ dysfunction caused by endotoxaemia in the rat. Eur J Pharmacol 300:99–104

Yukioka H, Bogod DG, Rosen M (1987) Recovery of bowel motility after surgery. Detection of time of first flatus from carbon dioxide concentration and patient estimate after nalbuphine and placebo. Br J Anaesth 59:581–584

Zittel TT, Reddy SN, Plourde V, Raybould HE (1994) Role of spinal afferents and calcitonin gene-related peptide in the postoperative gastric ileus in anesthetized rats. Ann Surg 219:79–87

What Dose of Neostigmine Is Effective for the Treatment of Postoperative Colonic Ileus? Lessons from Colonic Motility Studies

M. E. Kreis · T. T. Zittel · M. Kasparek · G. Thiers · A. Huge · H. D. Becker
E. C. Jehle

Chirurgische Abteilung, Universitätsklinik Tübingen, Waldhörnlestraße 22,
72072 Tübingen, Germany

Introduction

Inhibition of gastrointestinal motility is regularly seen following abdominal surgery. This so-called postoperative ileus may lead to patient discomfort, prolonged parenteral nutrition, or even relaparotomy. Thus, recovery from surgery may be impaired resulting in delayed discharge from hospital and increased health cost [2].

Efficient treatment of postoperative ileus is desirable, but difficult. Enemas or sennosides are frequently applied, with questionable success. For several decades, acetylcholinesterase inhibitors such as neostigmine have been used in order to stimulate postoperative gastrointestinal motility. Although this drug appears to have some effect, its efficacy in stimulating gastrointestinal motility during the postoperative period has never been investigated by gastrointestinal motility recordings. Furthermore, it is not precisely known what dose of neostigmine is required to stimulate the colon efficiently in the postoperative period [1, 3].

Postoperative ileus is most pronounced in the colon, lasting for several days, while the stomach and the small intestine have been reported to recover more rapidly [6]. Furthermore, some of the data available suggest that postoperative ileus is more pronounced in the distal colon, particularly if a left colonic anastomosis has been performed [4]. We, therefore, wished to investigate the effect of neostigmine on postoperative ileus by means of colonic motility recordings in patients following colorectal surgery and distal colonic anastomosis.

Methods

In all 11 patients were studied (7 women, 4 men, median age 60 years, range 39–71 years). All patients gave informed consent prior to their participation in the study, and the study protocol was approved by the ethics committee of the University of Tübingen, Germany. Before surgery, patients each ingested 3–4 l of a lavage solution (Klean-Prep, Norgine, Marburg, Germany). Patients underwent either anterior rectal resection ($n = 5$), sigmoid colon resection ($n = 5$) or reanastomosis following a previous Hartmann procedure (= 1). A complication requiring relaparotomy occurred in one patient who had a leaking anastomosis on day 4 following low anterior rectal resection.

Colonic motility recordings were performed with a combined barostat/manometry system. The barostat was operated by dedicated software installed on a personal computer (Barostat Model Distender Series II, Protocol Plus software, G&J Electronics,

M. K. Herbert et al. (Eds.), Problems of the
Gastrointestinal Tract in Anesthesia...

Toronto, Ont., Canada). It was connected to a custom-built catheter (Muy Scientific, Mississauga, Ont., Canada), which was 1.1 m long with four manometry channels and two barostat bags. The bags were highly compliant polyethylene bags tied to metal rings on the catheter. Barostat recordings were performed in parallel with water-perfused manometry (Arndorfer Perfusion Pump, Arndorfer Medical Specialities, Greendale, Wis.; Statham pressure transducers, Model P23XL, Spectramed, Oxnard, Calif.). Manometry data were recorded with a computer system (Combi-Interface, PC-Polygraf VIII, Synectics Medical, Frankfurt, Germany). For simultaneous analysis of barostat and manometry data, barostat signals were transmitted to the Synectics interface by a custom-built converter (Golden Gate, G&J Electronics).

After the completion of the colonic anastomosis, the recording catheter was introduced transanally and positioned by the surgeon with the distal barostat bag approximately 15 cm orad to the anastomosis. Recordings were performed once a day from postoperative day 1 to day 3. After a 30-min baseline recording period, neostigmine was given at a dose of 0.05 μg/kg body weight over 10 min intravenously. This period was followed by 10 min without neostigmine administration. Then, subsequent doses of 0.5 and 5 μg/kg body weight were given over 10 min each, with a 10-min period without neostigmine infusion between.

The motility for each neostigmine dose was evaluated from the beginning of the 10-min infusion to the end of the 10-min period without the infusion (total time 20 min). Mean barostat bag volumes were calculated for each neostigmine dose for comparison. Data are mean ± standard error of the mean (SEM) and were compared by the Signed Rank test and Bonferroni's correction for multiple testing. $P < 0.05$ was taken as significant.

Results

Neostigmine caused an increase in colonic motility (Fig. 1A). On day 1 after surgery, the colonic motility index of manometry recordings (area under the curve per minute) increased from 109 ± 52 mmHg/min at baseline to 671 ± 242 mmHg/min at 5 μg/kg body weight ($P < 0.05$) but did not increase significantly at lower doses. A similar pattern was observed on day 2 after surgery. However, on day 3 the motility index increased from 196 ± 69 mmHg/min at baseline to 321 ± 85 mmHg/min at 0.05 μg/kg, to 433 ± 110 at 0.5 μg/kg and to 919 ± 302 mmHg/min at 5 μg/kg body weight neostigmine ($P < 0.05$ for 0.5 and 5 μg/kg vs baseline; Fig. 1B).

The frequency of colonic contractions per minute increased on days 1 and 3 at 5 μg/kg neostigmine compared with baseline (day 1: 0.4 ± 0.2 vs 1.2 ± 0.2 min^{-1}, $P < 0.05$; day 2: 0.6 ± 0.2 vs 1.0 ± 0.2 min^{-1}, n.s.; day 3: 0.7 ± 0.2 vs 1.3 ± 0.2 min^{-1}, $P < 0.05$). The mean amplitude of colonic contractions was increased on days 2 and 3 following 5 μg/kg neostigmine compared with baseline (day 1: 6.7 ± 0.9 vs 12.2 ± 2.8 mmHg, n.s.; day 2: 7.4 ± 1.2 vs 12.6 ± 2.3 mmHg, $P < 0.05$; day 3: 7.9 ± 1.7 vs 18.2 ± 6.9 mmHg, $P < 0.05$). Barostat bag volumes decreased with increasing neostigmine doses in both bags. The decrease was more marked with increasing time after surgery (proximal barostat bag, baseline vs 5 μg/kg, day 1: 25 ± 6.7 vs 17 ± 5.8 ml, $P < 0.05$; day 2: 27 ± 6.9 vs 17 ± 6.3 ml, $P < 0.05$; day 3: 23 ± 2.6 vs 10 ± 0.5 ml; $P < 0.05$). A similar pattern was observed in the distal barostat bag at lower volumes.

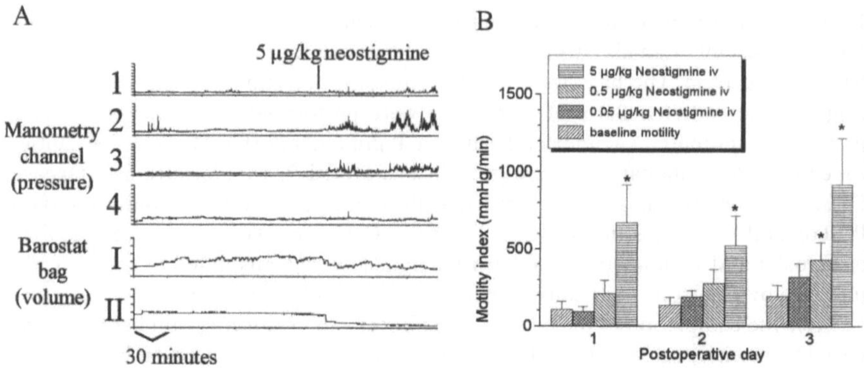

Fig. 1. A Representative recording of colonic motility recorded by a four-channel manometry system and two barostat bags following 5 µg/kg body weight neostigmine over a 10-min period. **B** Colonic motility index following 0.05, 0.5 and 5 µg/kg body weight neostigmine i.v. from postoperative day 1 to 3 ($n = 11$, $P < 0.05$ vs baseline)

Discussion

The present study demonstrates that 5 µg neostigmine/kg body weight infused intravenously over a 10-min period stimulates colonic motility from day 1 to 3 following colorectal surgery. On day 3 after surgery, one-tenth this dose of neostigmine was also effective in stimulating colonic motility. After neostigmine, an increase in both frequency and amplitude of colonic contractions was observed. The increase in colonic motility after neostigmine was accompanied by a reduction in barostat bag volumes, which indicate colonic tone.

Neostigmine has been investigated previously in combination with other drugs for the treatment of postoperative motility disorders [1, 3]. However, no data have become available to date describing dose-dependent effects of neostigmine on colonic motility. In previous studies clinical observation and the auscultation of bowel sounds were used to evaluate the effects of neostigmine. However, these methods do not allow selective study of gastrointestinal motility in different parts of the gut, as bowel sounds may originate from both the colon and the small intestine. Since colonic motility is usually limiting for the resolution of the postoperative inhibition of gastrointestinal motility, we focused our investigation on the colon. We did not apply any kind of "sympathicolytic treatment," so that the effect of neostigmine on the colon can be attributed solely to this drug and is not obscured by other drugs given concomitantly as in other studies.

Neostigmine has been reported to induce colonic decompression during colonic dilatation in Ogilvie's syndrome [5]. Although this report is merely based on clinical observation and plain radiographs, without any type of motility recording, it is in parallel with our finding that colonic tone is increased following neostigmine infusion. Neostigmine, therefore, seems not only to stimulate single colonic contractions but also to cause a general increase in colonic tone.

We conclude that 5 µg/kg body weight of neostigmine infused over 10 min is sufficient to stimulate colonic motility from day 1 to 3 after colorectal surgery. With increasing time after the operation, lower doses of neostigmine also appear to stimlu-ate colonic motility. Neostigmine should be useful in the treatment of postoperative inhibition of colonic motility. It remains to be determined, however, whether the neo-stigmine doses tested by us are sufficient to shorten the duration of postoperative ileus.

References

1. Grund KE (1982) Treatment of functional ileus: adrenergic blockade and stimulation. Dtsch Med Wochenschr 107:209–212
2. Livingston EH, Passaro EP (1990) Postoperative ileus. Dig Dis Sci 35:121–132
3. Petri G, Szénohradszky J, Pórszász-Gibiszer K (1971) Sympatholytic treatment of "paralytic" ileus. Surgery 70:359–367
4. Roberts JP, Benson MJ, Rogers J, Deeks JJ, Wiliams NS (1994) Characterization of distal colonic motility in early postoperative period and effect of colonic anastomosis. Dig Dis Sci 39:1961–1967
5. Stephenson BM, Morgan AR, Salaman JR, Wheeler MH (1995) Ogilvie's syndrome: a new approach to an old problem. Dis Colon Rectum 38:424–427
6. Waldhausen JHT, Shaffrey ME, Skenderis BS, Jones RS, Schirmer BD (1990) Gastrointestinal myo-electric and clinical patterns of recovery after laparotomy. Ann Surg 212:777–785

FREE COMMUNICATION

Small Bowel Transit Time in Intensive Care Unit Patients: Effect of Cisapride and Erythromycin

J. Barnert[1] · I. Röckl-Wiedmann[1] · C. Werner[1] · G. Neeser[1,2] · M. Wienbeck[1]

[1] Medizinische Klinik, Zentralklinikum Augsburg, Stenglinstrasse 2, 86156 Augsburg, Germany
[2] Klinik für Anästhesiologie und Operative Intensivmedizin, Zentralklinikum Augsburg, Stenglinstrasse 2, 86156 Augsburg, Germany

Introduction

Intestinal motility is often disturbed in intensive care unit (ICU) patients. This may result in increased morbidity, for example, by way of bacterial overgrowth. This problem may also delay the start of enteral feeding, which is actually considered to be quite important in intensive care unit patients. Although several motility drugs are used in clinical practice in this setting, few data exist concerning their efficiency.

The aim of our study was to answer the following questions:

1. Does cisapride, a prokinetic drug, shorten enteral transit time in ICU patients?
2. Does erythromycin, an antiobitic with strong effects on gastroduodenal motility, shorten enteral transit time in ICU patients?
3. Do the two drugs have effects on such clinical variables as bowel sounds and defecation?

Materials and Methods

Jejunocecal transit time was measured by the salazosulfapyridine method [1]. Salazosulfapyridine (SASP) is used for the treatment of inflammatory bowel disease. It is cleaved by colonic bacteria, which reduce the azo bond, releasing sulfapyridine (SP) and 5-aminosalicylic acid (Fig. 1). The SP released is immediately absorbed and can be assessed in the blood plasma by a spectrophometric method making use of the formation of a diazonium salt.

After an overnight fast, patients were given 2 g SASP with 20 ml of tap water through a commercial feeding tube. The tip of the feeding tube was placed at the duodenojejunal junction. This meant that the SASP solution was administered into the jejunum. The time between administration of SASP and the first detection of SP in the blood was used as marker of the jejeunocecal transit time.

The short-term effects of both drugs on clinical parameters were assessed by auscultation of the bowel and the number of defecations per day. The bowel sounds were graded as: none, audible, and strong. The observers of the clinical parameters did not know whether the drug or placebo had been given.

For statistical analysis the Mann-Whitney test for paired data was used.

M. K. Herbert et al. (Eds.), Problems of the Gastrointestinal Tract in Anesthesia ...

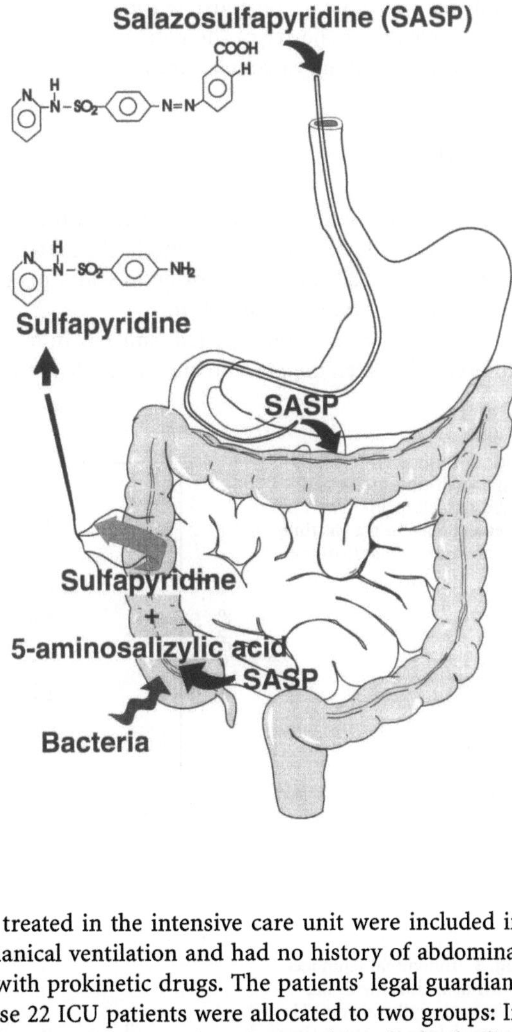

Fig. 1. Schematic illustrating the salazosulfapyridine (*SASP*) method

Patients

Twenty-two consecutive patients treated in the intensive care unit were included in our study. They all were on mechanical ventilation and had no history of abdominal surgery. None was being treated with prokinetic drugs. The patients' legal guardians gave their informed consent. These 22 ICU patients were allocated to two groups: In 12 ICU patients 20 mg of cisapride was given into the jejunum through the feeding tube three times a day. Placebo and cisapride were administered for 2 days through the nasojejunal feeding tube, to ensure a sufficiently high plasma level of cisapride, or no plasma cisapride in the placebo group. The other 10 ICU patients received erythromycin intravenously by continuous infusion. Erythromycin (250 mg) was infused for 3 h. On the second day of each period jejunocecal transit time was assessed by means of the SASP method described above. In both groups the study was performed using a cross-over design. In this way, the patients served as their own controls. The motility agent and placebo were administered in a randomized order. Half of the patients received the placebo first, while the other half received the drug first.

The ages of the patients and the underlying diseases were similar in both groups. In the cisapride group patients had been ventilated for 3.7 days on average and in the erythromycin group, for 5.3 days on average. In addition, cardiac and pulmonary problems were mainly responsible for the admissions to the intensive care unit. In both groups the majority of the patients received opioids for sedation and analgesia and were also taking catecholamines.

Results

Cisapride given into the jejunum shortened the jejunocecal transit time significantly (Fig. 2), a result seen in each patient. In the placebo period the mean transit time was 5.7 h, as against 3.9 h when cisapride was administered. Cisapride shortened the transit time by an average of one third.

The bowel sounds were graded similarly in both periods. There was no statistical difference between the placebo and cisapride periods. The number of defecations per

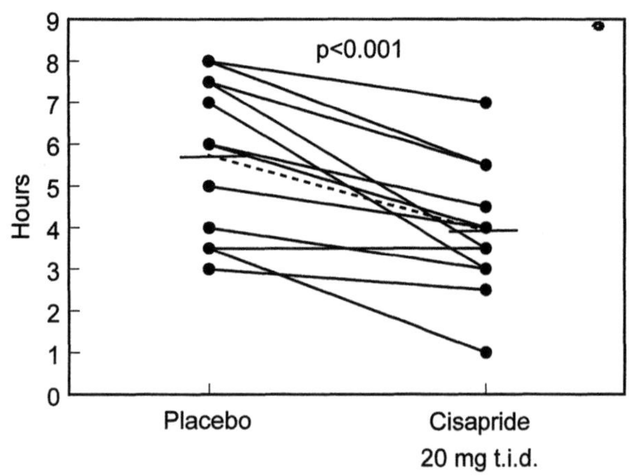

Fig. 2. Individual jejunocecal transit times with placebo and cisapride. The mean change in transit time is shown by the *dotted line*

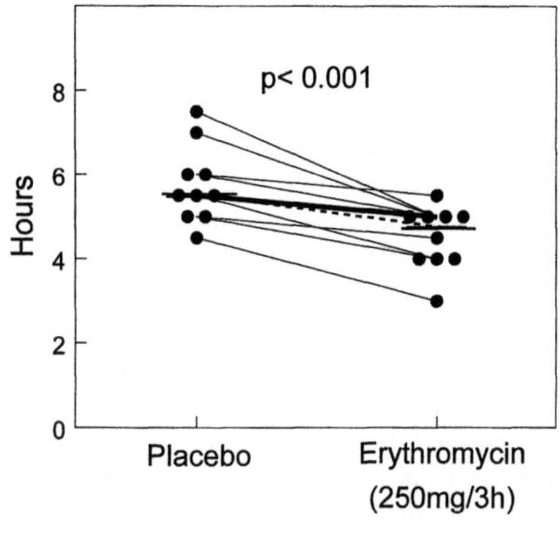

Fig. 3. Individual jejunocecal transit times with placebo and erythromycin. The mean change in transit time is shown be the *dotted line*

day was similar in both groups without any statistical difference. More than half of the patients in the study had no bowel movement in either period.

Erythromycin also shortened the jejunocecal transit time (Fig. 3). In the placebo period the mean transit time was 5.7 h, which was almost identical with the baseline value in the cisapride study. Infusion of erythromycin shortened the mean transit time to 4.5 h, that is by 21 %. This difference was also statistically significant. The graduation of bowel sounds was similar in the placebo and the erythromycin periods, and no statistical difference was seen. Most patients exhibited audible bowel sounds in both periods. Although there was a tendency towards more bowel movements during the infusion of erythromycin, this difference did not reach any statistical significance.

Discussion

Our study has shown that both cisapride and erythromycin shorten enteral transit time in ICU patients to a similar extent. For both drugs these are the first data on enteral transit time in ICU patients. In chronic idiopathic intestinal pseudoobstruction (CIPO) patients, Camillieri et al. [2] reported that cisapride shortened a prolonged intestinal transit time, although the effect of this prokinetic drug on symptoms was not significant. While erythromycin accelerates gastric emptying and induces MMC-like contractions in low dosages, its effects on intestinal transit time are ambiguous. Sarna et al. [3] observed an inhibition of jejunal and ileal motility after administration of 500 mg of erythromycin to fasting healthy subjects. On the other hand, it has been shown that erythromycin shortens intestinal transit time [4]. This study was also done in healthy controls. In the postprandial state erythromycin prolongs the intestinal transit time in normal subjects [5, 6].

The effects of both drugs on clinical variables were poor in our study. However, this issue should be examined in a study lasting several days and comprising considerably more patients. Bonacini et al. attempted to determine whether the administration of 250 mg of erythromycin every 8 h shortened the period of postoperative ileus [7], but the effect of erythromycin on clinical parameters was not significant. Using cisapride, Verlinden et al. [8] were able to shorten the postoperative atony of the bowel. Another group could not confirm this observation, although they observed an improvement of colonic motility after administration of cisapride [9].

References

1. Kellow JE, Borody TJ, Phillips SF, Haddad AC, Brown ML (1986) Sulfapyridine appearance in plasma after salicylazosulfapyridine. Another simple measure of intestinal transit. Gastroenterology 91:396–400
2. Camillieri M, Brown ML, Malagelada JR (1986) Impaired transit of chyme in chronic intestinal pseudoobstruction. Correction by cisapride. Gastroenterology 91:619–626
3. Sarna SK, Soergel KH, Koch TR, Stone JE, Wood CM, Ryan RP, Arndorfer RC, Cavanaugh JH, Nellans HN, Lee MB (1991) Gastrointestinal motor effects of erythromycin in humans. Gastroenterology 101:1488–1496
4. Gordin A, Lehtola J, Jauhonen P, Kesäniemi A, Wikberg R (1989) Erythromycin shortens transit time in healthy volunteers. Eur J Clin Pharmacol 36 [Suppl]:A330

5. Edelbroek MA, Horowitz M, Wishart JM, Akkermans LM (1993) Effects of erythromycin on gastric emptying, alcohol absorption and small intestinal transit in normal subjects. J Nucl Med 34:582–588
6. Landry C, Vidon N, Sogni P, Nepveux P, Chaumeil JC, Couturier D, Chaussade S (1995) Effects of erythromycin on gastric emptying, duodeno-caecal transit time, gastric and biliopancreatic secretion during continuous gastric infusion of a liquid diet in healthy volunteers. Eur J Gastroenterol Hepatol 7:797–802
7. Bonacini M (1993) Effect of intravenous erythromycin on postoperative ileus. Am J Gastroenterol 88:208–211
8. Verlinden M, Michiels G, Boghaert A, de Coster M, Dehertog P (1987) Treatment of postoperative gastrointestinal atony. Br J Surg 74:614–617
9. Clevers GJ, Smout AJPM, Akkermans LMA, Wittebol P (1988) Restoration of gastrointestinal transit and colonic motility after major abdominal surgery: effects of cisapride. Surg Res Commun 4:205–213

High-dose Catecholamines Diminish the Effect of Erythromycin on Antral Motility and Gastric Emptying in Intensive Care Unit Patients

J. Barnert[1] · J. Goebel[1] · G. Neeser[1, 2] · M. Wienbeck[1]

[1] III. Med. Klinik, Zentralklinikum Augsburg, Stenglinstrasse 2, 86156 Augsburg, Germany
[2] Klinik für Anästhesiologie und operative Intensivmedizin, Zentralklinikum Augsburg, Stenglinstrasse 2, 86156 Augsburg, Germany

Introduction

Gastric emptying is impaired in about half of all critically ill patients [1] . This may delay the start of enteral feeding and lead to large gastric residues. In addition, this situation may favor the occurrence of duodenogastric reflux, thereby predisposing the patient to colonization of the stomach by enteric bacteria. Several motility-enhancing drugs, such as metoclopramide or cisapride, are used in this setting, although their clinical effects are limited. Erythromycin is a macrolide antibiotic, which as a 'side effect' strongly stimulates gastroduodenal motility via stimulation of receptors for motilin, a gastrointestinal hormone [2, 3]. It has also been shown that erythromycin is effective in intensive care unit (ICU) patients [4]. Although erythromycin is increasingly used for improving gastric emptying in ICU patients, little is known about its interaction with other drugs often used in this setting, such as catecholamines or opiates, which delay gastric emptying. The aim of this study was to test for any influence of catecholamines on the effect of erythromycin concerning antral motility and gastric emptying.

Materials and Methods

Fifteen consecutive ICU patients (2 women/13 men) were studied. Their age covered a wide range, the mean being 62 years. They were all on mechanical ventilation and none had a history of abdominal surgery. None was taking prokinetic drugs. Their legal guardians gave informed consent on their behalf.

These 15 patients were divided into two groups according to the dose of catecholamines administered. Seven patients received no catecholamines or received dopamine only in a low dosage (<4 mg/kg per min). These were called the 'control group.' The other 8 patients received catecholamines such as dopamine, dobutamine, epinephrine and norepinephrine in higher doses. They were named the 'high-dose catecholamine group.' Although the Apache II score in the control group was lower on average (13 ± 6.5, mean ± SD) than in the high-dose catecholamine group (17.8 ± 8.9), this difference did not reach statistical significance (Mann-Witney test, P = 0.2716).

Motility of the gastric antrum was studied using water perfusion manometry. Six recording sites were placed in the gastric antrum, each 1 cm away from each of the others. Correct placement of the recording sites was checked by fluoroscopy. Data

M. K. Herbert et al. (Eds.), Problems of the Gastrointestinal Tract in Anesthesia...

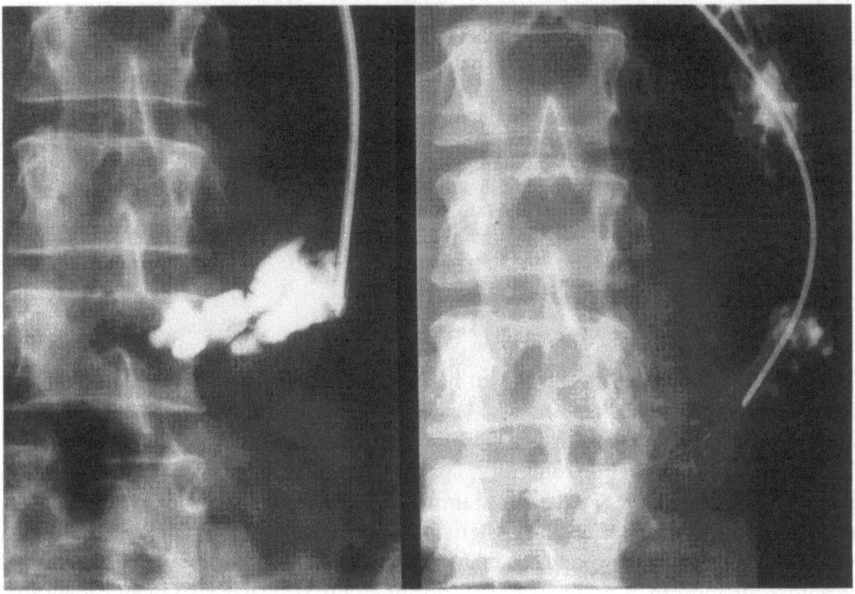

Fig. 1. X-ray picture during tube placement. The tip of the tube has reached the antrum. The inner stiffening wire has been pulled back and some contrast medium has been injected through the tube (seen on *left*). On the *right*, the tip of the tube has been advanced still further towards the pylorus

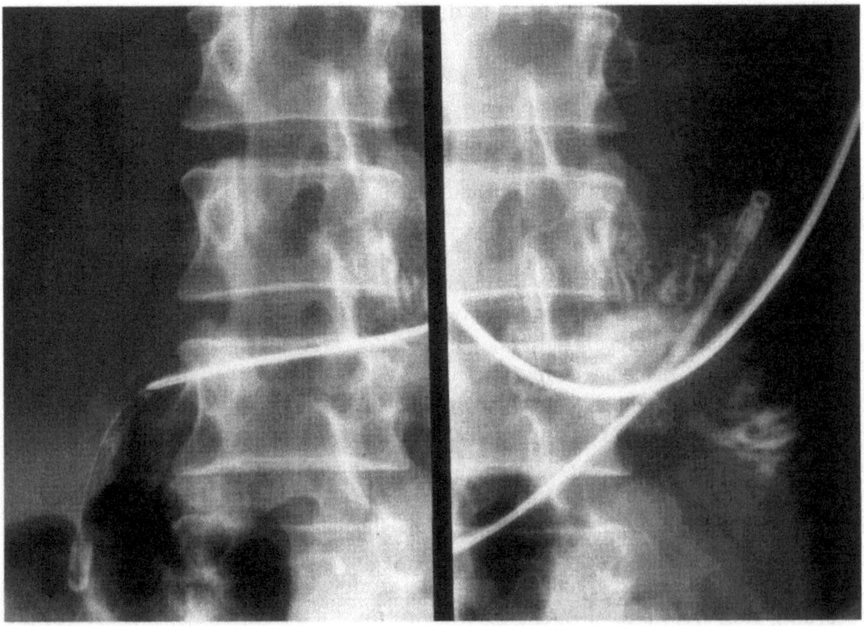

Fig. 2. The tip of the tube is shown on the *left* when it has just passed the pylorus and on the *right* when it has almost reached its final position beyond the duodenojejunal junction

First the feeding tube was advanced through the esophagus and the cardia until the wall of the gastric corpus was reached. Once in the corpus of the stomach the inner stiffening wire was pulled back by about 4 cm. Then a small amount of diluted contrast medium was given through the tube (Fig. 1). At this moment erythromycin was given i.v. The effect of erythromycin was seen immediately afterwards. Strong propulsive contractions began and pulled the tip of the tube forward. The contrast medium administered was also pushed forward. At this time the pyloric channel was visualized fluoroscopically. The smooth tip of the tube was advanced and passed the pylorus quite easily in most patients (Fig. 2, left). If this failed, the dose of erythromycin was increased step by step. Once beyond the pylorus the tip of the tube advanced easily and quickly through the duodenum (Fig. 2, right). The tube was considered to be in place once the tip was noted to be beyond the duodenojejunal junction.

Results

All 56 patients were evaluable. Successful tube placement at the duodenojejunal junction was achieved in 48 patients (86 %). In 8 patients transpyloric placement of the feeding tube failed.

The mean fluoroscopy time was 9.4 min, with a median of 8 min. The fluoroscopy time ranged from 1.8 to 40 min. (extremes recorded for 1 patient each).

The mean dose of erythromycin needed for successful tube placement was 368 mg, and the median dose needed amounted to 200 mg. In more than half of the patients 100–200 mg of erythromycin was sufficient for tube placement (Fig. 3). No untoward effects of erythromycin were seen.

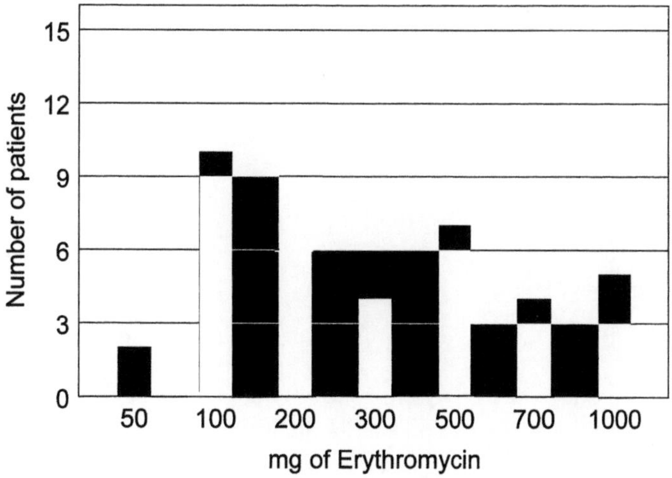

Fig. 3. Individual doses of erythromycin needed for successful placement of the nasojejunal feeding tube

Discussion

The effect of erythromycin on elimination of indigestible solids from the stomach can be used for transpyloric placement of an enteral feeding tube in ICU patients, as previously shown [1, 3]. Our study shows that the success rate may be increased by X-ray guidance, which was used in our study. However, further studies are needed to confirm this conjecture. In addition, X-ray guidance can easily demonstrate the correct position of the feeding tube. Immediately afterwards enteral feeding can be started. This seems to be important in ICU patients, who clearly benefit from early enteral nutrition. A major drawback is the long duration of fluoroscopy in some patients. In 15 of the 56 (27%) patients fluoroscopy took longer than 10 min. In these patients endoscopic placement of the feeding tube would have been faster.

An erythromycin dosage of 300 mg seems to be sufficient in many patients for transpyloric placement of the feeding tube. Thus, in clinical practice starting with a single intravenous dose of 300 mg is recommended. As our study demonstrates, the administration of erythromycin is well tolerated by ICU patients.

References

1. Barnert J, Dumitrascu D, Neeser G, Doesel S, Wienbeck M (1998) Gastric emptying of a liquid meal in intensive care unit patients. Gastroenterology 114:A865
2. Kalliafas S, Choban, PS, Ziegler D, Drago S, Flancbaum L (1996) Erythromycin facilitates postpyloric placement of nasoduodenal feeding tubes in intensive care unit patients: randomized, double-blinded, placebo-controlled trial. JPEN J Parenter Enteral Nutr 20:385–388
3. Stern MA, Wolf DC (1994) Erythromycin as a prokinetic agent: a prospective, randomized, controlled study of efficacy in nasoenteric tube placement. Am J Gastroenterol 89:2011–2013

High-dose Catecholamines Diminish the Effect of Erythromycin on Antral Motility and Gastric Emptying in Intensive Care Unit Patients

J. Barnert[1] · J. Goebel[1] · G. Neeser[1, 2] · M. Wienbeck[1]

[1] III. Med. Klinik, Zentralklinikum Augsburg, Stenglinstrasse 2, 86156 Augsburg, Germany
[2] Klinik für Anästhesiologie und operative Intensivmedizin, Zentralklinikum Augsburg, Stenglinstrasse 2, 86156 Augsburg, Germany

Introduction

Gastric emptying is impaired in about half of all critically ill patients [1] . This may delay the start of enteral feeding and lead to large gastric residues. In addition, this situation may favor the occurrence of duodenogastric reflux, thereby predisposing the patient to colonization of the stomach by enteric bacteria. Several motility-enhancing drugs, such as metoclopramide or cisapride, are used in this setting, although their clinical effects are limited. Erythromycin is a macrolide antibiotic, which as a 'side effect' strongly stimulates gastroduodenal motility via stimulation of receptors for motilin, a gastrointestinal hormone [2, 3]. It has also been shown that erythromycin is effective in intensive care unit (ICU) patients [4]. Although erythromycin is increasingly used for improving gastric emptying in ICU patients, little is known about its interaction with other drugs often used in this setting, such as catecholamines or opiates, which delay gastric emptying. The aim of this study was to test for any influence of catecholamines on the effect of erythromycin concerning antral motility and gastric emptying.

Materials and Methods

Fifteen consecutive ICU patients (2 women/13 men) were studied. Their age covered a wide range, the mean being 62 years. They were all on mechanical ventilation and none had a history of abdominal surgery. None was taking prokinetic drugs. Their legal guardians gave informed consent on their behalf.

These 15 patients were divided into two groups according to the dose of catecholamines administered. Seven patients received no catecholamines or received dopamine only in a low dosage (<4 mg/kg per min). These were called the 'control group.' The other 8 patients received catecholamines such as dopamine, dobutamine, epinephrine and norepinephrine in higher doses. They were named the 'high-dose catecholamine group.' Although the Apache II score in the control group was lower on average (13 ± 6.5, mean ± SD) than in the high-dose catecholamine group (17.8 ± 8.9), this difference did not reach statistical significance (Mann-Witney test, P = 0.2716).

Motility of the gastric antrum was studied using water perfusion manometry. Six recording sites were placed in the gastric antrum, each 1 cm away from each of the others. Correct placement of the recording sites was checked by fluoroscopy. Data

M. K. Herbert et al. (Eds.), Problems of the Gastrointestinal Tract in Anesthesia...

were recorded and analyzed using a computer software program (Polygram) provided by Synectics (Stockholm, Sweden). This computer program analyzes the number and amplitude of the contractions. It also calculates the area under the contractions. The area under the curve per second was taken as motility index. This motility index served as a marker of motility integrating the number and the amplitudes of the contractions.

Gastric emptying was measured by the dye dilution method first described by George [5]. Phenol red dissolved in 750 ml of tap water was used. In principle the volume of a fluid can be ascertained by determining the change in concentration of a dye produced by addition of a small concentrated dose of the same dye. Gastric volumes were calculated by George's equation as modified by Hurwitz [6]: $V_{n-1} = V_a[Z_{n-1}C_a - C_n)]/C_n - C_{n-1}$, where V is the volume to be determined, n is the number of volume determination cycle, C_n is the concentration of dye at the end of the nth cycle, V_a is the volume of added dye, C_a is the concentration of dye added in the first cycle, and Z is the multiplier of concentration of added dye. Statistical analysis was done using the Wilcoxon test for paired data. Data are given as mean ± standard deviation (SD).

Results

In the control group (no dopamine administration or low dose only) both dosages of erythromycin (EM) stimulated the motility index (Fig. 1, Table 1). The same applied to the amplitude (Fig. 1, Table 1) and the number of contractions (Table 1). Concerning gastric emptying, both doses of erythromycin decreased the gastric half-emptying time, 300 mg having a stronger effect than 50 mg of erythromycin (Fig. 2, Table 1)

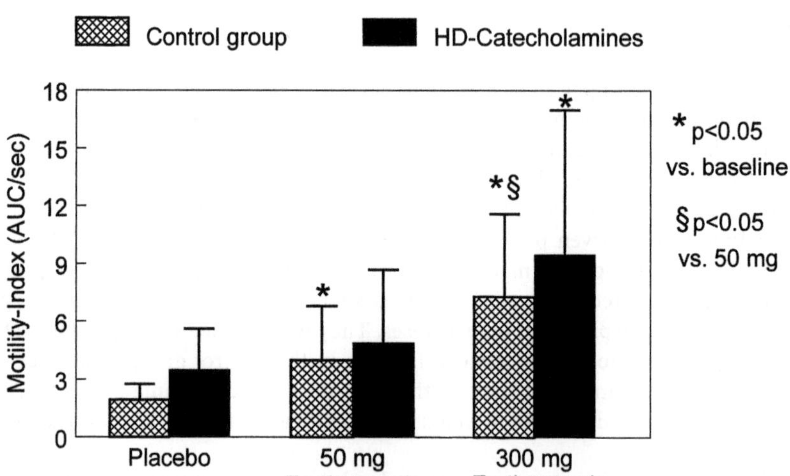

Fig. 1. Motility indices before and after administration of 50 and 300 mg of erythromycin (mean ± SD). The data are calculated for the whole recording session (0–180 min after administration of erythromycin)

Table 1. Number of contractions, mean amplitude of contractions, motility index and gastric emptying half-time ($T_{1/2}$) before and after erythromycin (*EM*) infusion at different doses (means ± SD). Motility data are calculated for the whole recording session (0–180 min after administration of erythromycin)

	Control group			High-dose catecholamine group		
	Baseline	50 mg EM	300 mg EM	Baseline	50 mg EM	300 mg EM
Motility index	1.9±0.8	4.0±2.8 (*)	7.3±4.3 *§	3.5±2.1	4.9±3.8	9.5±7.5*
Number of contractions/min	1.0±0.6	1.4±0.6	1.7±0.6*	0.9±0.7	1.0±0.6	2.0±1.1*§
Amplitude (mmHg)	32±19	45±21*	57±21*	31±12	36±15	53±24
$T_{1/2}$ (min)	16.4±3.5	10±2.5*	7.7±1.7*§	15.3±5.7	13.0±3.8	11.0±4,4

(*) $p = 0.05$, *$P < 0.05$ against baseline; § $p < 0.05$ against 50 mg EM

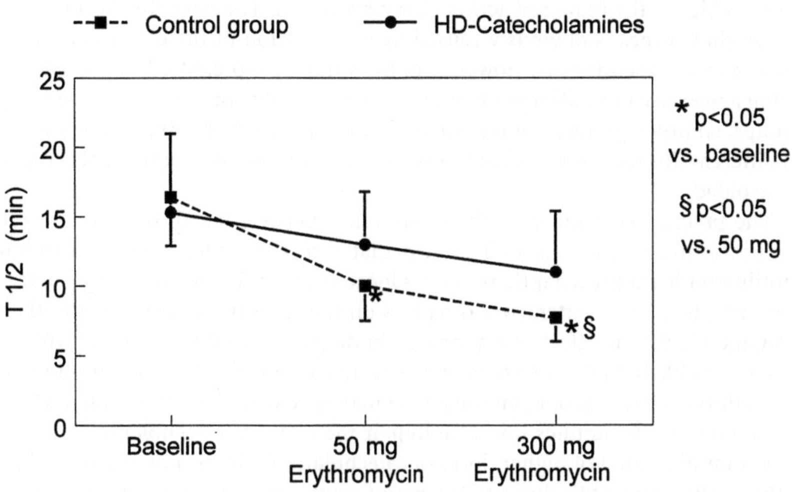

Fig. 2. Gastric emptying curve before and after administration of 50 and 300 mg of erythromycin

In the high-dose catecholamine group only 300 mg of erythromycin increased the motility index (Fig. 1, Table 1) as well as the amplitudes (Table 1) and the number of the contractions to a significant extent (Table 1). In this group a decrease in gastric emptying half-time was seen after administration of erythromycin (Fig. 2, Table 1), but this difference was statistically not significant.

Discussion

Several studies suggest that erythromycin acts as a motilin agonist working directly on motilin receptors [2, 3]. Administration of low doses of erythromycin (1–3 mg/kg per h) induces phase III activity (MMC) in the antrum of dogs and humans, which migrates to the duodenum. Higher doses (200–350 mg) administered to fasted human controls induce sustained bursts of contractions [7], which do not propagate to the duodenum. It was shown that a dosage of 200 mg of erythromycin increases the amplitude of antral contractions and improves antroduodenal coordination in the postprandial period also [8]. The Leuven group has shown that 200 mg of erythromycin accelerates gastric emptying of a solid meal in patients with diabetic gastroparesis [9]. In mechanically ventilated ICU patients 200 mg of erythromycin stimulated antral contractions and at the same time accelerated gastric emptying. The data recorded in our study confirm the effect of erythromycin in ICU patients. A dosage of 50 mg of erythromycin is effective, provided the patients do not receive catecholamines at higher doses. Higher doses of erythromycin have a more powerful effect on antral motility and gastric emptying in ICU patients with no catecholamines or low-dose dopamine administration. In ICU patients receiving higher doses of catecholamines the effect of erythromycin on antral motility and gastric emptying is impaired. One might wish to argue that other factors than catecholamines may be responsible for the impaired action of erythromycin. The need for the administration of catecholamines is obviously caused by a depression of the cardiovascular system, for example by septicemia. However, in the study now presented the Apache II score, being a measure of multiorgan failure, was statistically not different in the two patient groups. Another problem of our study is that the catecholamines were administered in different dosages and combinations, but in studies on ICU patients this bias cannot be avoided.

The precise mechanism of the interference between erythromycin and catecholamines is unknown. It is well known that catecholamines inhibit gastrointestinal motility both via presynaptic receptors located primarily on cholinergic enteric neurons and, to a lesser extent, via receptors on the smooth muscle. On the other hand, atropine blocks the effect of erythromycin on gastric motility in dogs [10]. It therefore seems likely that cholinergic mechanisms are involved in the motilin-like effect of erythromycin on gastric motility. One may speculate that inhibition of cholinergic stimuli by catecholamines may also impair the effect of catecholamines.

If administration of higher doses of catecholamines is considered for ICU patients, a therapeutic trial with doses of 300 mg of erythromycin and higher is warranted.

References

1. Barnert J, Dumitrascu D, Neeser G, Doesel S, Wienbeck M (1998) Gastric emptying of a liquid meal in intensive care unit patients. Gastroenterology 114:A865
2. Vantrappen G, Janssens J, Tack J, Muls E, Bouillon R, Peeters TL (1989) Erythromycin is a potent gastrokinetic in diabetic gastroparesis. Gastoenterology 96:525
3. Peeters TL, Matthijs G, Depoortere I, Cachet T, Hoogmartens J, Vantrappen G (1989) Erythromycin is a motilin receptor agonist. Am J Physiol 257:G470–474
4. Dive A, Miesse C, Galanti L, Jamart J, Evrard P, Gonzalez M, Installe E (1995) Effect of erythromycin on gastric motility in mechanically ventilated critically ill patients: a double-blind, randomized, placebo-controlled study. Crit Care Med 23:1356–1362
5. George JD (1968) New clinical method for measuring the rate of gastric emptying: the double sampling test meal. Gut 9:237–242
6. Hurwitz A (1981) Measuring gastric volumes by dye dilution. Gut 22: 85–93
7. Kawamura O, Sekiguchi T, Kusano M, Nishioka T, Itoh Z (1993) Effect of erythromycin on interdigestive gastrointestinal contractile activity and plasma motilin concentration in humans. Dig Dis Sci 38:870–876

8. Annese V, Janssens J, Vantrappen G, Tack J, Peeters TL, Willemse P, Van Cutsem E (1992) Erythromycin accelerates gastric emptying by inducing antral contractions and improved gastroduodenal coordination. Gastroenterology 102:823–828
9. Janssens J, Peeters TL, Vantrappen G, Tack JL, Urbain JL, De Roo M, Muls E, Bouillon R (1990) Improvement of gastric emptying in diabetic gastroparesis by erythromycin. N Engl J Med 322:1028–1031
10. Fox JE, Daniel EE, Jury J, Fox AE, Collins SM (1983) Sites and mechanisms of action of neuropeptides on canine gastric motility differ in vivo and in vitro. Life Sci 33:817–825

PART II

Dysfunction of the Gastrointestinal Tract in Shock, Sepsis and Critical Illness

INVITED ARTICLE

Gastrointestinal Secretion, Absorption, and Barrier Function

M. Fromm[1] · A. H. Gitter[1] · J.-D. Schulzke[1, 2]

[1] Institut für Klinische Physiologie, Universitätsklinikum Benjamin Franklin, Freie Universität Berlin, 12200 Berlin, Germany
[2] Medizinische Klinik I, Gastroenterologie und Infektiologie, Universitätsklinikum Benjamin Franklin, Freie Universität Berlin, 12200 Berlin, Germany

Introduction

Simple columnar epithelia cover the surfaces of the stomach and of the small and large intestines. They provide a boundary that acts not only as a selective barrier, but performs and controls the special secretory and absorptive functions of each segment of the gastrointestinal tract. This paper revisits basic transepithelial transport mechanisms. It is divided into four parts: (1) gastrointestinal secretion, (2) gastrointestinal absorption, (3) barrier function, and – as a specific topic related directly to anesthesia and intestinal transport – (4) effect of anesthesia on Na^+ and fluid transport in the distal colon.

Gastrointestinal Secretion

Two very basic secretory mechanisms are demonstrated, gastric HCl secretion and intestinal Cl^- (and K^+) secretion.

Gastric HCl Secretion: Controlled by an Apical Cl^- Channel

The gastric glands are composed of pepsin-producing chief cells and HCl secreting parietal, or oxyntic, cells, together with mucous neck cells and endocrine cells. The oxyntic cells possess long and narrow canaliculi opening to the apical, or luminal, side. In the schematic (Fig. 1) a single canaliculus is drawn short and wide for the sake of clarity. The central active mechanism in HCl secretion is an electroneutral ATP-driven K^+/H^+ exchange pump in the apical membrane (Sachs et al. 1976; Forte and Lee 1977). Thus, driven by 1 ATP molecule for each exchange cycle, H^+ and K^+ are transported in different directions in a 1:1 manner. Note that both ions are transported against electrochemical gradients, which means "uphill" with increasing electrochemical potential. This "primary active" (i.e., ATP-driven) antiport (or countertransport) can be blocked by omeprazole from the luminal side.

Almost all potassium taken up by the H^+/K^+-ATPase recirculates through an apical K^+ channel, so that there is virtually no net K^+ transport. However, since overall electroneutrality must be maintained in all epithelial transport processes, H^+ secretion is electrically coupled to the secretion of Cl^- through apical Cl^- channels. Indeed, the rate of H^+ secretion is controlled by the passive Cl^- conductance, rather than by activ-

M. K. Herbert et al. (Eds.), Problems of the Gastrointestinal Tract in Anesthesia...

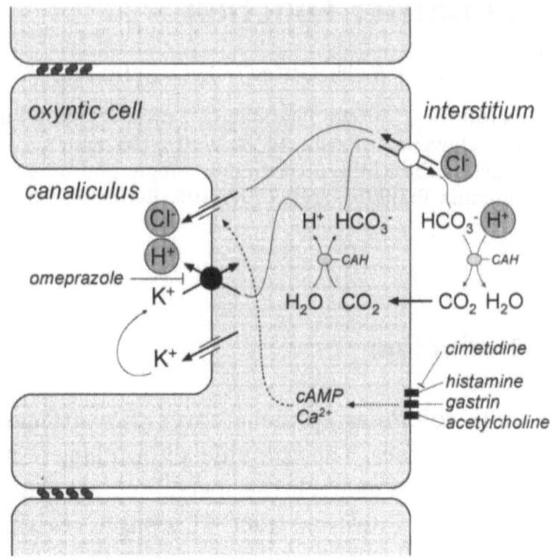

Fig. 1. Hydrogen ion and chloride secretion in the gastric gland

ity of the H^+/K^+-ATPase. Thus, if the Cl^- channels open, HCl secretion starts. On the basolateral side of the oxyntic cell, receptors for histamine, gastrin, and acetylcholine are located. Stimulation and inhibition of HCl secretion are mediated by G-proteins affecting the intracellular concentration of cyclic AMP and/or Ca^{2+}. Both intracellular second messengers cause the opening of the apical Cl^- channels.

As Cl^- leaves the oxyntic cell, the intracellular Cl^- concentration decreases, which facilitates the action of a Cl^-/HCO_3^- exchanger in the basolateral membrane. In order to make up for the loss of hydrogen ions (through the apical membrane) and bicarbonate (through the basolateral membrane), the intracellular enzyme carboanhydrase catalyzes the formation of H^+ and HCO_3^- from H_2O and CO_2. Owing to its lipophilic character, carbon dioxide does not rely on transmembranal carrier or channel proteins, but enters the cell through the phospholipid phase of the basolateral membrane. Outside the oxyntic cell CO_2 can, if necessary, be produced by the reaction of bicarbonate with hydrogen, again propelled by carboanhydrase. Note that basolateral uptake of hydrogen ions results, although no H^+ ion crosses the basolateral membrane.

Intestinal Cl^- and K^+ Secretion: A Unique Mechanism

In order to regulate the electrolyte composition of the stool, the intestine comprises mechanisms for secretion and absorption of anions and of cations. In health there is usually net absorption of chloride, but in secretory diarrhea an increase in Cl^- secretion, osmotically followed by water, causes the loss of intestinal fluid. This may reach excessive rates, e.g. in the case of cholera. Furthermore, mechanical distention of the intestine elicits secretion of Cl^- and water in a neuronal reflex pathway. The resulting lubrication of intestinal contents may represent a protective mechanism against ileus (Schulzke et al. 1995). Chloride secretion arises from a characteristic arrangement of transporters present in all segments of the intestine (Fig. 2).

Fig. 2. Intestinal chloride and potassium secretion (*CAH* carboanhydrase)

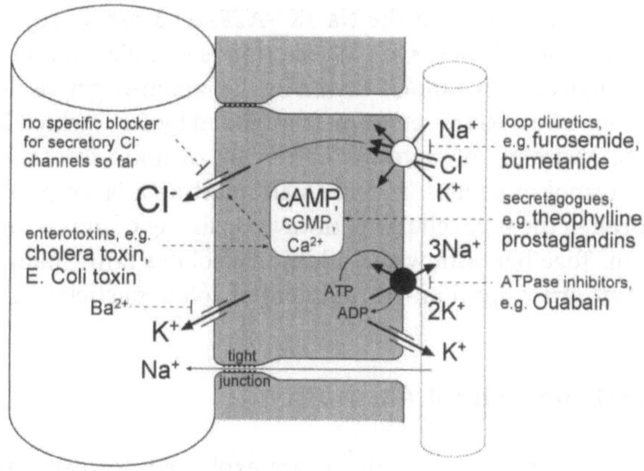

In the apical membrane resides a Cl^- channel, which – as in the oxyntic cells of the stomach – represents the rate-limiting step. There is evidence that this channel is identical with the "cystic fibrosis transmembrane conductance regulator" (CFTR), which is defective in cystic fibrosis. Consequently, cystic fibrosis leads to meconium ileus or distal intestinal obstruction syndrome. The Cl^- channel is stimulated via intracellular messengers cyclic AMP, cyclic GMP, and Ca^{2+} by such secretagogues as theophylline and prostaglandins, but also by enterotoxins such as cholera toxin and *E. coli* toxin, the latter two giving rise to the severe secretory diarrheas occurring in cholera and travelers' diarrhea, respectively. Unfortunately, at present no clinically useful blocker of this channel has been discovered.

At the basolateral side of the enterocyte, Cl^- is taken up by a symport carrier, which uses the steep electrochemical gradient of sodium. The Na^+ gradient, which is the conjugate driving force for the diffusional flow of Na^+, is built up and maintained by an ATP-driven exchange pump, the Na^+/K^+-ATPase. This primary active antiport, which is found in the basolateral membrane of all epithelia, can be blocked by ouabain from the contraluminal side. The free energy of the Na^+ gradient can be used to pull two chlorides and one potassium into the cell, together with one Na^+ ion, against their respective electrochemical gradients. The transport of Cl^- with the $Na^+K^+2Cl^-$ symport is defined as "secondary active," because it is uphill, but the metabolic energy (i.e. ATP) is consumed elsewhere, in the primary active Na^+/K^+-ATPase.

This arrangement of transporters providing chloride (and potassium) secretion is very common in epithelia (Fromm and Hierholzer 1997). This set of transporters is also present in Henle's loops of the kidney, but there the Cl^- channel is located basolaterally and the $Na^+K^+2Cl^-$ symport apically, so that Na^+ and Cl^- are absorbed. Furosemide and bumetanide, substances classified as "loop diuretics," block the $Na^+K^+2Cl^-$ symport in both kidney and gut. In nephrological applications there are no side effects in the intestine, because all diuretics are applied in a concentration that is not effective in the intestine. In the kidney these diuretics are filtered and then concentrated by water absorption and by secondary active secretion in the proximal tubule. Thus, in Henle's loop the diuretics arrive at concentrations about 30 times as high as in plasma Hierholzer and Fromm 1997).

Besides chloride, potassium is also secreted (Fig. 2): K^+ is taken up by the primary active mechanism of the Na^+/K^+-ATPase. Most K^+ recirculates through a basolateral K^+ channel. However, if Cl^- secretion is stimulated, an increased amount of K^+ leaves through apical channels driven by the lumen-negative electrical gradient produced by Cl^- exit. Potassium secretion is inhibited by Ba^{2+}, which blocks the apical K^+ channels. The secretion of water is driven by osmotic forces, about 1 l of water following 0.3 osmol of solutes. In the small intestine a large part of the secreted water passes through the paracellular pathway, consisting of intercellular spaces and the tight junction. Together with water, additional solutes flow (mainly Na^+ and Cl^-). This "solvent drag" arises from an entrainment of solute particles in the stream of solvent.

Gastrointestinal Absorption

Four absorptive mechanisms are explained: for carbohydrates, for amino acids and peptides, for sodium absorption in the proximal colon, and for sodium absorption in the distal colon and rectum.

Absorption of Carbohydrates

Absorption of carbohydrates follows two principles: (1) It takes place in the small intestine, but not in colonic segments, and (2) they are absorbed solely as monosaccharides, and not as disaccharides or even larger molecules (Fromm 1994). This means that dimers have to be split into monomers by disaccharidases, and if they are not – as in common lactose deficiency – these dimers will not be absorbed but will be metabolized by colonic bacteria. Two of the most important transport pathways are those for fructose and for glucose (and galactose) (Fig. 3, left).

Fructose is taken up through the apical cell membrane by a "uniport" carrier named GLUT5 (from *glu*cose *t*ransporter no. 5), which transports only with (not

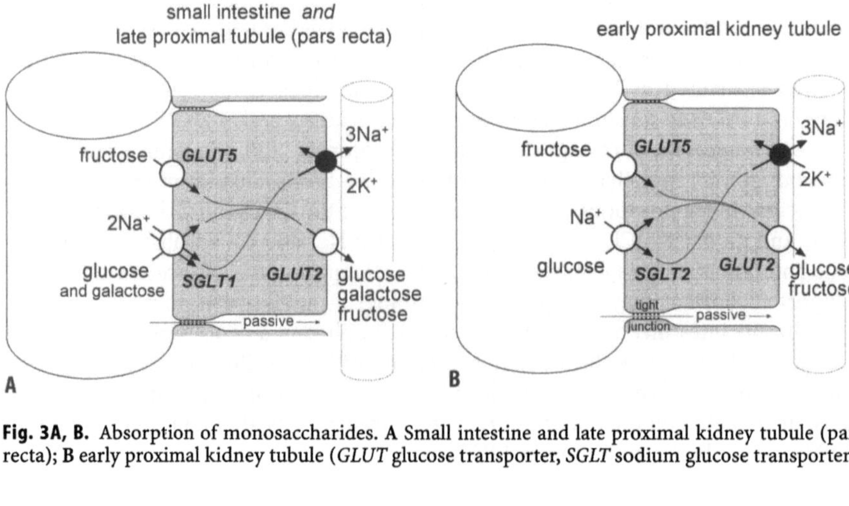

Fig. 3A, B. Absorption of monosaccharides. A Small intestine and late proximal kidney tubule (pars recta); B early proximal kidney tubule (*GLUT* glucose transporter, *SGLT* sodium glucose transporter)

against) the concentration gradient. Uniport-mediated transport processes used often to be referred to as facilitated diffusion. At the basolateral side fructose as well as all other sugars leave the enterocyte via a rather unspecific uniport carrier, GLUT2. Glucose and galactose are both taken up by a symport carrier, which employs the electrochemical gradient of two sodium ions for pulling one monosaccharide into the cell, even against a steep concentration gradient of the sugar. This transporter, SGLT1 (from *s*odium *gl*ucose *t*ransporter no. *1*), is well known (Wright 1993), but only recently was it discovered that it also carries about 210 molecules of water with each cycle (Meinild et al. 1998). This is remarkable, for it means that water transport is secondary active.

It is still an open question whether other sugar or amino acid carriers transport water in a similar way. The number of 210 molecules of H_2O per transport cycle of SGLT1 seems enormous, but in reality it is not: if water follows iso-osmotically (i.e. 290 mosmol per l water); even 570 H_2O have to follow each 2 Na^+ plus 1 glucose. Thus, 360 H_2O molecules pass the epithelium by other pathways. For the sake of completeness it should be mentioned that SGLT1 is also found in late proximal kidney tubule (pars recta). In the early proximal tubule, however, a similar but slightly different transporter, SGLT2, is located (Fig. 3, right). SGLT2 uses only one sodium for one glucose molecule (not galactose). It exhibits a higher transport capacity than SGLT1, but a lower affinity for glucose.

Absorption of Amino Acids and Peptides

Proteins are degraded to amino acids, or at least to tri- and dipeptides, before they are absorbed by several more or less specific carriers in the small intestine. Most of the amino acid carriers are symports with Na^+, but some, e.g. that for basic amino acids, are uniports. Others are more complex, e.g. that for acidic amino acids (Fig. 4).

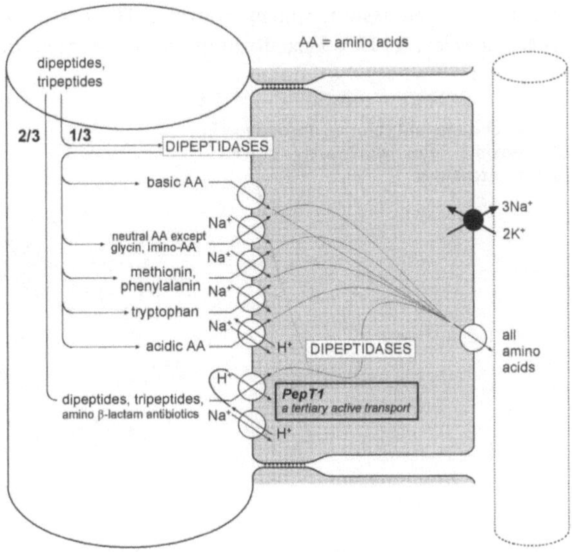

Fig. 4. Small intestinal absorption of amino acids and of di- and tripeptides (*PepT* peptide transporter)

Di- and tripeptides are apically taken up by a symport named PepT1 (for *pep*tide *t*ransporter no. *1*), which uses the electrochemical gradient of hydrogen ions for pulling the peptide uphill into the cell (Fei et al. 1994). The H^+ gradient is established by a secondary active Na^+/H^+-antiport. Since PepT1 is powered by a secondary active transport, it is referred to as a "tertiary active" carrier. PepT1 also accepts amino beta-lactam antibiotics. Intracellularly, the peptides are degraded by dipeptidases to single amino acids. All amino acids leave the enterocyte via uniport carriers in the basolateral cell membrane.

Sodium Absorption in the Proximal Colon

Sodium is absorbed in the proximal and distal segments of the colon by different mechanisms. In the ascending and transverse colon Na^+ is transported in a nearly 1:1 manner with Cl^- (Fig. 5). However, this is not done by a single Na^+Cl^- symport (as found in kidney distal tubule) but by an Na^+/H^+ antiport acting in parallel with a HCO_3^-/Cl^- antiport. Both transporters are loosely coupled by means of the stoichiometry of the carboanhydrase reaction, which provides equal amounts of H^+ and HCO_3^- (see above).

Sodium Absorption in the Distal Colon and Rectum

In the very distal parts of the colon (sigmoid and rectum) sodium is taken up from lumen by a channel named ENaC (for *e*pithelial *Na*$^+$ *c*hannel) (Fig. 6) in the apical membrane of the enterocyte. ENaC activity is under full control of aldosterone (Fromm et al. 1983). Through the basolateral membrane of the enterocyte, Na^+ is extruded against a steep electrochemical gradient by the Na^+/K^+-ATPase. ENaC can be blocked by amiloride. In the distal tubule and collecting duct of the kidney, amiloride acts as a potassium-sparing diuretic. The reason for this is an electrical coupling of Na^+ uptake and K^+ release through the apical membranes of kidney and colon cells.

Fig. 5. Sodium and chloride absorption in the proximal colon by a loosely coupled double exchanger

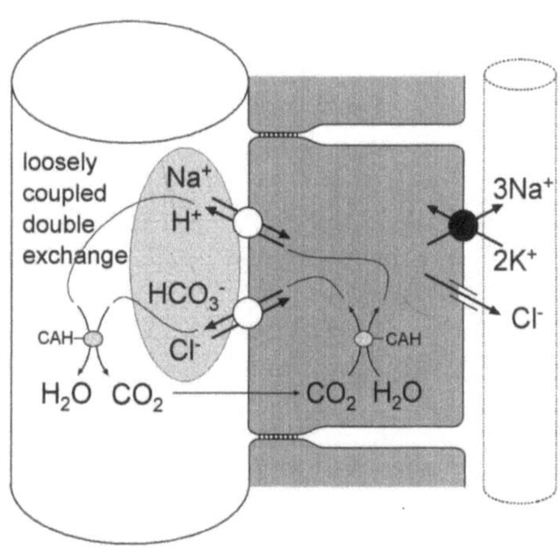

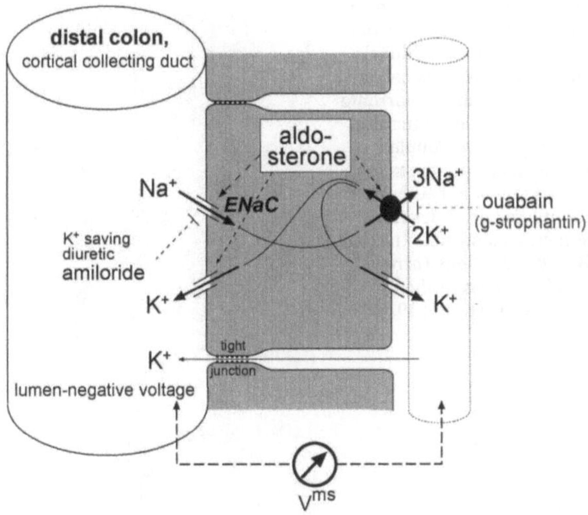

Fig. 6. Sodium absorption and potassium secretion in the distal colon and rectum (*ENaC* epithelial Na^+ channel)

Apical Na^+ uptake, via ENaC, results in the transfer of positive electrical charge, and therefore we refer to it as "electrogenic" or "rheogenic" (current-generating) transport. Thus, it decreases the apical membrane potential and generates a lumen-negative transepithelial potential of up to 100 mV. This is the driving force for K^+, which then leaves the cell via apical K^+ channels. From this it becomes clear that Na^+ absorption through ENaC is paralleled by K^+ secretion. If ENaC is blocked by amiloride, K^+ secretion also ceases. Hence, amiloride spares K^+. In therapeutic doses, amiloride acts preferably in the kidney cortical collecting ducts. The mechanisms, however, are present in the distal segments of colon and many other tubular epithelia (Fromm and Hierholzer 1997).

Barrier Function

Transepithelial solute and water transport is not only determined by the cellular transport mechanisms described above, but also by a barrier function preventing passive leakage. Indeed, there could be no lasting translocation, if all the solutes accumulated on one side were allowed to leak back across the epithelium. The resistance to electrolyte diffusion is essentially formed by (apical and basolateral) cell membranes and by the tight junctions, which seal the space between epithelial cells (Fig. 7). The tight junction is impermeable to molecules larger than disaccharides (for example), but it is – more or less – selectively permeable to certain small molecules, including water and small mono- and divalent ions. The permeability to small ions, as measured by electrical conductance (the reciprocal of resistance), is a reflection of the "leakiness" of an epithelium.

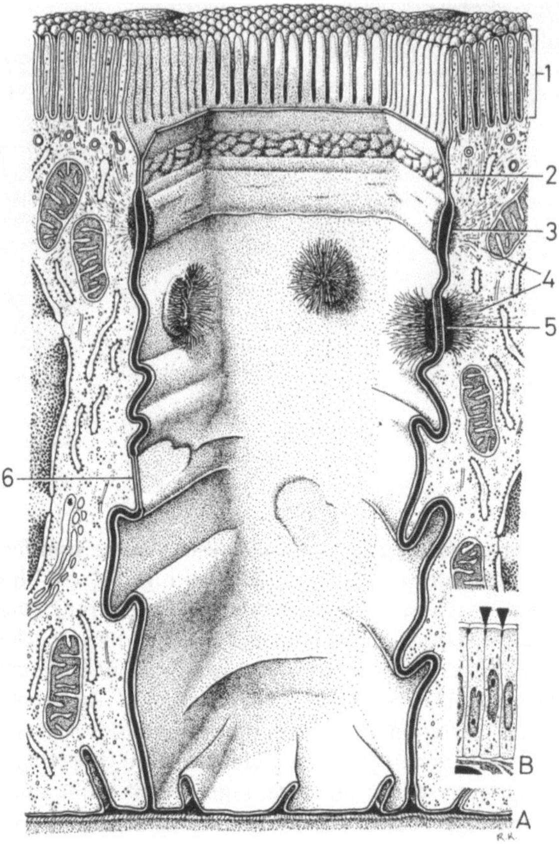

Fig. 7A, B. Cell junctions of a small intestinal epithelium. A The cell in the middle is shown devoid of its content. *1* Apical membrane forming microvilli, *2* tight junctions forming a web (zonula occludens), *3* adherens junctions (zonula adhaerens), *4* tonofilaments, *5* desmosomes, *6* connexons (nexus) B Tight junctions (*arrowheads*) as seen in the light microscope (Krstic 1976)

Leakiness Is Defined by the Ratio of Trans- to Paracellular Conductance

Two parallel routes of transepithelial transport exist, a transcellular route across the apical and basolateral cell membranes (which may pass through part of the intercellular space), and a paracellular route via the tight junction and through the full length of the lateral intercellular space. If the paracellular pathway is more conductive than the transcellular one (i.e., the tight junctions are more permeable to ions than are the cell membranes) the epithelium is classified as "leaky" (Table 1, first line). Leaky epithelia are found in the jejunum and ileum, but also in the kidney proximal tubule. They allow for large transport rates, but only against very small electrochemical gradients. Water follows iso-osmotically. The transport is enhanced by paracellular solvent drag (see above), a "forward leak," so to speak.

If the paracellular route is less conductive than the transcellular one (i.e., the tight junctions are less permeable to ions than the apical membrane) the epithelium is classified as "medium tight" (Table 1, line 2). Medium tight epithelia are found in the colon and rectum, but also in the kidney distal tubule and collecting duct. They allow only for small transport rates of solutes, although against large electrochemical gradi-

Table 1. Functional properties as determined by epithelial leakiness
G^{trans}/G^{para} = transcellular conductance divided by paracellular conductance

G^{trans}/G^{para}	Leakiness	Examples	Flux rates	Gradients	Function
< 1	Leaky	Ileum, proximal tubule	Large	Small	Mass transport
1–100	Medium tight	Colon, distal tubule	Small	Large	Fine regulation
> 100	Tight	Urinary bladder	Very small	Very large	Storage only

ents. Water follows by osmotic forces, but due to the lower paracellular permeability the luminal contents remain hyperosmolar relative to contraluminal (plasma) concentrations. In medium tight epithelia, transport rates are effectively controlled by hormones, e.g. aldosterone (see above) and, in the kidney, vasopressin.

Tubular Epithelia Share Segmental Strategy

From the segmental heterogeneities of transport and leakiness, which hold not only for the gastrointestinal tract and kidney tubules but also for other tubular epithelia (such as the ducts of salivary glands, sweat glands, and pancreas), a common strategy can be generalized. The main function of the leaky (proximal) segments of tubular epithelia is bulk transport of large amounts of solutes and water. On the other hand, the main function of the medium tight (distal) segments of tubular epithelia is accurate control of solute and water transport, in order to keep the electrolyte contents of the body at constant concentrations (homeostasis).

If the paracellular route is virtually not conductive at all (i.e., the tight junctions are really tight), the epithelium is defined as "tight" (Table 1, line 3). There is one epithelium in mammals proven to be tight, the urinary bladder. Here, transepithelial transport is practically zero and the only function of this epithelium is to store the urine. It remains possible, however, that there are other tight epithelia, e.g. in Reissner's membrane of the inner ear cochlea.

Barrier Function is Not Static: Tight Junctions Are Cellularly Controlled

Pathologic alterations of tight junction are caused by a variety of agents. These may act either on the luminal (or mucosal) side of the intestinal epithelium, and examples of such agents are bile salts, zonula occludens toxin (ZOT, a toxin of *Vibrio cholerae*), and toxins of *Clostridium difficile* (in pseudomembranous colitis), or on the contraluminal (serosal) side, an example being tumor necrosis factor-α (TNFα), which is elevated in intestinal bowel diseases, e.g. ulcerative colitis (Andus et al. 1991). Degradation of tight junctions increases paracellular ion permeability causing loss of electrolytes, which leads to "leak flux diarrhea." In order to illustrate the control of junctional permeability, we focus on the effect of TNFα on the ultrastructure of the tight junction. This example has been studied in our laboratory (Schmitz et al. 1999).

Surgically removed specimens of sigmoid colon from patients without intestinal inflammation exhibited a fully developed meshwork of tight junction strands, the linear elements that form the junctional seal (the strands run parallel to the epithelial

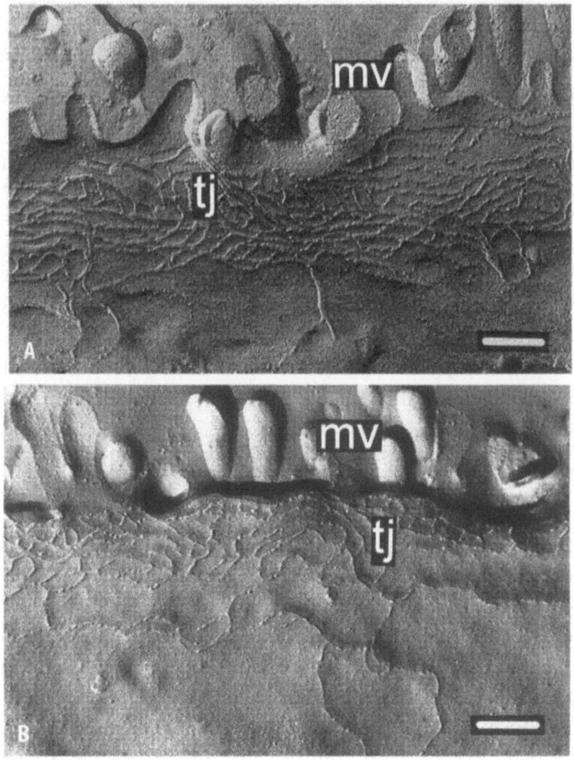

Fig. 8A, B. Freeze-fracture electron micrographs from the tight junctional region of colonic enterocytes. **A** Control sigma, **B** ulcerative colitis. (*mv* microvilli; *tj* tight junction strands). *Bar* 200 nm. Schmitz et al. (1999)

surface). In contrast, specimens from patients suffering from ulcerative colitis contain a reduced number of tight junction strands. Impairment of the seal may explain the leak flux diarrhea observed in this disease (Fig. 8, right). TNFα appears to be an important mediator of this alteration. For instance, in a colonic cell line (HT-29/B6) the cytokine elicits the same change, i.e. a decrease in the number of strands, as seen in ulcerative colitis (Schmitz et al. 1999).

Two Groups of Tight Junction Molecules, Occludin and the Claudins

The molecular structure of the tight junction is not yet fully known. Several intracellular molecules are associated with the tight junction, e.g. ZO-1, ZO-2 and cingulin (Fig. 9). The first membrane-spanning element, named occludin, was identified a few years ago by the group of Tsukita (Furuse et al. 1993). It is a 56-kDa protein with four transmembrane domains (Fig. 10) (Furuse et al. 1994). This protein was expected to form the strands, the structural correlate of the junctional barrier function. However, it was only 1998 when it turned out that tight junctional strands were also formed in the absence of occludin, because "occludin-deficient embryonic stem cells can differentiate into polarized epithelial cells bearing tight junctions" (the title of the paper published by Tsukita's group: Saitou et al. 1998).

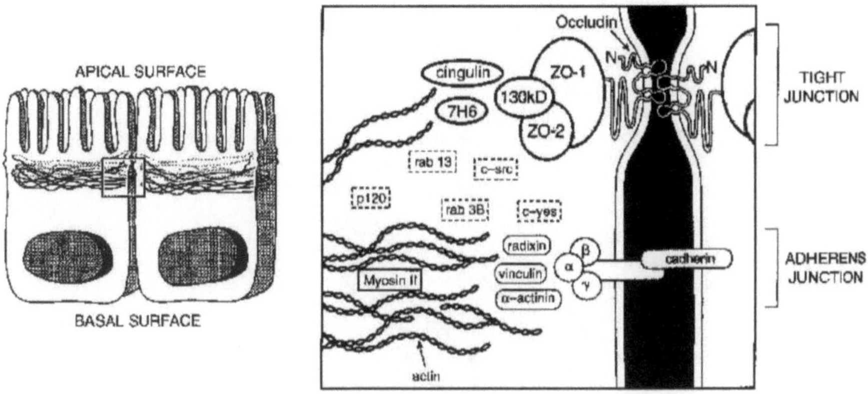

Fig. 9. Schematic illustrating tight junction-associated molecules. Mitic and Anderson (1998)

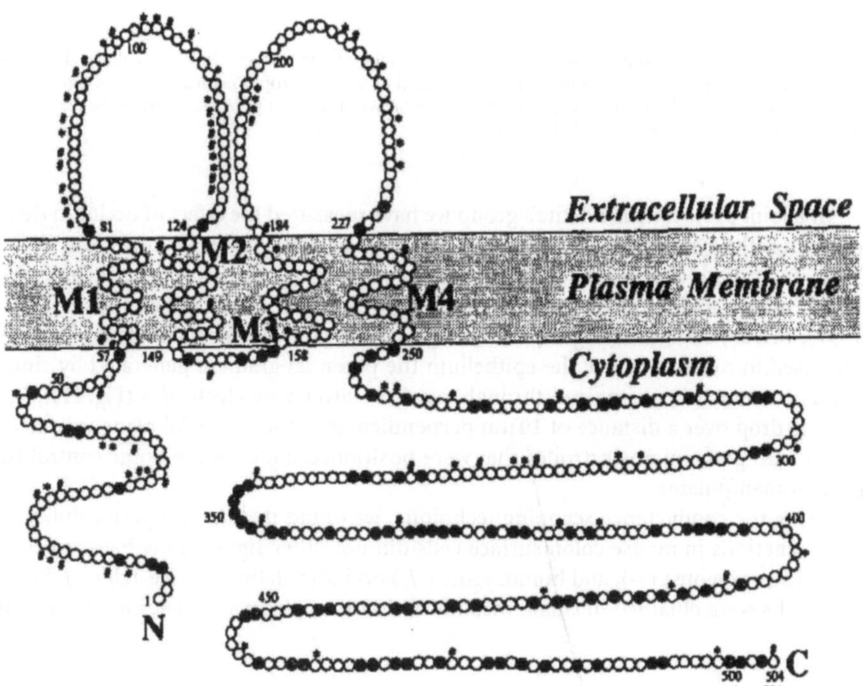

Fig. 10. Occludin, the first membrane-spanning component of the tight junction discovered. Furuse et al. (1993)

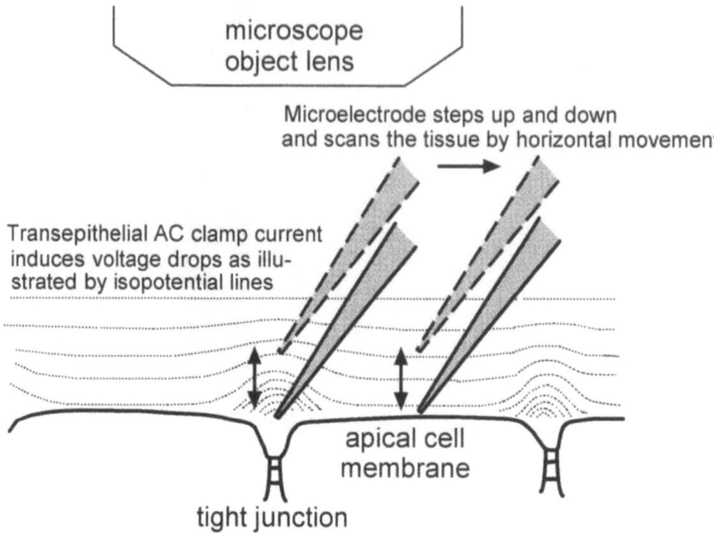

Fig. 11. Conductance scanning technique. Transepithelial clamp current induced voltage drops as illustrated by isopotential lines above the epithelium. The voltage drop was measured, at a tight junction or at an apical cell membrane, as the difference between the two potentials across the excursion of the scanning microelectrode. Gitter at al. (1997)

In a joint project with Tsukita's group we have measured the effect of occludin deficiency on the barrier function of tight junctions in distal colon in knock-out mice. This was possible with our recently developed "conductance scanning technique," which allows for direct measurements of tight junction conductance (Gitter et al. 1997). Briefly, an alternating current bridge system with synchronous demodulation was used to measure above the epithelium the potential gradient generated by sinusoidal current that was passed through a pair of silver wire electrodes (Fig. 11). The voltage drop over a distance of 10 μm perpendicular to the epithelial plane was measured with glass microelectrodes that were positioned under microscopic control by a micromanipulator.

Using the conductance scanning technique, we found that the ion permeability of tight junctions in mouse colon surface cells did not differ significantly between controls, heterozygote (+/-), and homozygote (-/-) occludin-deficient mice Table 2). Similar results were obtained in small intestine and in the urinary bladder, indicating that

Table 2. Total conductance of surface epithelium ($G^{surface}$), conductance of transcellular pathway (G^{cell}), and conductance of tight junctional pathway (G^{tj}) in late distal colon of occludin-deficient heterozygote (+/-) and homozygote (-/-) knock-out mice . Conductances are in mS/cm^2, referring to the gross tissue area; $G^s = G^{cell} + G^{tj}$. Data from Schulzke et al. (1999)

	G^s	G^{cell}	G^{tj}
Control	7.9	7.6	0.3
Occludin (+/-)	6.7	6.5	0.2
Occludin (-/-)	7.3	7.1	0.2

ccludin is not a necessary component of the seal in tight junctions of leaky, medium ight, and tight epithelia (Schulzke et al., 1999).

Very recently, "Claudin-1 and -2: novel integral membrane proteins localizing at ight junctions with no sequence similarity to occludin" were found (Furuse et al. 998). The claudins are 22 kDa proteins, also exhibiting 4 putative transmembrane lomains; the chain length of claudin-1 and claudin-2 is slightly different. The near uture will show whether the claudins are the barrier-forming components of the ight junctions.

:ffect of Anesthesia on Transepithelial Transport in Distal Colon

Nhile the above tight junction data were brand new, we turn now to some "classic" tudies, performed as long as two decades ago, dealing with the effect of anesthesia n solute and water transport in an aldosterone-sensitive epithelium. At that time ransport studies in rats were often performed on animals generally anesthetized vith thiobarbiturates (e.g. Inactin, 100 mg/kg b.w. i.p.). After cannulation and luminal erfusion of segments of the colon the transepithelial voltage could be measured for nany hours (Fig. 12).

To our surprise, the voltage in the rectum increased, after a lag of about 2 h, for everal hours, and reached a maximum after about 10–12 hours (Fromm and Hegel 1978). The simultaneously recorded transepithelial voltage of the upper colon emained constant (Fig. 12A). In contrast, if the adrenal glands were removed 1 week efore the experiment, no voltage increase occurred in the rectum. The voltage ncrease pattern was restored, however, after substituting the adrenalectomized aninal at the beginning of the experiment with a single dose of 40 µg/kg b.w. of aldoste-

Table 3. Aldosterone and corticosterone plasma concentrations and transepithelial voltage of rectal nucosa Anesthesia was always initiated with 3 % vapors of halothane. Cervical surgery (*Cerv*) ncluded cannulation of the trachea and placement of catheters both into the left carotid artery and he right jugular vein. Abdominal surgery (*abdom*) included a 4 – 5 cm ventral midline incision, canulation of the rectum, and placement of a catheter into the urinary bladder. Duration is total time lapsed between induction of anesthesia and decapitation. Transepithelial voltage (υ^{ms}) at the distal nd of the rectum was recorded immediately before decapitation. Adrenalectomized (ADX) rats were hronically maintained for 1 week on 15 ng/h aldosterone plus 50 ng/h dexamethasone and were lecapitated under short anesthesia. Data from Fromm et al. (1983)

Anesthesia	Surgery	Duration (min)	Aldosterone (ng/100 ml)	Corticosterone (µg/100 ml)	Rectal ψ^{ms} (mV)
None	–	–	11±2	17±2	–
Inactin	None	10	17±4	29±6	–
Inactin	Cerv + abdom	75	55±6	57±4	–12±3
Inactin	Cerv + abdom	300	91±12	44±3	–60±5
Inactin	Cerv only	300	39±8	28±4	–
Inactin	Cerv + abdom	400	101±15	38±2	–76±5
Inactin	Cerv + abdom	800	119±18	35±2	–87±8
Inactin	Cerv + abdom	1800	26±11	23±3	–83±8
Nembutal	Cerv + abdom	420	87±27	34±6	–72±9
(ADX + steroid substitution)			12±2	0.1±0.04	–

rone (Fig. 12B). These findings showed that the rectal voltage increase was dependent on aldosterone. Further, the similar time-courses of aldosterone-substituted adrenalectomized animals and intact controls suggested that in those controls a huge aldosterone release must have started at the beginning of the experiment.

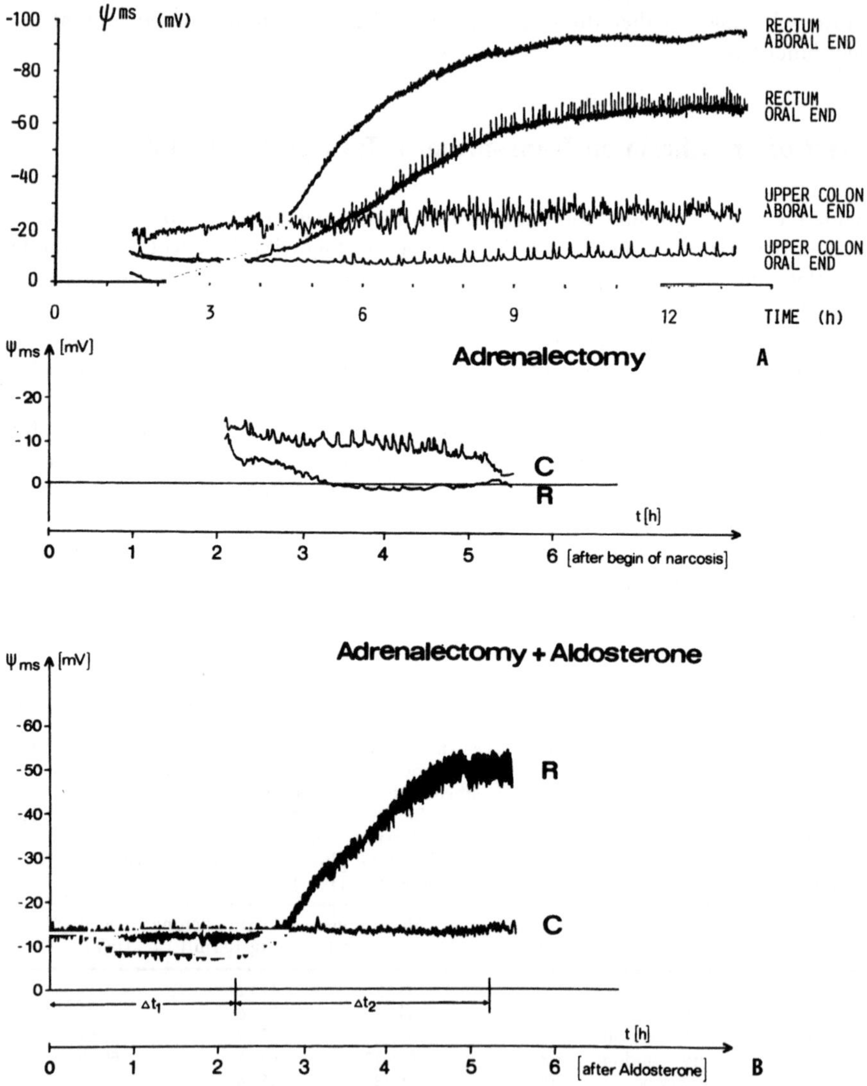

Fig. 12A, B. Transepithelial voltage in in vivo experiments. Rats were anesthetized with thiobarbital (Inactin), the abdomen opened, and the large intestine cannulated and perfused. A Spontaneous increase in controls; B adrenalectomy and adrenalectomy plus single-dose aldosterone substitution at beginning of the experiment. Fromm and Hegel (1978)

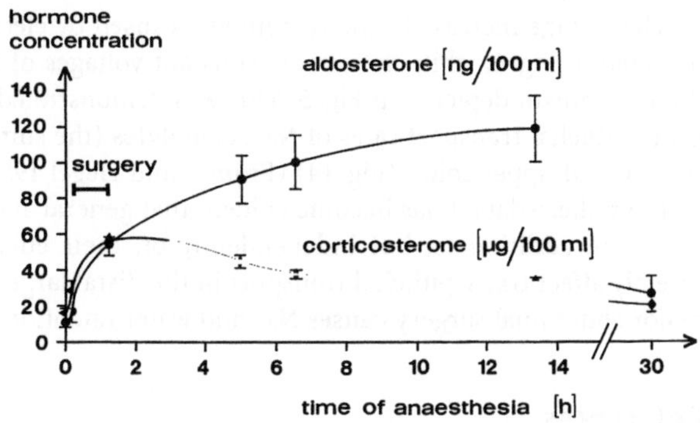

Fig. 13. Aldosterone and glucocorticoid plasma levels during general anesthesia and abdominal surgery. Fromm et al. (1983)

Indeed, measurements of plasma levels of aldosterone and corticosterone (the main glucocorticoid of rats) revealed that these hormones are released during general anesthesia and abdominal surgery (Fig. 13) (Fromm et al. 1983). A detailed survey is given in Table 3. General anesthesia without abdominal surgery produced a steroid increase that was about half that observed with abdominal surgery. Hence, the handling of the mesenterial radix had a pronounced effect on steroid release, although all surgical procedures were carried out very gently. The effect of increased steroid levels did not depend on the type of anesthetic. Nembutal gave results not significantly different from those obtained with Inactin.

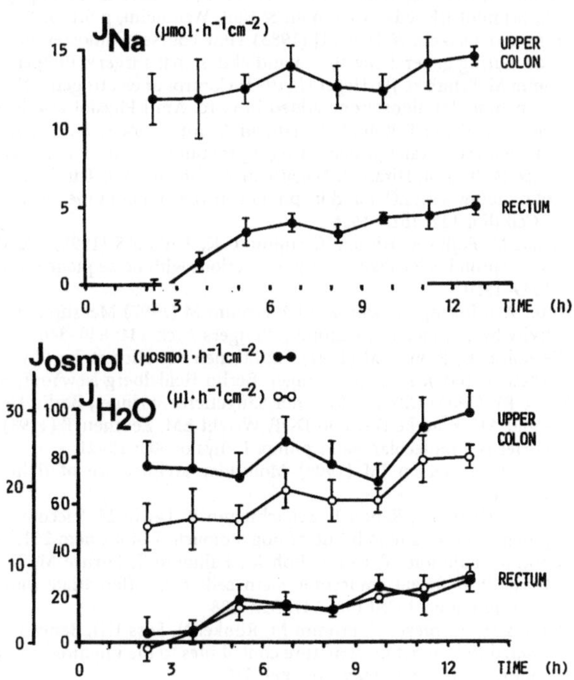

Fig. 14. Net absorption of Na^+, osmolytes (the sum of all solutes), and H_2O in upper colon and rectum. Fromm and Hegel (1987)

The voltage increase in the rectum was caused by electrogenic Na^+ absorption, as depicted in Fig. 6, while the almost constant voltages of the upper colon arose from the mechanism depicted in Fig. 5. This was demonstrated by direct measurements of transepithelial transport rates of Na^+, osmolytes (the sum of all solutes) and water in rectum and upper colon (Fig. 14) (Fromm and Hegel 1987).

From these data it has become evident that general anesthesia and abdominal surgery – in addition to, but independently of, their effects on intestinal motility – directly affect transepithelial transport in the distal large intestine. This explains how major abdominal surgery causes Na^+ and water retention in the postoperative phase.

References

Andus T, Gross V, Casar I, Krumm D, Hosp J, David M, Schölmerich J (1991) Activation of monocytes during inflammatory bowel disease. Pathobiology 59: 166–170

Fei YJ, Kanai Y, Nussberger S, Ganapathy V, Leibach FH, Romero MF, Singh SK, Boron WF, Hediger MA (1994) Expression cloning of a mammalian proton-coupled oligopeptide transporter. Nature 368: 563–566

Forte JG, Lee HC (1977) Gastric adenosine triphosphatases: a review of their possible role in HCl secretion. Gastroenterology 73: 921–926.

Fromm M (1994) Störungen der Verdauung und des epithelialen Transports. In: Hierholzer K, Schmidt RF (eds) Pathophysiologie des Menschen. Chapman & Hall, Weinheim, pp 6.28–6.38

Fromm M, Hegel U (1978) Segmental heterogeneity of epithelial transport in rat large intestine. Pflügers Arch 378: 71–83

Fromm M, Hegel U (1987) Net ion fluxes and zero flux limiting concentrations in rat upper colon and rectum during anaesthesia-induced aldosterone liberation. Pflügers Arch 408: 185–193

Fromm M, Hierholzer K (1997) Epithelien. In: Schmidt RF, Thews G (eds) Physiologie des Menschen, 27th edn. Springer, Berlin Heidelberg NewYork, pp 719–736

Fromm M, Hegel U, Wiederholt M (1994) Epithelien. In: Pathophysiologie des Menschen, Hierholzer K, Schmidt RF (eds), Chapman & Hall, Weinheim, p 5.1–5.19

Fromm M, Oelkers W, Hegel U (1983) Time course of aldosterone and corticosterone plasma levels in rats during general anesthesia and abdominal surgery. Pflügers Arch 399: 249–254

Fromm M, Schulzke JD, Hegel U (1993) Control of electrogenic Na^+ absorption in rat late distal colon by nanomolar aldosterone added in vitro. Am J Physiol 264: E68–E73

Furuse M, Hirase T, Itoh M, Nagafuchi A, Yonemura S, Tsukita S, Tsukita S (1993) Occludin: a novel integral membrane protein at tight junctions. J Cell Biol 123: 1777–1788

Furuse M, Itoh M, Hirase T, Nagafuchi A, Yonemura S, Tsukita S, Tsukita S (1994) Direct association of occludin with ZO-1 and its possible involvement in the localization of occludin at tight junctions. J Cell Biol 127: 1617–1626

Furuse M, Fujita K, Hiiragi T, Fujimoto K, Tsukita S (1998) Claudin-1 and -2: novel integral membrane proteins localizing at tight junctions with no sequence similarity to occludin. J. Cell Biol. 141: 1539–1550

Gitter AH, Bertog M, Schulzke JD, Fromm M (1997) Measurement of paracellular epithelial conductivity by conductance scanning. Pflügers Arch 434: 830–840

Hierholzer K, Fromm M (1997) Funktionen der Nieren. In: Physiologie des Menschen. Schmidt RF, Thews G (eds), 27th ed, Springer, Berlin Heidelberg NewYork, p 737–777

Krstic RV (1987) Ultrastruktur der Säugetiere. Springer, Berlin Heidelberg New York

Meinild AK, Klaerke DA, Loo DDF, Wright EM, Zeuthen T (1998) The human Na^+-glucose cotransporter is a molecular water pump. J Physiol 508: 15–21

Mitic LL, Anderson JM (1998) Molecular architecture of tight junctions. Annu Rev Physiol 60: 121–142

Sachs G, Chang H, Rabon E, Schackmann R, Lewin M, Saccomani G (1976) A non-electrogenic H^+ pump in plasma membrane of hog stomach. J Biol Chem 251: 7690–7698

Saitou M, Fujimoto K, Doi Y, Itoh M, Fujimoto T, Furuse M, Takano H, Noda T, Tsukita S (1998) Occludin-deficient embryonic stem cells can differentiate into polarized epithelial cells bearing tight junctions. J Cell Biol 141: 397–408

Schmitz H, Barmeyer C, Fromm M, Runkel N, Foss HD, Bentzel CJ, Riecken EO, Schulzke JD (1999) Altered tight junction structure contributes to the impaired epithelial barrier function in ulcerative colitis. Gastroenterology 116: 309–310

INVITED ARTICLE

The Human Intestinal Microflora: Physiology and Pathophysiology

I. B. Autenrieth

Max von Pettenkofer-Institut für Hygiene und Medizinische Mikrobiologie,
Ludwig Maximilians Universität, Pettenkoferstrasse 9a, 80336 München, Germany

Introduction

The mucosal surfaces of the human body, including the gastrointestinal, the respiratory and the urogenital tract, have a total surface area of more than 400 m^2 (Neutra and Kraehenbuhl 1992). All these surfaces are colonized by a normal intestinal bacterial microflora (designated as indigenous microflora) that consists of more than 400 different bacterial species and subspecies with a total number of 10^{14} bacterial cells. As the human body consists of 10^{13} cells and is colonized by 10^{14} bacteria, there are actually 10 bacteria for each cell of the body! Both fungi and protozoa may also occur as part of the indigenous microflora. However, due to their low number, eukaryotic microorganisms do not play a significant role. The surface of the gastrointestinal tract is about 200–300 m^2 and colonized by 10^{13-14} bacteria with more than 400 bacterial species and subspecies.

The indigenous microflora in its steady state represents a physiological ecological system exerting various beneficial effects on the host. Both bacteria–bacteria interactions as well as host–bacteria interactions are involved in and required for this critical balance. In fact, the balance of this system is crucial for the host physiology. Alterations of the host or bacterial factors may result in dysbalance and subsequent pathophysiological clinical manifestations. Both physiology and pathophysiology of the bacterial flora and its clinical implications are discussed herein.

The Intestinal Microflora

In a stable gastrointestinal ecosystem, all available habitats are probably occupied by indigenous microorganisms. Therefore, practically any microbial species acquired from the environment (food, water, etc.) will usually not colonize. Instead, most microbial species will rapidly pass through the gastrointestinal tract or will be killed by host or bacterial factors.

The indigenous flora is not just randomly distributed in various compartments of the gastrointestinal tract. In fact, there is a characteristic distribution of microorganisms in each particular region of the gastrointestinal tract (Table 1) (Autenrieth 1998; Berg 1996; Lee 1985; Simon and Goa Bach 1995). The microflora of the oral cavity is comprised of about 200 bacterial species with a density of 10^9 bacteria per ml fluid or tissue from oral surfaces (teeth, tongue, cheeks). Dental plaques, for instance, contain even higher bacterial populations (up to 10^{11} bacteria/g). The colonization of the

M. K. Herbert et al. (Eds.), Problems of the
Gastrointestinal Tract in Anesthesia...

INVITED ARTICLE

The Human Intestinal Microflora: Physiology and Pathophysiology

I. B. Autenrieth

Max von Pettenkofer-Institut für Hygiene und Medizinische Mikrobiologie,
Ludwig Maximilians Universität, Pettenkoferstrasse 9a, 80336 München, Germany

Introduction

The mucosal surfaces of the human body, including the gastrointestinal, the respiratory and the urogenital tract, have a total surface area of more than 400 m^2 (Neutra and Kraehenbuhl 1992). All these surfaces are colonized by a normal intestinal bacterial microflora (designated as indigenous microflora) that consists of more than 400 different bacterial species and subspecies with a total number of 10^{14} bacterial cells. As the human body consists of 10^{13} cells and is colonized by 10^{14} bacteria, there are actually 10 bacteria for each cell of the body! Both fungi and protozoa may also occur as part of the indigenous microflora. However, due to their low number, eukaryotic microorganisms do not play a significant role. The surface of the gastrointestinal tract is about 200–300 m^2 and colonized by 10^{13-14} bacteria with more than 400 bacterial species and subspecies.

The indigenous microflora in its steady state represents a physiological ecological system exerting various beneficial effects on the host. Both bacteria–bacteria interactions as well as host–bacteria interactions are involved in and required for this critical balance. In fact, the balance of this system is crucial for the host physiology. Alterations of the host or bacterial factors may result in dysbalance and subsequent pathophysiological clinical manifestations. Both physiology and pathophysiology of the bacterial flora and its clinical implications are discussed herein.

The Intestinal Microflora

In a stable gastrointestinal ecosystem, all available habitats are probably occupied by indigenous microorganisms. Therefore, practically any microbial species acquired from the environment (food, water, etc.) will usually not colonize. Instead, most microbial species will rapidly pass through the gastrointestinal tract or will be killed by host or bacterial factors.

The indigenous flora is not just randomly distributed in various compartments of the gastrointestinal tract. In fact, there is a characteristic distribution of microorganisms in each particular region of the gastrointestinal tract (Table 1) (Autenrieth 1998; Berg 1996; Lee 1985; Simon and Goa Bach 1995). The microflora of the oral cavity is comprised of about 200 bacterial species with a density of 10^9 bacteria per ml fluid or tissue from oral surfaces (teeth, tongue, cheeks). Dental plaques, for instance, contain even higher bacterial populations (up to 10^{11} bacteria/g). The colonization of the

M. K. Herbert et al. (Eds.), Problems of the
Gastrointestinal Tract in Anesthesia...

Table 1. The indigenous gastrointestinal microflora (*ae* aerobic, *aa* anaerobic)

Distribution/localization	Bacterial numbers	Frequent species
Oral cavity	10^9/ml saliva	*Streptococcus* spp., *Neisseria* spp., *Veillonella* spp., *Bacteroides* spp., *Prevotella* spp.
Stomach	$0–10^5$/g	See oral cavity (transient): Lactobacilli (ae)[a], gram-positive cocci (ae)
Duodenum	10^3/g	See stomach
Jejunum	10^5/g	Lactobacilli (ae), *Streptococcus* spp. (ae), few anaerobic bacteria
Ileum	10^{8-9}/g	Gram-positive cocci (e.g., *Enterococcus* spp. (ae), Enterobacteriaceae[a] (ae), *Bacteroides spp.* (aa[a]), other anaerobic bacteria)
Colon[b]	10^{10-11}/g	*Bacteroides* spp. (aa), *Clostridium* spp. (aa), *Bifidobacterium* spp. (aa), *Eubacterium* (aa), lactobacilli (ae), Enterobacteriaceae (ae), *Fusobacterium* spp. (aa), *Peptostreptococcus* spp. (aa), *Enterococcus* spp. (ae)

[a]Enterobacteriaceae: *Escherichia coli, Klebsiella* spp., *Enterobacter* spp, *Proteus* spp.
[b]Yeasts and protozoa may occur in low numbers

stomach varies considerably depending on nutrition factors and comprises 10^1 – 10^5 bacteria per ml gastric contents. Clearly, the gastric acid exerts bactericidal effects on the microflora. One third of the human world population is colonized in the stomach with *Helicobacter pylori* (Moayyedi and Axon 1995). Only in a small subpopulation *H. pylori* causes actually disease. Nevertheless, although it is not yet clear, *H. pylori* should not be considered as part of the indigenous microflora.

In the upper part of the small intestine (duodenum, jejunum) there are 10^3–10^4 bacteria per ml intestinal contents. The relatively low number is due to the low pH of the intestinal contents resulting from gastric acid production and the relatively high peristalsis of the small bowel. The most frequent microorganisms are lactobacilli and streptococci. In the lower part of the small intestine 10^8–10^9 microorganisms per ml intestinal contents are present. Lactobacilli, streptococci and Enterobacteriacae including *Escherichia coli* are found. The higher bacterial numbers in the ileum are associated with a lower peristalsis and lower oxidation–reduction potentials.

The colon contains 10^{11}–10^{12} bacteria/g intestinal contents comprising more than 400 bacterial species. More than 99 % of the colonic microflora are obligate anaerobes such as *Bacteroides* spp., *Eubacterium, Bifidobacterium* and *Clostridium* spp. In fact, *Clostridium difficile* and *Clostridium perfringens* may also occur as part of the normal indigenous microflora. About 10^8/g intestinal contents facultative anaerobes including *Escherichia coli* and other coliforms as well as up to 10^3/g yeast may occur. The high number of microorganisms in the colon contents are due to the very low intestinal motility with transit times of up to 60 h and the very low oxidation-reduction potentials. Moreover, it is important to note that many bacterial species are not yet known or characterized as they are noncultivable and cannot be grown on agar plates in vitro (Fig. 1). Furthermore, the microflora located in the lumen of the colon might differ from that associated with the glycocalyx of the intestinal epithelial cells. Thus, the microorganisms found in stool specimens may not necessarily closely reflect the actual composition of the colonic flora.

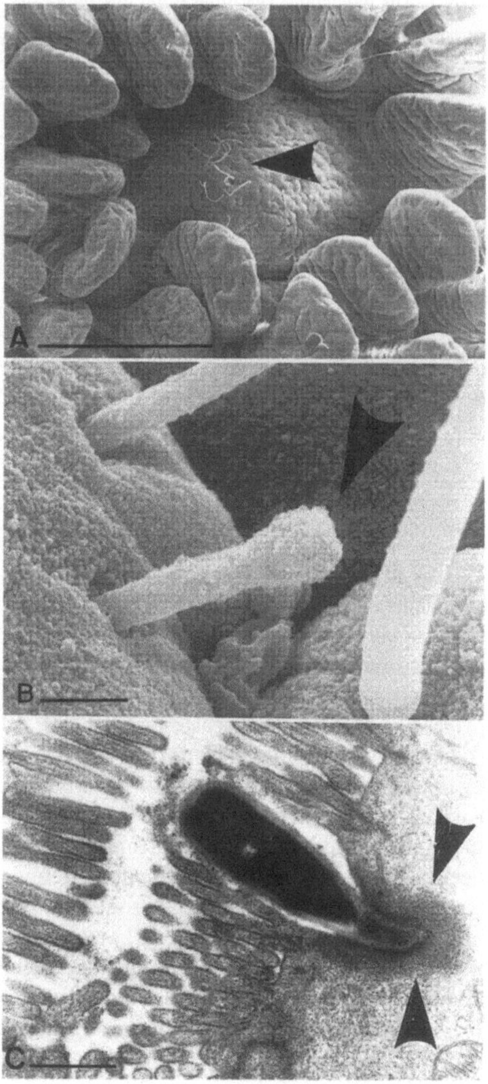

Fig. 1A–C. Scanning electron microscopy of the small intestine of a mouse. A Villi and follicle-associated epithelium (FAE; center) overlying Peyer's patches. Segmented filamentous bacteria (SFB; *arrow*) attached to the FAE are part of the normal microflora of rodents and cannot be grown in vitro. *Bar* 200 μm. **B** Higher magnification of the FAE with SFB (*arrow*). *Bar* 5 μm. C Transmission electron microscopy of SFB sticking within an enterocyte. The dark area (*arrow*) around the bacterium is due to F-actin accumulation within the cell, indicating a bacterial--host cross-talk. *Bar* 1 μm

The composition of the indigenous microflora of the intestine depends on several host factors such as age and nutrition factors (Simon and Goa Bach 1995). A fiber-rich or a vegetarian beef-reduced diet appears to favor colonization with aerobic bacteria while a beef-rich diet favors colonization with anaerobic bacteria. While it is not yet clear, whether a specific intestinal microflora may be associated with the development of colonic cancer, there is striking evidence that *Helicobacter pylori* may be associated with gastric tumors.

Beneficial Effects Exerted on the Host by the Indigenous Intestinal Microflora

Under normal circumstances the normal indigenous microflora in its steady state represents a physiological system which is dependent on both bacteria-bacteria and host-bacteria interactions. In this situation, the microflora exerts several beneficial effects on the host including colonization resistance, promotion of epithelial cell metabolism and peristalsis as well as stimulation of the mucosa-associated lymphoid tissue (Figs. 2, 3).

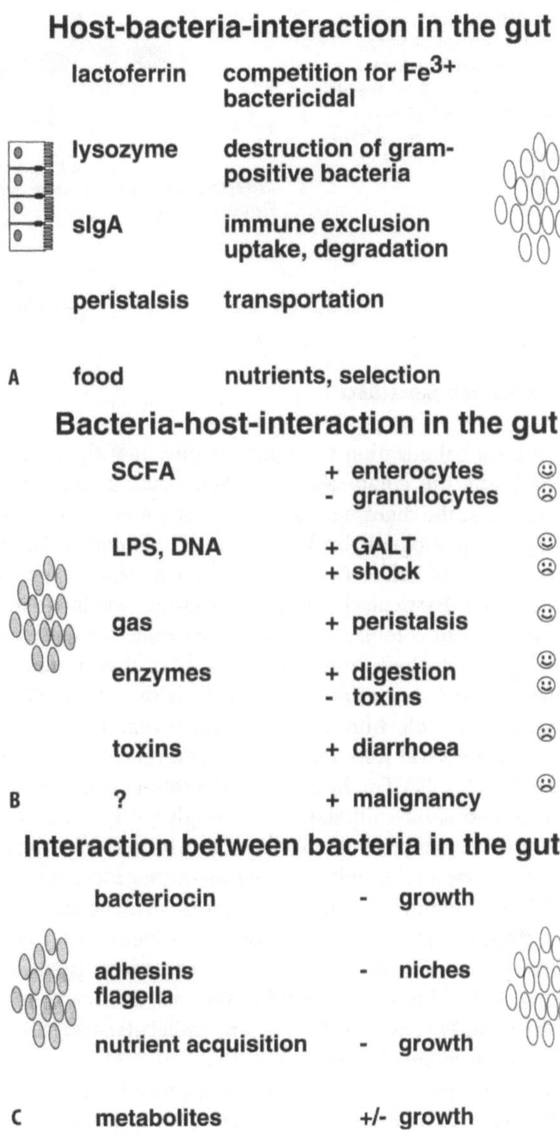

Fig. 2A–C. Interactions between the indigenous intestinal microflora and the host. A The flora is regulated by host factors. B Moreover, the microflora can exert both beneficial and harmful effects on the host. C The microflora regulates itself by bacteria--bacteria interactions

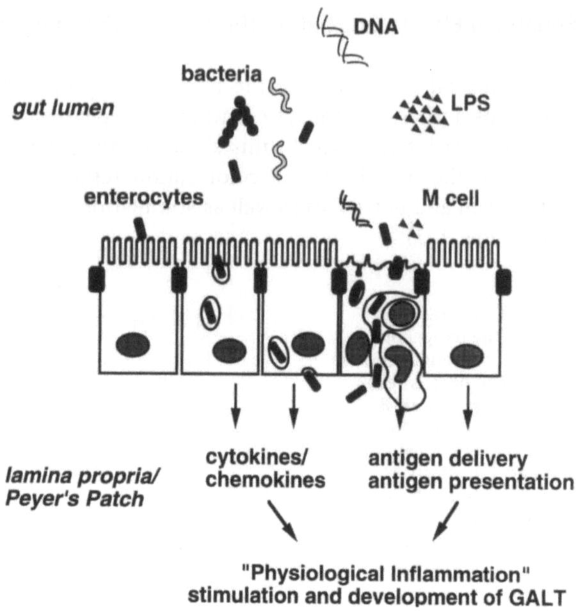

Fig. 3. The indigenous microflora stimulates the development of the mucosa-associated lymphoid tissue (MALT). The content of the intestine, including bacteria and their products, such as LPS or DNA, stimulates the development of the MALT. Enterocytes are part of the MALT and may produce cytokines and chemokines in response to bacterial stimulation, which leads to the recruitment of phagocytes and lymphocytes. Most bacteria cannot invade via enterocytes but are translocated into the Peyer's patches selectively via M cells

Colonization Resistance

The term colonization resistance implies that the indigenous microflora of the intestine limits the colonization of exogenous, potentially pathogenic (mostly aerobic) bacteria in the digestive tract (Vollaard and Clasener 1994). In fact, the susceptibility for enteropathogenic bacteria such as *Salmonella, Shigella,* enteropathogenic *E. coli,* or *Yersinia* as well as *Clostridium difficile* depends on the presence of the indigenous microflora. Particularly obligate anaerobes, such as *Bacteroides* spp., are required for promotion of colonization resistance, while facultative anaerobic bacteria such as *E. coli* appear to have only a minor role in this process. Similarly, anaerobic bacteria may prevent bacterial overgrowth with potentially pathogenic microorganisms including *E. coli.* Although the mechanisms that are involved in colonization resistance are not yet fully understood, several events are obviously involved in this process (Fig. 2.): (1) The indigenous microflora occupies niches and receptors for bacterial adhesins on epithelial cells, the glycocalyx or in the mucus. (2) The indigenous microflora produces metabolites and bacteriocins toxic for other bacterial species. Bacteriocins are antibiotic proteins or peptides which act as DNases, RNases or via inhibition of murein synthesis. There is evidence that c. 50 % of freshly isolated bacteria from the intestinal tract produce bacteriocins. (3) There is competition for substrates, vitamins, growth factors. Many microorganisms have developed highly efficient, high-affinity iron uptake systems to survive in iron-restricted environments (Bagg and Nylands 1987). The low-molecular-weight iron-chelating compounds designated as siderophores are secreted and after iron-chelation are taken up by specific transport systems of the microorganisms. Although certain bacteria do not produce siderophores on their own, they can take up siderophores produced by other bacterial species in the gut, in order to compete for Fe^{3+} with lactoferrin produced by host cells. Interestingly, siderophores may have a dual role in the pathogenesis of infections: hence, siderophores may also suppress immune responses of the host (Autenrieth et al. 1991). (4) The indigenous microflora may destroy bacterial toxins. (5) The pH and the oxidation–reduction potentials are modulated.

Apart from bacteria–bacteria interaction, a number of host factors exert a profound impact on the microflora. Thus, host factors such as secretory IgA, lactoferrin, defensins, lysozyme and complement may regulate the intestinal microflora, thereby influencing the susceptibility for infections with exogenous microorganisms (Fig. 2).

The Mucosa-associated Lymphoid Tissue Is Stimulated by the Indigenous Microflora

The gastrointestinal tract contains about 25 % of all lymphocytes. These immune cells are part of the so-called mucosa-associated lymphoid tissue (MALT), which consists of the organized lymphoid tissue (e.g., Peyer's patches) and the diffuse lymphoid tissue (e.g., lamina propria lymphocytes, intraepithelial lymphocytes). Studies with germ-free animals and subsequent reconstitution experiments demonstrated the essential role of the indigenous microflora for development of the MALT. Germ-free animals exhibit only very small Peyer's patches. Moreover, the composition of gastrointestinal lymphocytes population including IEL are changed in germ-free animals (Imaoka et al. 1996). Consequently, germ-free animals exhibit an increased susceptibility for infections with both facultative-pathogenic as well as obligate pathogenic microorganisms.

It is well established that microorganisms can trigger the production of proinflammatory chemotactic cytokines including chemokines (e.g. IL-8) (Eckmann et al. 1995; Schulte and Autenrieth 1998). Therefore, it is believed that intestinal epithelial cells are part of the innate immune system (Fig. 3) (Eckmann et al. 1995). Consequently, microbial products may stimulate epithelial and other immune cells to produce cytokines which may promote the development of the MALT and the recruitment of (polymorphonuclear) leukocytes. The intestinal T cell population, however, is down-modulated or appears to be tolerant of the antigens of the intestinal flora. Similarly, intestinal macrophages appear to be down-regulated by the local microenvironment.

A further example of positive effects of the flora on the host is that the metabolism of bacteria of the indigenous microflora results in production of short-chain fatty acids (SCFA). SCFA including particularly n-butyrate, account for 40–70 % of the energy source of colonic epithelial cells. Furthermore, SCFA stimulate the colonic peristalsis and shorten transit times significantly.

Bacterial Translocation

The term translocation has been defined as the passage of bacteria from the gastrointestinal tract to extraintestinal sites such as mesenteric lymph nodes or blood. More recently, Berg has proposed to define bacterial translocation as the passage of viable indigenous bacteria from the gastrointestinal tract to extraintestinal sites (Berg

1995). There is evidence that three major mechanisms promote bacterial translocation (Berg 1995; Pasquale et al. 1994): (1) intestinal bacterial overgrowth, (2) deficiency in host immunity, and (3) increased permeability or damage of the intestinal mucosal barrier. Paradoxically, the presence of a balanced indigenous microflora prevents bacterial translocation to a certain degree. Nevertheless, bacterial translocation probably occurs physiologically continuously on a low level even in healthy individuals. In this situation, however, the mucosa-associated lymphoid tissue including cells of the reticulo-endothelial system kill the translocated microorganisms and may give rise to production of (for example) proinflammatory cytokines. These events may contribute to a state termed as "physiological inflammation" in the gastrointestinal tract, which is beneficial for the development of the MALT.

Alterations in bacteria–bacteria or bacteria–host interactions in the gastrointestinal tract, such as bacterial overgrowth syndrome, host defense deficiency, and breakdown of the intestinal epithelial barrier, may lead to increased bacterial translocation with subsequent abscesses in lymph nodes, liver, and spleen, as well as septicemia. Although the rate of bacterial translocation correlates directly with the number of microorganisms present in the lumen of the gastrointestinal tract, microorganisms including *Pseudomonas aeruginosa, Klebsiella* spp., *E. coli* and *Proteus mirabilis* translocate more efficiently than *Staphylococcus* spp. or *Lactobacilli. Bacteroides* spp. and *Fusobacteria* translocate even less efficiently from the gastrointestinal tract to extraintestinal sites. Moreover, it should be stressed that most microorganisms cannot invade or be translocated via normal intestinal epithelial cells such as enterocytes, but only be translocated via specialized cells within the follicle-associated epithelium of Peyer's patches, the so-called M cells (Neutra and Kraehenbuhl 1992; Schulte and Autenrieth 1998). The M cells are specialized in that they take up antigens or bacteria from the intestinal lumen and transport them to the Peyer's patches, thereby stimulating immune responses of the MALT. Paradoxically, microorganisms such as *Yersinia, Salmonella* and *Shigella* exploit these cells in order to get access to the host tissue.

In addition, the indigenous microflora has a tremendous metabolic activity, including synthesis of vitamins (e.g., K, B complex), metabolism of bile acid, etc. Moreover, bacteria may produce and secrete enzymes including proteases, nitroreductases, and sulfatases, which might contribute to activation or inactivation of drugs (e.g., inactivation of antibiotics) as well as detoxification of toxins.

Owing to the many desirable effects of the microflora on the host, it is a consequent and rational approach to use bacteria as probiotics to support the protective function of the flora. However, it is not yet clear whether probiotics can efficiently prevent infections with exogenous enteropathogenic microorganisms or bacterial translocation, although several studies with promising results have been published in the past few years (Berg 1998).

Disturbance of the Indigenous Microflora and Harmful Consequences for the Host

Intestinal peristalsis and production of bactericidal gastric acid are probably the two most important host factors that account for regulation of the intestinal flora. The continuous transport of the flora by the peristalsis prevents bacterial overgrowth syndrome, the colonization of the proximal small intestine with anaerobes and increased bacterial translocation. Patients with achlorhydria suffer from bacterial overgrowth of the small intestine and the stomach. Moreover, these patients exhibit an increased susceptibility to infections with enteropathogenic bacteria.

The microflora might be harmful to the host if the net translocation rate is increased. This might occur following disruption of the intestinal barrier or in patients with compromised host defense mechanisms. Subsequently, septicemia and abscesses caused by organisms among the indigenous flora, such as *E. coli*, may occur. Moreover, certain bacterial products might be harmful to the host and may disturb wound healing, for example (Autenrieth 1994). Short chain fatty acids stimulate the peristalsis and the metabolism in epithelial cells of the intestine. However, on the other hand, SCFA may inhibit the bactericidal activity of polymorphonuclear leukocytes owing to proton shuttling into to the cytosol, which subsequently may lead to intracellular acidification resulting in cellular dysfunction (Rothstein 1993). In addition, bacterial products and enzymes such as collagenases, peptidases, hyaluronidases, lipases and IgA proteases may damage host tissues, cells and humoral factors (Autenrieth 1994).

Antimicrobial Agents May Disrupt the Microflora

Treatment with antimicrobial agents may disrupt the intestinal flora which may result in increased susceptibility of the host for infection with exogenous pathogens. In mice treated with streptomycin susceptibility to infection with enteropathogenic *E. coli* is 1,000- to 100,000-fold that in mice that have not been so treated. Moreover, antibiotic-associated diarrhea and pseudomembranous colitis attributable to *Clostridium difficile* are well-known complications of the alterations of the indigenous flora that are caused by administration of antimicrobial agents (Kelly et al. 1994). Furthermore, antibiotics may induce endotoxin release from gram-negative bacteria, which may cause a systemic inflammatory response syndrome (Crosby et al. 1994, Prins et al. 1994). Recently, however, several novel approaches to prevention or treatment of bacterial translocation have been described (Berg 1998; Berger et al. 1996; Chandra et al. 1992; Zapata-Sirvent et al. 1994).

Inflammatory Bowel Disease Is Triggered by the Indigenous Microflora

In the past few years, mouse models with transgenic immunodeficient mice have provided evidence that the normal indigenous flora may have a crucial role in the development of chronic inflammatory bowel disease (MacDonald 1994). Thus, knock-out mice such as interleukin-2-deficient mice spontaneously develop a chronic inflammatory bowel disease resembling ulcerative colitis in humans. IL-2deficient knock-out mice kept in a completely germ-free environment, however, do not develop chronic inflammatory bowel disease (Sadlack et al. 1993). On the basis of these observations, it is now clear that the normal indigenous flora triggers the manifestation of chronic inflammatory bowel disease based on a dysregulated immune system of the host. The mechanisms by which the indigenous flora triggers inflammatory bowel disease are not yet known. However, there is evidence that intestinal epithelial cells, in addition to their absorptive functions, are an important part of the mucosa-associated immune system. Thus, intestinal epithelial cells may secrete proinflammatory cytokines in response to bacterial stimulation. Moreover, bacterial DNA has been recognized as a potent immunostimulatory compound. Certain prokaryotic, but not eukaryotic, DNA motifs (e.g., GC motifs with altered methylation) may induce the production and secretion of proinflammatory cytokines such as tumor necrosis factor-α, interleukin-1 in macrophages or production of interferon-γ and other cytokines in lymphocytes, giving rise to lethal shock in mice (Sparwasser 1997). Furthermore, foreign DNA might be taken up and expressed in the host (Dörfler 1997). Thus, although it is purely speculative, it might well be that the microflora stimulates epithelial intestinal cells that initiate an inflammatory response, which in the absence of appropriate regulatory mechanisms might result in colitis.

Concluding Remarks

The intestinal microflora is a complex ecosystem that is not yet fully understood. Nevertheless, there is substantial evidence showing that there can be both beneficial and harmful effects of the microflora on the host, depending on a number of known and unknown host-bacteria and bacteria-bacteria interactions. As a substantial number of bacteria from the microflora cannot be grown in vitro, novel approaches, including molecular tools, are required for further elucidation of the physiology and pathophysiology of the indigenous microflora.

References

Autenrieth IB, Hantke K, Heesemann J (1991) Immunosuppression of the host and delivery of iron to the pathogen: a possible dual role of siderophores in the pathogenesis of microbial infections? Med Microbiol Immunol 180:135–141

Autenrieth IB (1994) Molekuläre und infektionsbiologische Aspekte von Wundheilungsstörungen durch bakterielle Infektionen. Dtsch Zahnarztl Z 49:1021–1027

Autenrieth IB (1998) Physiologie und Pathophysiologie der intestinalen Flora. Wien Klin Wochenschr 110 [Suppl 1]:16–20

Bagg A, Neylands J (1987) Molecular mechanisms of regulation of siderophore-mediated iron assimilation. Microbiol Rev 51:509–518

Berg RD (1995) Bacterial translocation from the gastrointestinal tract. Trends Microbiol 3:149–154

Berg RD (1996) The indigenous gastrointestinal microflora. Trends Microbiol 4:430–435

Berg RD (1998) Probiotics, prebiotics or 'conbiotics'? Trends Microbiol 6:89–92

Berger D, Bölke E, Hiki N, Lissner R, Arnold A, Hausmann F, Seidelmann N, Beger HG (1996) Perioperative endotoxin leakage from the gastrointestinal tract can be prevented by enteral application of an immunoglobulin enriched colostral milk preparation. Ninth European Congress on Intensive Care Medicine, Glasgow, UK, pp 439–443

Chandra RH, Wang S, Au B (1992) Enriched feeding formular and immune responses in outcome after *Listeria monocytogenes* challenge in mice. Nutrition 8:426–429

Crosby HA, Bion JF, Penn CW, Elliott TS (1994) Antibiotic-induced release of endotoxin from bacteria. J Med Microbiol 40:23–30

Dörfler W, Schubbert R (1997) Fremde DNA im Säugersystem. Dtsch Arzteblatt 95:2537–2542

Eckmann L, Kagnoff M, Fierer J (1995) Intestinal epithelial cells as watchdogs for the natural immune system. Trends Microbiol 3:118–129

Imaoka A, Matsumoto S, Setoyama H, Okada Y, Umesaki Y (1996) Proliferative recruitment of intestinal intraepithelial lymphocytes after microbial colonization of germ-free mice. Eur J Immunol 26:945–948
Kelly CP, Pothoulakis C, LaMont JT (1994) *Clostridium difficile* colitis. N Engl J Med 330:257–262
Lee A (1985) Neglected niches – the microbal ecology of the gastrointestinal tract. In: Marshal KC (ed) Advances in microbal ecology, vol 8. Plenum, New York, pp 115–162
MacDonald TT (1994) Gastrointestinal inflammation: inflammatory bowel disease in knockout mice. Curr Biol 4:261–263
Moayyedi P, Axon A (1995) *Helicobacter pylori*: the research explosion. Curr Opin Infect Dis 8:374–379
Neutra MR, Kraehenbuhl J-P (1992) Transepithelial transport and mucosal defence. I. The role of M cells. Trends Cell Biol 2:134–138
Pasquale MD, Cipolle MD, Cerra FB (1994) Bacterial translocation: myth versus reality. In: Reinhart K, Eyrich K, Sprung C (eds) Sepsis. Springer, Berlin Heidelberg New York, pp 86–106
Prins JM, van Deventer SJH, Kuijper EJ, Speelman P (1994) Clinical relevance of antibiotic-induced endotoxin release. Antimicrob Agents Dis 38:1211–1218
Rothstein OD (1993) Interactions between leukocytes and anaerobic bacteria in polymicrobal surgical infections. Clin Infect Dis 16:190–194
Sadlak B, Merz H, Schorle H, Schimpel A, Feller AC, Horak I (1993) Ulcerative colitis like disease in mice with a disrupted interleukin-2 gene. Cell 75:253–261
Schulte R, Autenrieth IB (1998) *Yersinia enterocolitica*-induced interleukin-8 secretion by human intestinal epithelial cells depends on cell differentiation. Infect Immun 66:1216–1224
Simon GL, Goa Bach SL (1995) Normal alimentary tract microfloral. In: Blazer MJ, Smith PD, Ruvdin JI, Greenberg HB, Guerrant RL (eds) Infections of the gastrointestinal tract, chap 4. Raven Press, New York, pp 53–69
Sparwasser T, Miethke T, Lipford G,. Borschert K, Häcker H, Heeg K, Wagner H (1997) Bacterial DNA cause septic shock. Nature 386:336–337
Vollaard EJ, Clasener HAL (1994) Colonization resistance. Antimicrob Agents Chemother 38:409–414
Zapata-Sirvent RL, Hansbrough JF, Ohara MM, Rice-Asaro N, Nyhan WL (1994) Bacterial translocation in burned mice after administration of various diets including fiver and glutamin enriched enteral formulars. Crit Care Med 22:690–696

Clinical Strategies for Prevention of Bacterial Translocation

W. Druml

Department of Medicine III, Division of Nephrology, Vienna General Hospital,
Währinger Gürtel 18–20, 1090 Vienna, Austria

Introduction

For decades the gastrointestinal tract was more or less a neglected organ system in intensive care medicine. This has considerably changed during recent years, because it has been recognized that the gut can play a critical role in the pathophysiology of various disease states, is not only a "victim" of systemic illness but can be a "mover," being able to initiate and perpetuate systemic infections and the multiple organ dysfunction syndrome (MODS), and has a crucial function in the modulation of the inflammatory response of the organism to infections. The maintenance of intestinal functions has been identified as a prerequisite for survival and has consequently become a cornerstone of treatment of intensive care patients.

Bacterial Translocation

The concept of intestinal tract as a source of systemic infections is not new. Even more than 100 years ago, Fränkel demonstrated in elegant experimental and clinical studies that luminal bacteria can permeate through the intestinal wall and cause infections [1, 2]. He concluded that "both in the presence of an intact intestinal tube or with various alterations and especially with local inflammation, furthermore in all states with exclusion of intestinal loops and/or in which the transport of luminal contents is impaired and which are associated with growth of bacteria, all can as a consequence cause permeation of those from the intestines...." [2].

In the early 1950s Fine rediscovered this phenomenon and formulated a "leaky gut hypothesis" with the demonstration of bacterial dissemination after hemorrhagic shock [3]. Irreversibility of a shock state was characterized by the influx of endotoxin into systemic circulation through the intestinal wall.

Gut decontamination has been used in hematology for decades during cytoreductive therapy to prevent the development of gut-derived infections during the neutropenic phase of chemotherapy. In intensive care medicine, this concept – at least for some years – has been experiencing a revival in the form of "selective digestive decontamination" (SDD).

The most compelling evidence of the permeation of intact microorganisms from the intestinal lumen through an intact intestinal mucosa into the systemic circulation (now termed "translocation") was demonstrated in an impressive self-experiment as long ago as in the late 1960s: Krause drank a suspension of *Candida albicans*, and

M. K. Herbert et al. (Eds.), Problems of the
Gastrointestinal Tract in Anesthesia...

Table 1. Determinants of bacterial translocation

Luminal factors	Type and load of bacteria, motility, bile acids, fiber, etc.
Mucosal factors	"Permeability of the intestinal wall", i.e., atrophy, inflammation, direct insults, impaired lymphatic clearance, etc.
Systemic factors	Immunocompetence of the organism, nutritional state, etc.

30 min later he experienced chills and the blood and urinary cultures became positive for *Candida* [4]. This experiment illustrates the three major determinants of translocation: a luminal factor (number of organisms, gastrointestinal motility), a wall factor (barrier function) and, finally, the immunocompetence of the organism (Table 1).

Translocation of microorganisms, endotoxin or other macromolecules is a physiological phenomenon and also occurs in the intact organism; it must be stressed that it certainly does not represent a "physiological defect," but is a phenomenon crucial for the development and maturation of the gastrointestinal immune system and the immunocompetence of the whole organism [5]. However, if the bacterial count is low and the immunocompetence of the subject is maintained and if the microorganisms are cleared by the lymphatic system and/or the liver, no systemic infection will evolve.

These findings ultimately led, in the 1980s, to the formulation of the "Gut Hypothesis" of the development of systemic infections and/or septicemia [6, 7]. This concept postulates that both local factors (direct injury to the mucosal wall) and systemic insults (such as hypotension) impair the cellular integrity and barrier function of the intestinal wall and cause the spread of viable microorganisms into the lymphatic system and ultimately into the systemic circulation. As a consequence, systemic infections and septicemia, but also MODS, may evolve, and the gut has been designated the "cause or motor" of MODS [8, 9].

Most experiments on bacterial translocation have been performed in rodents, an animal order with a high degree of translocation, and the criticism that the findings recorded in such studies cannot necessarily be extrapolated to the human situation has been leveled repeatedly. However, both earlier [2, 4] and recent investigations [10–12] have provided compelling evidence that the concept of bacterial translocation is relevant for humans and also in the clinical situation.

Strategies aimed at maintaining intestinal functions and supporting the intestinal barrier and at preventing or reducing bacterial translocation have become one of the pillars of the treatment of intensive care patients. In this chapter those factors that contribute to the impairment of intestinal functions and therapeutic concepts by which the breakdown of the mucosal barrier function can be prevented and the extent of bacterial translocation can be reduced are summarized.

Therapeutic Strategies Aimed at Local Factors that Promote Bacterial Translocation

Local insults, such as inflammation of the intestinal wall and direct injury by immunosuppressive drugs and/or radiation, can compromise the barrier function of the intestinal wall (Table 2). These factors usually cannot be modified directly. Nevertheless, a broad spectrum of strategies have been evaluated to improve the mucosal bar-

Table 2. Local factors promoting bacterial translocation

Ischemia
Inflammation of the gut wall
Cytotoxic medications
Radiation injury
Bacterial overgrowth
Impairment of motility

rier function and/or reduce the extent of translocation by increasing the tolerance of the mucosal wall to local insults and by modifications of the luminal contents.

A first approach is the provision of specific substrates that can help to maintain intestinal integrity and functions. Among these, glutamine has received considerable interest during recent years [13, 14]. There is compelling evidence that provision of glutamine can increase the tolerance of animals to detrimental effects of radiation or cytotoxic agents [15]. Also, supplementation of an enteral diet with arginine can – potentially by serving as a precursor of nitric oxide – reduce radiation injury to the intestinal wall [16]. Other potential substrates are nucleotides and also short chain fatty acids, which present important nutrients for proliferation of colonic mucosa [17].

Bacterial overgrowth caused by inappropriate antibiotic treatment and/or bacterial selection induced by intestinal decontamination can result in an increase in bacterial translocation [18]. When gram-negative bacteria were eliminated by decontamination overgrowth and increased translocation of gram-positive species were demonstrable [19].

Stasis of intestinal juice in blind loops or by decreased gastrointestinal motility can also promote bacterial translocation. This is especially important in the presence of obstructive or of paralytic ileus [20]. In this scenario the gut has also been depicted as an "undrained abscess" serving as a constant reservoir for spreading of intestinal bacteria [21]. The preservation of intestinal motility must thus be one of the first and most important goals in the maintenance of intestinal functions.

Reduction of bacterial counts by whole-body wash-out using an intestinal lavage solution (Golytely) decreased febrile response and improved respiratory function in patients with severe sepsis [22]. Furthermore, it has been suggested that intestinal colonization with exogenous nonpathogenic bacteria or yeasts such as *Lactobacilli* or *Saccharomyces boulardii* reduces translocation of pathogenic microorganisms [23].

Selective digestive decontamination (SDD) was originally introduced to reduce respiratory tract infections that might be caused by silent aspiration of ascending intestinal microorganisms in intensive care patients. SDD, certainly, should restricted to specific indications in selected patient groups and cannot be generally recommended for intensive care patients. Nevertheless, there have been some reports that SDD might reduce the evolution of systemic infections not only by reducing the local spread of bacteria but also by diminishing the amount of translocated microorganisms [24, 25].

Luminal modifications, such as the addition of fiber to enteral nutrition (see below), or the type of ulcer prophylaxis may also affect the process of bacterial translocation. At least in the animal experiment sucralfate can reduce the number of microorganisms permeating the intestinal wall after hemorrhagic or septic shock

[26]. Enteral supplementation with immunoglobulins can reduce necrotizing enterocolitis in newborns, but also the degree of postoperative endotoxinemia in surgical patients. Furthermore, enteral lactulose has been shown to reduce bacterial translocation [27].

Therapeutic Strategies Aimed at Systemic Factors that Promote Bacterial Translocation (Tables 3, 4)

Impaired Intestinal Perfusion and/or Oxygenation

Mesenteric vasculature is specifically sensitive to various types of stress situations and all disease states associated with hemodynamic instability in which it responds with a disproportionate decrease in intestinal perfusion [28]. This can be aggravated by pharmacologic interventions used in circulatory support in intensive care patients, such as constant infusion of suprarenin. Moreover, mucosal tissue is also extremely vulnerable to hypoxia [29]. Thus, preservation and optimization of intestinal perfusion and oxygenation by volume resuscitation, circulatory support and artificial ventilation is of the utmost importance also for maintaining intestinal integrity and functions.

Unspecific Effects of Stress

In contrast to generally accepted concepts that skeletal muscle is the main source of amino acids during stress states and catabolic disease, recent investigations have clearly demonstrated that after exhaustive exercise, in stress reactions and also dur-

Table 3. Systemic factors promoting bacterial translocation

Any type of circulatory shock
Hypoxia, hypotension
Any type of severe stress state
Systemic infections/SIRS/MODS
Endotoxinemia
Malnutrition
Burn injury
Immunosuppressive agents
Parenteral nutrition

Table 4. Therapeutic strategies to prevent/reduce bacterial translocation

Avoid direct mucosal injury
Optimize gastrointestinal perfusion/ oxygenation
Maintain gastrointestinal motility
ENTERAL NUTRITION (even "minimal") (without/with specific substrates i.e. glutamine, etc.)
Adapt/reduce antibiotic medications
Modifications of parenteral nutrition (additions of glutamine, arginine, SCFA etc.)
Luminal interventions (sucralfate, lactulose, bile acids, etc.)
Selective digestive decontamination?
Specific systemic interventions? (oxygen radical scavengers, etc.)

ing systemic inflammatory response syndrome (SIRS) it is the intestinal protein that is mobilized and released during the acute phase, at least for the first 48–72 h [30]. Immediate postoperative feeding can prevent this acute intestinal protein loss and help to maintain intestinal barrier function during this insult phase, which has been identified as a critical period for the further course of disease [31].

Malnutrition

Accumulating evidence both in animal experiments and the clinical situation has convincingly shown that nutritional depletion results in an atrophy of the intestinal mucosa, impairs intestinal functions, increases permeability and thus, promotes translocation [32, 33]. In turn, the prevention of development of nutritional depletion can also help to prevent this cascade of events and preserve intestinal integrity [31].

Parenteral Nutrition

Parenteral nutrition per se and/or the lack of luminal nutrients can be an important factor in the evolution of mucosal atrophy or an impairment of intestinal defense mechanisms and in promotion of translocation of microorganisms and/or endotoxins. This has been illustrated by an elegant animal experiment, in which three types of nutrition were provided: oral standard chow, enteral infusion of a parenteral nutrition solution and intravenous infusion of this mixture [34]. Whereas there was virtually no bacterial colonization in mesenteric lymph nodes (MLNs) with oral standard chow, 33 % of the MLNs were colonized during enteral feeding of the parenteral nutrition solution and 66 % of the MLNs during strictly parenteral nutrition.

These observations provide evidence, first, for the fact that parenteral nutrition is inadequate for maintaining intestinal defense functions, but secondly they also indicate that currently available parenteral nutrition solutions are incomplete, obviously not containing all substrates required for preservation of intestinal functions.

This realization has stimulated investigations aimed at finding whether modifications of the nutrient solution and the addition of specific nutritional substrates can help to make the solutions more complete in the sense of covering the nutrient requirements of the intestines. Among the specific parenteral substrates considered to support intestinal functions, glutamine has received widespread interest during the last decade.

Glutamine, which conventionally was termed a “nonessential” amino acid, has been shown to fulfill crucial physiological functions: glutamine is a regulator of nitrogen homeostasis and is an essential nutritional substrate both for immunocompetent cells and for rapidly proliferating cells, such as intestinal mucosal cells [13, 14]. Supplementation of parenteral nutrition with glutamine can help to improve nitrogen balance, to stimulate immunocompetence of the organism and also to preserve intestinal integrity and barrier function. In the clinical situation a reduction of intestinal permeability and of the incidence of nosocomial infections, a reduction in the length of hospital stay and an improvement in long-term survival of patients have been demonstrated [35, 36].

Enteral Nutrition

The first and by far the most important and most effective means of maintaining intestinal functions and of reducing and/or preventing bacterial translocation is enteral nutrition ("use it or lose it"). In fact, the current boom of enteral nutrition was precipitated by the recognition of its effect on preservation of the integrity of the gut and the reduction of bacterial translocation [37].

Several investigations have compared the effects of enteral versus parenteral nutrition on the evolution of various complications, and especially on the incidence of infections in intensive care patients. Most but not all studies have reported a weakening of the inflammatory response reaction and a reduction of the incidence of infectious complications during enteral nutrition [38, 39].

It must not be forgotten that the effect of enteral nutrition is not confined to the local provision of luminal substrates required for mucosal proliferation. Enteral nutrition exerts a broad pattern of beneficial effects on various aspects of intestinal functions (Table 5).

The most obvious function of enteral nutrition is the provision of nutritional substrates for mucosal cells, which not only support the barrier function but also help to prevent the development of mucosal lesions and erosions [40, 41]. Among other effects of enteral nutrition are the improvement of intestinal perfusion, the stimulation of motility, of bile flow and pancreatic secretions, the release of gastrointestinal hormones and trophic factors (Table 5).

Addition of fibers to enteral nutrition is a further possibility when it is desired to modify bacterial translocation [17]. Potentially, this is mediated by adsorption of endotoxin and/or bacteria or by the release of trophic substances such as short chain fatty acids. Increasing the luminal volume load by the addition of fibers may also contribute to an improvement of motility and/or release of gastrointestinal hormones.

It is important to note that enteral nutrition exerts its beneficial effects on gastrointestinal functions not only if given at a rate at which the nutrient requirements of the whole organism are covered. In patients who need to be fed parenterally for other reasons, the supplementary provision of even small amounts of luminal nutrients can help to maintain barrier function. Between 10 % and 25 % of requirements provided by the enteral route is sufficient to support the barrier function and decrease intestinal permeability [42].

Similarly to the situation in parenteral nutrition, several studies have investigated the effect of supplementation of the enteral diet with specific substrates, which might be especially important for the support and maintenance of intestinal functions. In this respect, again, glutamine has received the widest interest, and a reduction in nosocomial infections was also demonstrated with enteral glutamine supplementation [43]. Further investigations have focused on the effect of enteral diets enriched with

Table 5. Effects of enteral nutrition on the intestinal tract

Improves intestinal perfusion by local vasodilatation
Stimulates mucosal cell proliferation
Stimulates enteric nervous system and motility
Decreases bacterial overgrowth
Stimulates secretion of trophic intestinal hormones
Portal substrate flux improves substrate utilization

arginine, nucleotides and ω-3 fatty acids ("immunonutrition"), and again, a reduction in the incidence of local and systemic infections and an improvement of the outcome of the patients was documented [44, 45].

Specific Interventions

In addition to these more or less unspecific and general measures that can be applied to improve various aspects of intestinal function and reduce the extent of bacterial translocation, a broad spectrum of more specific and focused pharmacological interventions have been evaluated. Among those, antioxidants and oxygen radical scavengers, inhibitors of inducible nitric oxide synthase, anti-cytokine antibodies, antibodies to endotoxin, recombinant bactericidal/permeability-increasing protein were all effective at least in the experimental situation in improving or stabilizing intestinal barrier functions in sepsis [8, 46, 47]. These investigations have added greatly to our understanding of the process of intestinal injury in various disease states but, at least for the time being, have not generated results that are relevant to humans. In the clinical situation general measures such as optimization of perfusion, oxygenation, preservation and stimulation of motility and, especially, enteral nutrition are much more important than specific pharmacological interventions.

In several studies in catabolic disease states the effect of growth factors such as growth hormone or insulin-like growth factor-1 on nitrogen balance and nutritional state was evaluated. The studies were also extended in part to the investigation of mucosal proliferation and intestinal translocation. In a burn model in rats receiving total parenteral nutrition, therapy with IGF-1 prevented intestinal translocation of endotoxin [48].

Conclusions

The intestines – long neglected in intensive care medicine – are a crucial organ system in critically ill patients. There is compelling evidence that the phenomenon of bacterial translocation is also of the utmost importance in humans. The gastrointestinal tract is a source of systemic infections, can be the origin of the initiation and maintenance of sepsis and multiple organ dysfunction syndrome, and modulates the inflammatory response reaction of the organism.

The restoration and maintenance of intestinal functions has become one of the cornerstones of treatment for intensive care patients. In this respect unspecific measures and the general management of the patient, such as maintenance of perfusion, oxygenation and motility, avoidance of inappropriate antibiotic therapy and, especially, the early initiation of enteral nutrition, are of the utmost importance. The avoidance of exclusively parenteral nutrition and the early initiation of enteral nutrition, which stimulates and supports a broad pattern of intestinal functions, has become a central therapeutic approach in the management of critically ill patients. In contrast – but as in the therapy of sepsis – more specific pharmacological interventions, which have been very valuable in extending our understanding of the pathophysiology of the process of translocation, have not so far achieved any major importance for the clinical situation, and it cannot be expected that a "magic bullet" that will make it possible to eliminate the problem of intestinal translocation will be identified in the near future.

References

1. Druml W (1996) Darm und Sepsis. Wien Klin Wochenschr 108:309–310
2. Fraenkel A (1891) Über peritoneale Infektion. Wien Klin Wochenschr 4:285–289
3. Fine J (1954) Bacterial factor in experimental hemorrhagic shock. Am J Physiol 179:532–540
4. Krause W, Matheis H, Wulf K (1969) Fungaemia and funguria after oral administration of *Candida albicans.* Lancet I:599–601
5. Stallmach A, Zeitz M (1998) Der Darm als immunologisches Organ. Wien Klin Wochenschr 110:72–78
6. Wilmore DW, Smith RJ, O'Dwyer ST, Jacobs DO, Ziegler TR, Wang XD (1988) The gut: a central organ after surgical stress. Surgery 104:917–923
7. Deitch EA (1990) The role of intestinal barrier failure and bacterial translocation in the development of systemic infection and multiple organ failure. Arch Surg 125:403–404
8. Bahrami S, Redl H, Schlag G (1998) Der Darm als Ursache von Sepsis und Multiorganversagen. Wien Klin Wochenschr 110 [Suppl 1]:2–10
9. Nieuwenhuijzen GAP, Deitch EA, Goris RJA (1996) Infection, the gut and the development of multiple organ dysfunction syndrome. Eur J Surg 162:259–273
10. Doig CJ, Sutherland LR, Sandham JD, Fick GH, Verhoef M, Meddings JB (1998) Increased intestinal permeability is associated with the development of multiple organ dysfunction syndrome in critically ill ICU patients. Am J Respir Crit Care Med 158:444–451
11. Sedman PC, MacFie J, Sagar P, Mitchell CJ, May J, Mancey-Jones B, Johnstone D (1994) The prevalence of gut translocation in humans. Gastroenterology 107:643–649
12. Brathwaite CEM, Ross SE, Nagele R, Mure AJ, O'Malley KF, Garcia-Perez FA (1993) Bacterial translocation occurs in humans after traumatic injury: evidence using immunofluorescence. J Trauma 34:586–590
13. Souba WW, Klimberg VS, Plumley DA, Salloum RM, Flynn TC, Bland KI, Copeland EM (1990) The role of glutamine in maintaining a healthy gut and supporting the metabolic response to injury and infection. J Surg Res 48:383–391
14. Roth E, Spittler A, Oehler R (1996) Glutamin: Wirkungen auf das Immunsystem, auf Eiweißhaushalt und Darmfunktionen. Wien Klin Wochenschr 108:669–676
15. Souba WW, Klimberg VS, Hautamaki RD, Mendenhall WH, Bova FC, Howard RJ, Bland KI, Copeland EM (1990) Oral glutamine reduces bacterial translocation following abdominal radiation. J Surg Res 48:1–5
16. Gurbuz AT, Kunzelmann J, Ratzer EE (1998) Supplemental dietary arginine accelerates intestinal mucosal regeneration and enhances bacterial clearance following radiation enteritis in rats. J Surg Res 74:149–153
17. Mao Y, Nobaek S, Kasravi D, Adawi D, Stenram D, Molin G, Jeppson D (1996) The effects of lactobacilli strains and oat fiber on methotrexate induced enterocolitis in rats. Gastroenterology 111:334–344
18. Berg RD, Wommak E, Deitch EA (1988) Immunosuppression and intestinal bacterial overgrowth synergistically promote translocation. Arch Surg 123: 1359–1364
19. Jackson RJ, Smith SD, Rowe MI (1990) Selective bowel decontamination results in gram-positive translocation. J Surg Res 48:444–447
20. Deitch EA (1989) Simple intestinal obstruction causes bacterial translocation in man. Arch Surg 124:899–701
21. Marshall JC, Christou NV, Meakins JL (1993) The gastrointestinal tract: the "undrained abscess" of multiple organ failure. Ann Surg 218: 111–119
22. Alverdy J, Piano G (1997) Whole gut washout for severe sepsis: review of technique and preliminary results. Surgery 121:89–94
23. Scheppach W, Dusel G, Kuhn T, Loges C, Karch H, Barton HP, Richter F, Christl SU, Kasper H (1994) Effect of L-glutamine and *n*-butyrate on the restitution of rat colonic mucosa after acid induced injury. Gut 38:878–885
24. Sorkine P, Szold O, Halpern P, Gutman M, Greemland M, Rudik V, Goldman G (1997) Gut decontamination reduces bowel ischemia-induced lung injury in rats. Chest 112:491–495

25. Späth G, Kirner A (1998) Microbial translocation and impairment of mucosal immunity induced by an elemental diet in rats is prevented by selective decontamination of the digestive tract. Eur J Surg 164:223–238
26. Georgopoulos A, Feistauer SM, Makristathis A, Burgmann H, Laggner AN (1996) Influence of stress ulcer prophylaxis on translocation of bacteria from the intestinal tract in rats. Wien Klin Wochenschr 108: 321–325
27. Ozaslan C, Turkcapas AG, Kesenci M, Karayalan K, Yerdel MA, Bengisum S, Toruner A (1997) Effect of lactulose on bacterial translocation. Eur J Surg 163:463–467
28. Fink MP, Kaups KL, Wang H, Rothschild HR (1991) Maintenance of superior mesenteric arterial perfusion prevents increase mucosal permeability in endotoxic pigs. Surgery 110:154–161
29. Gennari R, Alexander JW (1996) Effects of hyperoxia on bacterial translocation and mortality during gut-derived sepsis. Arch Surg 131:57–62
30. Molina PE, Ajmal M, Abumrad NN (1998) Energy metabolism and fuel mobilization: from the perioperative period to recovery. Shock 9:241–248
31. Carr CS, Ling E, Boulos P, Singer M (1996) Randomized trial of safety and efficacy of immediate postoperative enteral feeding in patients undergoing gastrointestinal resection. BMJ 312:869–871
32. Reynolds JV, O'Farrelly CO, Feighery C, Murchan P, Leonard N, Filton G, O'Moran C, Keane FBV, Tanner WA (1996) Impaired gut barrier function in malnourished patients. Br J Surg 83:1288–1291
33. Van der Hulst RRWJ, von Meyenfeldt MT, van Kreel BK, Thunnissen FBJM, Brummer RJM, Arends JW, Soeters PB (1998) Gut permeability, intestinal morphology, and nutritional depletion. Nutrition 14:1–6
34. Alverdy JC, Aoys E, Moss GS (1988) Total parenteral nutrition promotes bacterial translocation from the gut. Surgery 104:185–190
35. Van der Hulst RRWJ, van Kreel BK, von Meyenfeldt MT, Brummer RJM, Arends JW, Deutz NEP, Soeters PB (1993) Glutamine and the preservation of gut integrity. Lancet 334:1363–1365
36. Griffiths RD, Jones C, Palmer TE (1997) Six-months outcome of critically ill patients given glutamine-supplemented parenteral nutrition. Nutrition 13:295–302
37. Mochizuki H, Trocki O, Domionini L, Brackett KA, Joffe SN, Alexander JW (1984) Mechanism of prevention of postburn hypermetabolism and catabolism by early enteral feeding. Ann Surg 200:297–310
38. Kudsk KA, Croce MA, Fabian TC, Minard G, Tolley EA, Poret A, Kuhl MR, Brown RO (1992) Enteral versus parenteral feeding. Effects on septic morbidity after blunt and penetrating abdominal trauma. Ann Surg 215:503–513
39. Moore FA, Feliciano DV, Andrassy RJ, McArdle AH, McL Booth FV, Morgenstein -Wagner TB, Kellum JM, Welling RE, Moore EE (1992) Early enteral feeding, compared with parenteral, reduces postoperative septic complications. The results of a meta-analysis. Ann Surg 216:172–183
40. Sriram K, Abrahamian V, Kaminski MV, Santiago GC (1987) Efficacy of enteral diets in the prevention of stress-induced gastric erosions in rats. J Am Coll Nutr 6:165–168
41. Ephgrave KS, Kleiman-Wexler RL, Adair CG (1990) Enteral nutrients prevent stress ulceration and increase intragastric volume. Crit Care Med 18: 621–624
42. Sax HG, Illig KA, Ryan CK, Hardy DJ (1996) Low-dose enteral feeding is beneficial during total parenteral nutrition. Am J Surg 171:587–590
43. Houdijk APJ, Rijnsburger ER, Jansen J, RIC Wesdorp, Weiss JK, McCamish MA, Teelink T, Meuwissen SGM, Haarman HJTM, Thijs LG, van Leeuwen PAM (1998) Randomized trail of glutamine-enriched enteral nutrition on infectious morbidity in patients with multiple trauma. Lancet 352:772–776
44. Bower RH, Cerra FB, Bershadsky B, et al (1995) Early enteral administration of a formula supplemented with arginine, nucleotides, and fish oil in intensive care patients: Results of a multicenter, prospective, randomized, clinical trial. Crit Care Med 1995; 23: 436–449
45. Braga M, Gianotti L, Cestari A, Vignali A, Pellegatta F, Dolci A, Di Carlo V (1996) Gut function and immune and inflammatory responses in patients perioperatively fed with supplemented enteral formulas. Arch Surg 131:1257–1265
46. Alican I, Kubes P (1996) A critical role for nitric oxide in intestinal barrier function and dysfunction. Am J Physiol 270:G225–G237
47. Bahrami S, Yao Y-M, Leichtfried G, Redl H, Schlag G, Di Padova FE (1997) Monocloncal antibody to endotoxin attenuates hemorrhage-induced lung injury and mortality in rats. Crit Care Med 25:1030–1036
48. Sugiura T, Tashiro T, Yamamori H, Morishima Y, Otsubo Y, Hayashi N, Furukawa K, Nitte H, Nakajiama N, Ishizuka T, Tabuma M, Ino H, Ito I (1997) Effects of insulin like growth factor-1 on endotoxin translocation in burned rat receiving total parenteral nutrition. Nutrition 13:783–787

Reduction of Perioperative Endotoxin Leakage from the Gastrointestinal Tract by Enteral Application of Immunoglobulin-enriched Colostral Milk Preparation

E. Bölke · D. Berger · K. Buttenschön · R. Lissner · A. Arnold · F. Hausmann
M. Seidelmann · H.G. Beger

Department of General Surgery, University of Ulm, Steinhövelstrasse 9, 89075 Ulm, Germany

Introduction

The pathogenetic role of endotoxin in gram-negative sepsis is generally accepted [1, 2]. In septic diseases the role of intestinal endotoxin reaching the bloodstream was experimentally demonstrated by Cuevas and Fine more than 20 years ago [3]. In recent studies endotoxemia has been observed during and after major surgical procedures such as vascular, abdominal and cardiac operations [4–9]. In the case of abdominal surgery there is clear evidence of a pathogenetic role of endotoxin in terms of an association of endotoxemia and the occurrence of infectious complications [4]. In patients who had had cardiac surgery the endotoxin plasma levels correlated with the catecholamines needed to obtain adequate hemodynamic conditions at the end of cardiopulmonary bypass [9]. Martinez et al. demonstrated in cardiac patients that the severity of endotoxemia could be reduced by preoperative selective decontamination of the gastrointestinal tract, supporting the relevance of endotoxin translocation from the gastrointestinal tract [10].

The enteral application of an IgA-enriched immunoglobulin preparation reduced the incidence of necrotizing enterocolitis in premature babies [11]. The pathophysiological basis of that disease is the well-known barrier dysfunction of the immature gut, which leads to an inflammatory process in the gut wall [12]. Obviously, feeding with immunoglobulins may support the gut barrier and prevent the entrance of bacteria and bacterial products into the bowel wall [13].

The favorable effect of immunoglobulin feeding in premature babies and the clearly demonstrated gut barrier dysfunction after major surgery prompted the question as to whether the enteral application of an immunoglobulin-enriched colostral preparation might prevent the peri- and postoperative endotoxin translocation. A further question concerned the influence of eventually reduced endotoxemia on the clinical course as checked by sequential analysis of the APACHE-II score.

Patients, Materials and Methods

Forty patients, 22 male and 18 female, who were scheduled to undergo major surgical procedures on the stomach or pancreas, were enrolled in the study. Their mean age ± SD was 58 ± 15 years. No demographic differences between control and verum group could be observed. After randomization, patients in the verum group were treated with 56 g of the colostral preparation (Biotest, Dreieich, Germany) for 3 days preoper-

M. K. Herbert et al. (Eds.), Problems of the Gastrointestinal Tract in Anesthesia...

atively. The exact description of the purification and content of the verum preparation is given elsewhere [14]. Control patients did not receive any treatment. Further enteral pretreatment was restricted to an enema on the day before the operation in both groups. Major gastric procedures were performed in 6 patients in each group; pancreatic surgery was done in 13 patients in the verum group and 14 patients in the placebo group. In the case of 1 patient in the verum group laparotomy only was performed, because of unresectable cancer.

Exclusion criteria were based on immunosuppression and reduced liver and bowel function. Chronic inflammatory diseases of the gut would also have precluded enrollment in the study. The study was approved by the local review board.

The clinical course was monitored by daily determination of the APACHE-II score. Blood was taken pre- and perioperatively at time points defined by the surgical procedure and daily until day 10 after the operation. The blood samples were anticoagulated with heparin (10 IU/ml) and stored frozen at –70 °C for up to 4 weeks after the preparation of platelet-poor plasma.

The determination of endotoxin and endotoxin neutralizing capacity (ENC) was done by using a chromogenic modification of the Limulus amebocyte lysate test and is described elsewhere [4, 9, 15]. Interleukin-6 levels were determined by an ELISA obtained from Immunotech (Hamburg, Germany). CRP (C-reactive protein) was measured nephelometrically.

Statistical analysis was performed by comparing the area under the curve (AUC) by means of the Mann-Whitney U-test.

Results and Conclusion

Endotoxin Plasma Levels

As expected from previous studies, the endotoxin plasma levels increased in both groups of patients. The AUC calculated for the verum group was significantly lower than that in patients receiving no treatment ($P < 0.05$). The main increase in endotoxin levels was observed later, and endotoxemia was found only on the day of the operation in patients treated with the colostral preparation. Control patients had endotoxemia until the 1st postoperative day, and the maximal values were higher.

Time-course of ENC

The ENC changed significantly in terms of a loss of plasma ENC. Even immediately after the induction of anesthesia ENC was reduced in patients in the control group, whereas the pretreatment delayed the fall of ENC until after mobilization of the organ to be resected. Maximal loss of ENC was reduced and recovery was accelerated by the colostral preparation. Comparison of AUC showed a significant improvement of ENC in the verum group ($P < 0.006$).

Time-course of Acute Phase Parameters

Plasma levels of interleukin-6 increased to maximal median values of 288 pg/ml and 384 pg/ml in the verum and control groups 4 h after the operation. The tendency to lowered IL-6 levels was observed throughout the whole observation period, but owing to the wide variance of the individual values statistical significance could not be calculated. The determination of CRP did not reveal any difference between the two groups.

Clinical Course

No difference was seen in the APACHE-II score during the observation period, and nor was the incidence of clinically obvious infectious complications reduced in patients in the verum group. However, the maximal APACHE-II score amounted to only 9.0 and 8.0 on day 2 in the verum and control groups, respectively. Also the incidence of infectious complications was too low to allow detection of any differences between treatment and control groups in this pilot study.

The study clearly demonstrates significant endotoxemia during and after elective abdominal surgery. The occurrence of endotoxin in the bloodstream was associated with a loss of the endogenous ENC. The enteral pretreatment with an immunoglobulin-enriched preparation of bovine colostral milk significantly reduced the amount of endotoxemia and shortened the duration of endotoxemia. A similar improvement in the plasma ENC was observed in patients receiving the treatment. These results support the hypothesis that peri- and postoperative endotoxemia is caused by endotoxin translocation from the gastrointestinal tract, which can be reduced by the enteral pretreatment with the preparation described. The question as to whether reduced endotoxin translocation is associated with reduced acute phase fraction and further improvement of the clinical course, however, remains to be elucidated in patients with a higher incidence of infectious complications.

References

1. Sibbald WJ (1976) Sepsis – the Wayne State University Symposium. III. Bacteremia and endotoxemia: a discussion of their roles in the pathophysiology of gram-negative sepsis. Heart Lung 5:765–771
2. Hurley JC (1993) Reappraisal of the role of endotoxin in the sepsis syndrome. Lancet 341:1133–1135
3. Cuevas P, Fine J (1972) Role of intestinal endotoxin in death from peritonitis. Surg Gynecol Obstet 134:935–957
4. Berger D, Schmidt UM, Ott S, Seidelmann M, Martin R, Beger JG (1995) Incidence and pathophysiological relevance of postoperative endotoxemia. FEMS Immunol Med Microbiol II:285–290
5. Roumen RM, Frieling JT, van Tits HW, van der Vliet JA, Goris RJ (1993) Endotoxemia after major vascular operations. J Vasc Surg 18:853–857
6. Soong CV, Blair PH, Halliday ML, McCaigue MD, Campbell GR, Hood JM, Rowlands BJ, Barros DS (1993) Endotoxaemia, the generation of the cytokines and their relationship to intramucosal acidosis of the sigmoid colon in elective abdominal aortic aneurysm repair. Eur J Vasc Surg 534–539
7. Andersen LW, Landow L, Baek L, Jansen E, Baker S (1993) Association between gastric intramucosal pH and splanchnic endotoxin, antibody to endotoxin, and tumor necrosis factor-alpha concentrations in patients undergoing cardiopulmonary bypass. Crit Care Med 21:210–217

8. Casey WF, Hauser GJ, Hannallah RS, Midgley FM, Khan WN (1992) Circulating endotoxin and tumor necrosis factor during pediatric cardiac surgery. Crit Care Med 20:1090–1096
9. Berger D, Bölke E, Högel H, Seidelmann M, Hannekum A, Beger HG (1995) New aspects concerning the regulation of the postoperative acute phase reaction during cardiac surgery. Clin Chim Acta 239:121–130
10. Martinez-Pellus AE, Merino P, Bru M, Conejero R, Seller G, Munoz C, Fuentes T, Gonzalez G, Alvarez B (1993) Can selective digestive decontamination avoid the endotoxemia and cytokine activation promoted by cardiopulmonary bypass? Crit Care Med 21:1684–1691
11. Eibl MM, Wolf HM, Furnkranz H, Rosenkranz A (1990) Prophylaxis of necrotizing enterocolitis by oral IgA-IgG: review of a clinical study in low birth weight infants and discussion of pathogenic role if infection. J Clin Immunol 10:72–77
12. Go LL, Ford HR, Watkins SC, Healey PJ, Albanese CT, Donhalek A, Simmons RL, Rowe MI (1994) Quantitative and morphologic analysis of bacterial translocation in neonates. Arch Surg 129:1184–1190
13. Albanese CT, Smith SD, Watkins S, Kurkchubasche A, Simmons RL, Rowe MI (1994) Effect of secretory IgA on transepithelial passage of bacteria across the intact ileum in vitro. J Am Coll Surg 179:679–688
14. Stephan W, Dichtelmüller H, Lissner R (1990) Antibodies from colostrum in oral immunotherapy. J Clin Chem Biochem 28:19–23
15. Berger D, Ott S, Schmidt UM, Bölke E, Seidelmann M, Beger HG (1996) Determination of endotoxin-neutralizing capacity of plasma in postsurgical patients. Eur Surg Res 28:130–139

Bacterial Translocation and Endotoxemia During Aseptic Surgery

E. Bölke · D. Berger · N. Hiki · B. Poch · A. Beier · M. Graf
M. Seidelmann · H. G. Beger

Department of Vascular Surgery, University of Ulm, Steinhövelstrasse 9, 89075 Ulm, Germany

Introduction

Bacterial translocation following gut barrier dysfunction is a well-documented phenomenon after major trauma and burn injury [1–5]. The clinical relevance, however, has yet to be elucidated. The same question applies to the recently observed bacterial translocation during abdominal surgery [6]. Similarly, circulating endotoxin has been described after trauma, burn and major surgical procedures, again indicating gut barrier dysfunction [1, 7–12]. Therefore, the severity of perioperative endotoxemia could be diminished by selective decontamination of the gastrointestinal tract before cardiac surgery, supporting the view of endotoxemia originating from the gastrointestinal tract [13]. Although some pathogenetic sequelae leading to the translocation of whole bacteria, such as the role of radical formation and preceding endotoxemia, are understood, no definite explanation of the mechanisms of bacterial and endotoxin translocation exists [14].

The aim of our study was to evaluate (1) the incidence of bacterial and endotoxin translocation during surgery and (2) the time sequence of gut barrier dysfunction and changes of pHi in order to obtain information about the role of disturbances of the microcirculation correlating with gut barrier dysfunction [15].

Patients, Materials and Methods

A group of 27 patients with a median age of 46 years (range 27–84 years) underwent surgical treatment of benign diseases of the thyroid gland. A further 56 patients with a median age of 56 years (range 33–77 years) underwent resection of the stomach ($n = 9$), pancreatic resection ($n = 23$), or resection of the colon or rectum ($n = 3$). The exclusion criteria were any signs of an inflammatory process existing pre- or intraoperatively, pre-existing immunosuppression, and lack of informed consent.

Patients who were to undergo colonic surgery were prepared by antibiotic-free orthograde lavage of the gastrointestinal tract. All other patients had an enema on the day before the operation was planned.

Preoperative selective decontamination was not performed. The differentiation of endotoxin plasma levels between patients with and without orthograde lavage did not reveal any influence of bowel preparation. No patient enrolled in the study died. Minor infectious complications occurred in 2 patients.

M. K. Herbert et al. (Eds.), Problems of the Gastrointestinal Tract in Anesthesia...

The schedule of blood sampling was dictated by the surgical procedure: (1) preoperatively, (2) after the induction of anesthesia, (3) after skin incision, (4) after exposure of the situs, (5) after mobilization of the organ, before opening of any hollow viscera, (6) before wound closure, (7) 2 h postoperatively, (8) 6 h postoperatively. The blood samples were anticoagulated by adding 10 IU heparin per ml of blood. After centrifugation plasma was stored at –70 °C for up to 4 weeks. Quantitative measurements of endotoxin plasma levels were done by a chromogenic modification of the *Limulus* amebocyte lysate test as described earlier [11].

The technique used for microbiology of lymph nodes, which were obtained from the ileocecal mesentery at time point 5, has also already been described elsewhere [16].

The measurement of intramucosal pH was performed by introducing a tonometer (gastric tonometer and sump, "NGS" manufactured by Tonometric, Mass., USA) into the patient's stomach after the induction of anesthesia. When partial or total gastrectomy was planned a sigmoid tonometer was used. The correct placement was controlled intraoperatively. The intramucosal pH was assessed according to the method described by Fiddian-Green, using 0.9 % saline for filling the balloon and an equilibration time of 30 min [15, 17].

Longitudinal statistical analysis was done by using the Friedman or the Kruskal-Wallis test. Chi-square analysis was used for comparison of bacteriology and the ratio of increased endotoxin plasma levels. Usually median values ± quartiles were given, because of lacking normal distribution. Only pHi values could be demonstrated as mean ± SD.

Results

Bacterial Translocation

Lymph nodes from the ileocecal mesentery could be sampled in 34 patients during abdominal surgery after the mobilization of the organ that was to be resected and before any hollow viscera had been opened. Bacterial growth was detected in 12 samples. In 3 samples pure gram-positive rods were cultured (Staphylococcus epidermidis in 2, S. aureus in 1), indicating probable exogenous contamination. Bacterial growth in 12 out of 34 samples means a 35 % incidence of bacterial translocation from the gastrointestinal tract to mesenteric lymph nodes.

Endotoxin Translocation

After thyroid surgery endotoxin plasma levels changed significantly during the observation period. After skin incision the levels of endotoxemia started to increase, remaining elevated until time point 7. During abdominal surgery increased endotoxin plasma levels were detected after the induction of anesthesia (0.04 EU/ml preoperatively to 0.13 EU/ml). Peak values were observed before closure of the abdominal wall. Endotoxemia was followed until the end of the observation period. The endotoxin plasma levels changed significantly, as checked by the Friedman test. At time point 5, 50 out of 56 patients had higher endotoxin levels than preoperatively, indicating a 90 % incidence of endotoxin translocation, which is significantly greater than the described incidence of bacterial translocation.

Intramucosal pH

The intramucosal pH started to decrease significantly in patients after abdominal and thyroid surgery at the second measurement point, which corresponded to the skin incision. No difference was observed between the two groups. It should be pointed out that a preanesthetic pHi determination was not available.

Conclusion

In conclusion, the incidence of endotoxemia may be much higher than the incidence of translocation of viable bacteria. Furthermore, endotoxin appeared in the bloodstream very early. This observation supports the previously published view that the gut barrier represents a very sensitive system, which is influenced by even minor changes in homeostasis [11, 18, 19]. The splanchnic microcirculation is also disturbed very early in the course of an operative procedure. The lack of any pHi difference between patients who underwent thyroid and patients undergoing abdominal surgery showed tonometry to be only a gross method compared with the determination of endotoxin plasma levels.

References

1. Van Leeuwen PA, Boermeester MA, Houdijk AP, Ferwerda CC, Cuesta MA, Meyer S, Wesdorp RL (1994) Clinical significance of translocation. Gut 35:S28-S34
2. Kudsk KA, Croce MA, Fabian TC, Minard G, Tolley EA, Poret HA, Kuhl MR, Brown RO (1992) Enteral versus parenteral feeding. Effects on septic morbidity after blunt and penetrating abdominal trauma. Ann Surg 215:503–513
3. Reed LL, Martin M, Manglano R, Newson B, Kocka F, Barrett J (1994) Bacterial translocation following abdominal trauma in humans. Circ Shock 42:1–6
4. Deitch EA, Berg RD (1987) Endotoxin but not malnutrition promotes bacterial translocation of the gut flora in burned mice. J Trauma 27:161–166
5. Deitch EA (1990) Intestinal permeability is increased in burn patients shortly after injury. Surgery 107:411–416
6. Sedman PC, Macfie J, Sagar P, Mitchell CJ, May J, Mancey-Jones B, Johnstone D (1994) The prevalence of gut translocation in humans. Gastroenterology 107:643–649
7. Rush BF Jr, Sori AJ, Murphy TF, Smith S, Flanagan JJ Jr, Machiedo GW (1988) Endotoxemia and bacteremia during hemorrhagic shock. The link between trauma and sepsis? Ann Surg 207:549–554
8. Winchurch RA, Thupari JN, Munster AM (1987) Endotoxemia in burn patients: levels of circulating endotoxins are related to burn size. Surgery 102:808–812
9. Roumen RM, Frieling JT, van Tits HW, van der Vliet JA, Goris RJ (1993) Endotoxemia after major vascular operations. J Vasc Surg 18:853–857
10. Andersen LW, Landow L, Baek L, Jansen E, Baker S (1993) Association between gastric intramucosal pH and splanchnic endotoxin, antibody to endotoxin and tumor necrosis factor-alpha concentrations in patients undergoing cardiopulmonary bypass. Crit Care Med 21:210–217
11. Berger D, Bölke E, Hügel H, Seidelmann M, Hannekum A, Beger HG (1995) New aspects concerning the regulation of the postoperative acute phase reaction during cardiac surgery. Clin Chim Acta 239:121–130

12. Hiki N, Berger D, Buttenschoen K, Bölke E, Seidelmann M, Strecker W, Kinzl L, Beger HG (1995) Endotoxemia and specific antibody behaviour against different endotoxins following multiple injury. J Trauma 38:794–801
13. Martinez-Pellus AE, Merino P, Bru M, Conejero R, Seller G, Munoz C, Fuentes T, Gonzalez G, Alvarez B (1993) Can selective digestive decontamination avoid the endotoxemia and cytokine activation promoted by cardiopulmonary bypass? Crit Care Med 21:1684–1691
14. Deitch EA, Specian RD, Berg RD (1991) Endotoxin-induced bacterial translocation and mucosal permeability: role of xanthine oxidase, complement activation and macrophage products. Crit Care Med 19:785–791
15. Groeneveld AB, Kolkman JJ (1994) Splanchnic tonometry: a review of physiology, methodology and clinical applications. J Crit Care 9:198–210
16. Brinkmann A, Wolf CF, Berger D, Kneitinger E, Neumeister B, Büchler M, Radermacher P, Seeling W, Georgieff M (1999) Perioperative endotoxemia and bacterial translocation during major abdominal surgery: evidence for the protective effect of endogenous prostacyclin? Crit Care Med (in press)
17. Fiddian Green RG (1995) Gastric intramucosal pH, tissue oxygenation and acid-base balance. Br J Anaesth 74:591–606
18. Berger D, Schmidt UM, Ott S, Seidelmann M, Martin R, Beger HG (1995) Incidence and pathophysiological relevance of postoperative endotoxemia. FEMS Immunol Med Microbiol 11:285–290
19. Berger D, Bölke E, Stanescu A, Buttenschoen K, Vasilescu C, Seidelmann M, Beger HG (1995) Endotoxemia and mediator release during colonoscopy. Endoscopy 27:671–675

Antiendotoxin Antibody Production of Mononuclear Cells in Multiply Injured Patients

K. Buttenschön · D. Berger · K. Stenzel · T. Piper · H. G. Beger
Department of Surgery, University of Ulm, Steinhoevelstrasse 9, 89075 Ulm, Germany

Introduction

In 1990 the definition of 'translocation' was expanded to include the passage of both viable and nonviable microbes and microbial products across an intact intestinal barrier [1]. Damage to the intestinal barrier causes increased permeability, which is responsible for bacterial components (e.g., endotoxins) entering the circulation [2–4]. Endotoxin is accepted as a potent trigger of the mediator cascade which can cause systemic inflammatory response syndrome (SIRS) and multiple organ failure. Multiply injured patients suffer from temporary endotoxemia, which is most probably due to translocation of endotoxin through the intestinal barrier [5, 6]. Endotoxins are T cell-independent antigens and can stimulate B cells directly [7]. Although there is an acquired immunological deficit after trauma [8], endotoxins are capable of stimulating the synthesis of antiendotoxin antibodies, increasing the amount of the specific IgM antibodies against endotoxins in the serum [5, 6]. However, the concentration of any substance in the blood is a result of production (synthesis or delivery into the blood) and consumption (degradation or removal from the blood). Therefore, this study examined the effect of temporary endotoxemia on peripheral mononuclear cells cultured after blood collection.

Methods

Blood was collected from 14 patients (mean age 40 ± 4 years) with multiple injury (mean injury severity score 25±4) directly after their admission to the hospital and again 3, 5, 7 and 12 days later. Mononuclear cells were isolated by Ficoll and cultured for 9 days. Endotoxin was determined by the *Limulus* amebocyte lysate test with a chromogenic modification [9]. Specific antibodies against endotoxins in the cell culture supernatant were measured by ELISA [6]. Antibodies against the following endotoxins were determined: lipid A of *E. coli*, lipopolysaccharide (LPS) of *E. coli* and LPS of *Vibrio cholerae*.

Results

Endotoxemia peaked 0–3 h post injury (0.1 ± 0.02 EU/ml) and decreased continuously thereafter to 0.04 ± 0.02 EU/ml) at day 12. The isolated mononuclear cells synthesized antibodies against all tested endotoxins, with a peak at/between day 5 and day 7. The

M. K. Herbert et al. (Eds.), Problems of the Gastrointestinal Tract in Anesthesia...

Table 1. Significant increases ($P < 0.05$) of IgA antibodies and IgM antibodies against lipid A of *E. coli* (*LA*), LPS of *E. coli* (*EC*) and LPS of *Vibrio cholerae* (*VC*) in the cell culture supernatant produced by mononuclear cells of multiply injured patients (arbitrary units; average ± standard error)

Time	LA (IgA)	EC (IgA)	VC (IgA)	LA (IgM)
0–3 h	34 ± 7	37 ± 7	39 ± 19	218 ± 36
5 days	69 ± 17	86 ± 21	93 ± 25	489 ± 73
7 days	98 ± 24	113 ± 30	141 ± 61	300 ± 50

increase was significant for specific IgA antibodies and for IgM antibodies against lipid A of *E. coli* (Table 1). However, there was only a slight increase in the total IgM concentration (day 7, but $P = 0.23$) and only fluctuations of the total IgA and IgG concentration in the supernatant without any tendency.

Conclusion

Multiply injured patients show temporary endotoxemia, which is most probably due to translocation from the gastrointestinal tract. B cells were stimulated to synthesize specific antibodies against endotoxins. However, these antibodies cross-react with LPS of *Vibrio cholerae*, an endotoxin that was very probably not present in the gut of the patients studied. Hence, cross-reactivity of the synthesized antibodies and/or polyclonal stimulation is assumed to be responsible.

Discussion

An injury to the intestinal barrier increases the passage of substances from the lumen of the gut into the circulation. Multiply injured patients suffer from temporary endotoxemia [5, 6]. One of the major factors in host defense is the immune system, which is impaired in injured patients [10, 11]. Transient depression in numbers of B cells, depression of immunoglobulin synthesis, depression of T lymphocytes, and increased activity of T suppressor cells have been reported [8, 12]. On the other hand, some investigations have shown that endotoxins are potent activators of B cells [13, 14]. The immune consequences of translocation are not completely disclosed yet and endotoxemia in humans with multiple injury is not generally accepted [15, 16]. The aim of this study was to describe the kinetics of endotoxemia in multiply injured patients up to the 12th day after trauma and the investigation of the time-course of specific antiendotoxin antibody production (IgM, IgA, IgG) in the supernatant of cultured mononuclear cells after blood collection.

This study showed the highest concentration of endotoxin shortly after injury, at admission of the patients to the hospital. Thereafter the concentration of endotoxin decreased. These results confirm earlier findings [5, 6], but the peak concentration in this study was not as high.

Earlier investigations dealt with the time-course of antiendotoxin antibodies in the serum. However, a concentration of a substance in the serum reflects the dynamic equilibrium between production and consumption. Therefore, this study examined the effect of temporary endotoxemia on peripheral mononuclear cells, which were cultured after blood collection because there is no consumption of proteins in the cell culture supernatant. The amounts of specific antibodies were compared with the total immunoglobulin concentration of the corresponding immunoglobulin class. Specific IgA response to endotoxins peaked at/between days 5 and 7 after trauma. The immune response was detectable after a proper time lack. Earlier investigations [5, 6] revealed only an increase in IgM antibodies against endotoxins in the serum. However, the main sphere of activity of IgA antibodies is the mucosa. It could be speculated that there is a transport of specific IgA antibodies against endotoxins to the surface of the intestinal mucosa. This mechanism counteracts increasing IgA levels in the serum despite increased IgA production of mononuclear cells.

Vibrio cholerae is a gram-negative bacterium, and it may be assumed that it does not occur in the gut of normal humans living in the geographical area around our university. A stay abroad was excluded. Under these conditions the immune response to *Vibrio cholerae* can act as a control for cross-reactivity. The similarities in the lipid A moiety between different LPS molecules forms the basis for the wide cross-reactions [17]. The results show a significant increase in specific antibodies against *Vibrio cholerae* (IgA), most probably due to cross-reactivity.

There was no clear tendency and only minor fluctuations of the total immunoglobulin concentrations (IgM, IgA and IgG). Hence, the significant increase in antibodies against endotoxins is specific and not a general phenomenon.

References

1. Alexander JW, Boyce ST, Babcock GF (1990) The process of microbial translocation. Ann Surg 212:496–512
2. Baker JW, Deitch EA, Li M, Berg R, Specian R (1988) Hemorrhagic shock induces bacterial translocation from the gut. J Trauma 28:896–906
3. Deitch EA, Morrison J, Berg R, Specian RD (1990) Effect of hemorrhagic shock on bacterial translocation, intestinal morphology, and intestinal permeability in conventional and antibiotic-decontaminated rats. Crit Care Med 18:529–536
4. Van Leeuwen PA, Boermeester MA, Houdijk AP, et al (1994) Clinical significance of translocation. Gut 35:S28-S34
5. Hiki N, Berger D, Buttenschoen K, et al (1995) Endotoxemia and specific antibody behavior against different endotoxins following multiple injuries. J Trauma 38:794–801
6. Buttenschoen K, Berger D, Hiki N, Strecker W, Seidelmann M, Beger HG (1996) Plasma concentrations of endotoxin and antiendotoxin antibodies in patients with multiple injuries: a prospective clinical study. Eur J Surg 162:853–860
7. Feldmann M, Male D (1991) Zellkooperation bei der Antikörperantwort. In: Roitt IM, Brostoff J, Male DK (eds) Kurzes Lehrbuch der Immunologie. Thieme, Stuttgart New York, pp 90–115
8. Ninnemann JL (1989) The immune consequences of trauma: an overview. In: Faist E, Ninnemann JL, Green D (eds) Immune consequences of trauma, shock, and sepsis. Springer, Berlin Heidelberg New York, pp 1–8
9. Berger D, Marzinzig E, Marzinzig M, Beger HG (1988) Quantitative endotoxin determination in blood – chromogenic modification of the limulus amebocyte lysate test. Eur Surg Res 20:128–136
10. Machiedo GW, Deitch EA (1991) Case 21: bacteremia of unknown origin. Postgrad Gen Surg 3:147–150
11. Walker RI (1978) The contribution of intestinal endotoxin to mortality in hosts with compromised resistance: a review. Exp Hematol 6:172–184
12. O'Mahony JB, Palder SB, Wood JJ, et al (1984) Depression of cellular immunity after multiple trauma in the absence of sepsis. J Trauma 24:869–875
13. Levitt D, Stull DD, Lawton AR (1981) T-cell-dependent and independent plasma cell differentiation induced by *Escherichia coli* lipopolysaccaride in human peripheral blood lymphocytes. Clin Immunol Immunopathol 18:309–321

14. Izui S, Eisenberg RA, Dixon FJ (1981) Subclass-restricted IgG polyclonal antibody production in mice injected with lipid A-rich lipopolysaccarides. J Exp Med 153:324–338
15. Caridis DT, Reinhold RB, Woodruff PWH, Fine J (1972) Endotoxaemia in Man. Lancet II:1381–1386
16. Moore FA, Moore EE, Poggetti R, et al (1991) Gut bacterial translocation via the portal vein: a clinical perspective with major torso trauma. J Trauma 31:629–638
17. Galanos C, Freudenberg MA, Jay F, et al (1984) Immunogenic properties of lipid A. Rev Infect Dis 6:546–552

Multivariate Analysis of Parameters Predicting Lethal Outcome in a Porcine Model of Abdominal Sepsis

T. Strate[1] · C. G. Schneider[1] · M. Wolf[1, 2] · J. R. Izbicki[1] · C. Bloechle[1]

[1] Department of Surgery, University Hospital of Hamburg, Martinistr. 52, 20246 Hamburg, Germany
[2] Department of Internal Medicine, University Hospital of Hamburg, Germany

Introduction

Despite advances in resuscitation, new potent antibiotics and organ support systems, the survival of patients with multiple organ failure syndrome (MOF) has not dramatically improved since Baue first described it in the early 1970s [2, 17]. It is still the leading cause of death in U.S. intensive care units (ICU) [3]. Infection, trauma, hemorrhage, pancreatitis etc. can lead to or augment the disastrous self-destructing mechanism [7]. Since mortality is high even though modern treatment options are available, one mechanism of breaking through this vicious circle might be early recognition of the disease entity, followed by timely correction of inadequate tissue oxygenation [14].

To find variables that allow early identification of patients at risk, many measurements and calculations have been suggested [4, 10]. These parameters have not been subjected to multivariate analysis including the aspects of both lethal outcome and timely recognition (MEDLINE search 1980 to September 1998).

The aim of this study was to find independent parameters closely related to lethal outcome in severe abdominal sepsis.

Materials and Methods

A total of 24 pigs were randomly allocated into two groups: sham group ($n = 6$) and treatment group ($n = 18$). The treatment group underwent standardized gastrotomy under general anesthesia to induce peritonitis. In addition, an arterial line and a Swan-Ganz catheter were inserted. After 12 h, a gastric tonometry catheter was inserted, the defect was oversewn and the abdomen was lavaged thoroughly.

In the sham group a gastrotomy was not performed and no defect was repaired, but otherwise the two operations were performed in a similar way with special regard to a similar timing.

Shortly before the definitive repair and 30 min afterwards the following parameters were retrieved:

- QT, SVR, CVP using a Swan-Ganz catheter
- MAP and HR using an arterial line
- pHi (gastric mucosal pH) using gastric air tonometry
- pH using standard blood gas analysis
- Endotoxin, TNF-α, leukocytes, HKT using blood aliquots.

M. K. Herbert et al. (Eds.), Problems of the Gastrointestinal Tract in Anesthesia...

During the operation animals were given Ringer's lactate for resuscitation, continuous ketamine and midazolam infusion for anesthesia and analgesia, and at the end of the operation tramadol 100 mg was administered i.m. for postoperative analgesia. Intraoperatively Ringer's lactate was infused at a maximum rate of 1500 ml/h to keep CVP > 3 mmHg, MAP > 60 mmHg, and HR < 140 min^{-1}. No additional therapy was instituted. All animals were allowed free access to water and were fed a standard diet on postoperative day 1. The main outcome was survival 48 h postoperatively. All parameters were subjected to the Spearman rank correlation test. The parameters that correlated best with mortality ($r > 0.8$, $P < 0.01$) were subjected to multivariate analysis.

Results

In the treatment group 7 of the 18 pigs (39 %) died within the 48-h observation period. Data were obtained before the initiation of therapy (T1, $index_1$) and 30 min later (T2, $index_2$). These time points representing admission and early intervention were completed for trends [admission value minus value at early intervention (Δ)]. Nine parameters fulfilled the criteria for strong correlation and were entered on multivariate analysis (Table 1).

Endotoxin levels 30 min after initiation of therapy and the trend in pHi (Δ-pHi = pHi1–pHi2) had the highest predictive value for mortality.

When the cut-off level for endotoxin was set at 50 EU/ml, it accurately predicted lethal outcome with a specificity and sensitivity of 100 %.

When therapy had no positive effect on pHi (increase or avoidance of further decrease) during the first 30 min, the animals died. An increase in pHi was equivalent to survival (specificity and sensitivity = 100 %).

Table 1. Multivariate discriminant analysis of significant variables correlating with mortality after Spearman rank correlation ($r > 0{,}8$ and $P < 0.01$); $index_1$ before and $index_2$ 30 min after initiation of therapy in 18 cases (7 nonsurvivors, 11 survivors): 2 class levels, 9 variables, significance level to stay 0.05. Numbers in parentheses are excluded by multivariate analysis (Δ admission value minus value at early intervention, *F*, *P*, *TNF* tumor necrosis factor)

Parameter	Number	F at entry	P at entry	Survivors mean (± SD)	Deaths mean (± SD)
$Endotoxin_2$ (EU/ml)	1	143.0	0.000	17.9 (± 12.1)	110.8 (± 21.0)
Δ-pHi	2	103.2	0.017	−0.15 (± 0.011)	0.039 (± 0.013)
QT_2	(3)	67.3	0.294	6.9 (± 0.2)	7.9 (± 0.2)
Δ-QT (l/min)	(4)	51.4	0.299	−0.28 (± 0.21)	−1.11 (± 0.36)
TNF-α_2 (pg/ml)	(5)	40.1	0.441	84.4 (± 37.7)	458.3 (± 324.6)
$Leukocytes_2$ (G/l)	(6)	32.1	0.494	23.0 (± 3.2)	35.2 (± 4.5)
TNF-α_1 (pg/ml)	(7)	25.6	0.659	101.7 (± 26.9)	511.7 (± 222.0)
Δ-Endotoxin (EU/ml)	(8)	20.3	0.805	11.1 (± 10.8)	−73.6 (± 24.4)
PHi_2	(9)	16.1	0.899	7.20 (± 0.01)	7.15 (± 0.02)

Discussion

Since abdominal sepsis is an important disease entity often followed by MOF and subsequent death, this experimental setting compares most of the sepsis-relevant variables with reference to their predictive value for lethal outcome in abdominal sepsis. The time interval has been chosen to be short and between only two measurements to identify early changes indicating clinical deterioration.

Interestingly, ΔpHi and endotoxin level evaluated at 30 min after the beginning of the operation were the parameters that best predicted lethal outcome according to multivariate analysis. An important role has been attributed to the gut in the development of MOF. It is thought that the splanchnic blood supply is especially susceptible to microcirculatory deficit because of its countercurrent blood flow [17]. A splanchnic microcirculatory deficit can be found in severe diseases (e.g., trauma, infection, hemorrhage) [1, 8, 9, 11, 13, 16]. This could potentially lead to mucosal hypoxia and ischemia, especially in the mucosa, which serves as the main barrier against bacterial translocation. If the mucosa is damaged by the mechanisms outlined, more bacteria and/or endotoxin can translocate and start a systemic cascade of response (macrophages, cytokines, effector organs-liver, blood vessels, kidney, lungs, etc.).

Mucosal ischemia can be measured indirectly with the use of gastric tonometry. The potential advantages are: (1) it could be readily available in any setting, since only a nasogastric tube needs to be inserted, (2) it has little potential for complications, and (3) it seems to be an accurate and early predictor of lethal outcome in abdominal sepsis, which has been shown in this experimental setting, and is best explained by the cascade of the "gut hypothesis" outlined above. If splanchnic mucosal injury happens early in the course of abdominal sepsis, and if the same mechanism is followed by potentially deleterious bacterial translocation, timely recognition of mucosal ischemia by gastric tonometry before the breakdown of the protective barrier and institution of counterregulatory therapy could possibly break the imminent vicious circle. Furthermore, tonometric data can be retrieved almost continuously, allowing almost immediate reflection of the splanchnic mucosal status. This would be its main advantage over endotoxin serum determination, for which the probes in special non-pyrogenic containers need to be put on ice and processed in a complicated way using the limulus amebic lysate test. The earliest results are available 2 h later and parameters cannot be monitored continuously. This test is not available in every hospital, and its use requires a special laboratory, whereas tonometry is easy to use, can be applied after 5 min introduction time and yields results that are simple to interpret.

Even though hemodynamic variables did not correlate very well with mortality in this multivariate analysis, they are of great clinical importance for monitoring hemodynamic stability. Its use is common in many ICUs. Perhaps our data should have been complemented with DO_2 and VO_2 calculations as indicators of oxygen delivery and consumption in the periphery. But Ivatory et al. demonstrated in a prospective randomized trial that tonometry is a better predictor of sufficient resuscitation and lethal outcome in severely traumatized patients with MOF than VO_2 and DO_2 [12]. Also, after the report of Connors et al. of a higher 30-day hospital mortality in a group of ICU patients monitored by a right heart catheter than in patients in whom a Swan-Ganz catheter was not inserted during the first 24 h in the ICU [5], the use of right heart catheters underwent a critical appraisal. Connors prospectively analyzed two well-matched groups (matched-pair analysis, $n = 5735$). Potential causes for the increased mortality could be (1) early (operative) and (2) late (infectious) complications, or (3) the complexity of the data retrieved using a Swan-Ganz catheter, so misdiagnosis is a potential hazard especially in inexperienced hands [6, 15].

In conclusion, based on the results of this study, tonometry is certainly a valuable and early predictor of a lethal outcome in experimental abdominal sepsis and should therefore have more clinical recognition.

References

1. Antonsson JB, Boyle CC, Kruithoff KL, Wang H, Sacristan E, Rothschild HR, Fink MP (1990) Validation of tonometric measurement of gut intramural pH during endotoxemia and mesenteric occlusion in pigs. Am J Physiol 259:G519–G523
2. Baue AE (1975) Multiple, progressive or sequential systems failure: a syndrome of the 1970's. Arch Surg 110:779–781
3. Beal AL, Cerra FB (1994) Multiple organ failure syndrome in the 1990s: systemic inflamatory response and organ dysfunction. JAMA 271:226–223
4. Bone RC (1992) Towards an epidemiology and natural history of SIRS (systemic inflammatory response syndrome). JAMA 268:3452–3455
5. Connors AF Jr, Speroff T, Dawson NV, Thomas C, Harrell FE Jr, Wagner D, Desbiens N, Goldman L, Wu AW, Califf RM, Fulkerson WJ Jr, Vidaillet H, Broste S, Bellamy P, Lynn J, Knaus WA (1996) The effectiveness of right heart catheterization in the initial care of critically ill patients. JAMA 276:889–897
6. Dalen JE, Bone RC (1996) Is it time to pull the pulmonary artery catheter? JAMA 276:916–918
7. Deitch EA (1992) Multiple organ failure. Pathophysiology and potential future therapy. Ann Surg 216:117–134
8. Gomersall CD, Joynt GM, Ho KM, Young RJ, Buckley TA, Oh TE (1997) Gastric tonometry and prediction of outcome in the critically ill. Arterial to intramucosal pH gradient and carbon dioxide gradient. Anaesthesia 52:619–623
9. Hartmann M, Montgomery A, Joennson K, Haglund U (1991) Tissue oxygenation in hemorrhagic shock measured as transcutaneous oxygen tension, subcutaneous oxygen tension and gastrointestinal intramucosal pH in pigs. Crit Care Med 19:205–210
10. Hasselgren PO (1998) Intestinal cytokines during sepsis and endotoxinaemia. In: Schein M, Wise L (eds) Cytokines and the abdominal surgeon. Landes, Austin, pp 202–207
11. Heinonen PO, Jousela IT, Blomqvist KA, Olkkola KT, Takkunen OS (1997) Validation of air tonometric measurement of gastric regional concentrations of CO_2 in critically ill septic patients. Intensive Care Med 23:524–529
12. Ivatury RR, Simon RJ, Havriliak D, Garcia C, Greenbarg J, Stahl WM (1995) Gastric mucosal pH and oxygen delivery and oxygen consumption indices in the assessment of adequacy of resuscitation after trauma: a prospective, randomized trial. J Trauma 39:128–136
13. Ivatury RR, Simon RJ, Islam S, Fueg A, Rohman M, Stahl WM (1996) A prospective randomized study of end points of resuscitation after major trauma: global oxygen transport indices versus organ-specific gastric mucosal pH. J Am Coll Surg 183:145–154
14. Krafte-Jacobs B, Carver J, Wilkinson JD (1995) Comparison of gastric intramucosal pH and standard perfusional measurements in pediatric septic shock. Chest 108:220–225
15. Leibowitz AB (1996) Do pulmonary artery catheters improve patient outcome? No. Crit Care Clin 12:559–568
16. Montgomery A, Almquist P, Arvidsson D, Lindgren S, Haglund U (1990) Early detection of gastrointestinal mucosal ischemia in porcine *E. coli* sepsis. Acta Chir Scand 156:613–620
17. Pastores SM, Katz DP, Kvetan V (1996) Splanchnic ischemia and gut mucosal injury in sepsis and the multiple organ dysfunction syndrome. Am J Gastroenterol 91:1697–1710

INVITED ARTICLE

Gastric Mucosal Tonometry

M. V. Chapman · M. G. Mythen

The University College London Hospitals, Mortimer Street, London W1N 8AA, UK

Introduction

Gastrointestinal (GI) tonometry has become established as an effective technique for the assessment of splanchnic perfusion in the clinical setting. Despite the many studies performed that have shown tonometrically derived variables to be both predictive of patient outcome and useful in the guidance of therapeutic interventions, it does not enjoy widespread use as a monitoring tool, probably because the saline method used until recently is labor intensive, requires long equilibration times and is prone to measurement errors.

A new automated on line gas based system, The Tonocap (Datex-Engstrom, Tonometrics Division, Instrumentarium, Helsinki, Finland) has solved many of these practical problems. Its introduction as a bedside monitor should allow further clinical assessment and evaluation in the field of GI tonometry.

Rationale Behind GI Tonometry

It would be difficult to disagree with the principle that maintaining end-organ perfusion should be a fundamental goal in the practice of anesthesia and intensive care. Many of the tools available to help us achieve this goal, e.g., the pulmonary artery catheter, mixed venous oxygen saturations and blood lactate levels, not only have inherent problems of accuracy and measurement but also tend to reflect the global situation, with normal or near-normal values masking poor blood flow to individual tissue capillary beds.

It has been known since the early part of this century that tissue CO_2 diffuses from regional blood vessels into the lumen of hollow visci [1]. The measurement of luminal PCO_2 can therefore be taken to correspond to tissue PCO_2 and as such reflects the balance between CO_2 production by both aerobic and anaerobic metabolism and CO_2 removal by perfusion and blood flow [2]. This constitutes the basis of GI tonometry: the measurement of gastric luminal PCO_2 ($PgCO_2$) can be used to monitor end-organ perfusion of the gastrointestinal bed.

The measurement of luminal PCO_2 is not restricted to the GI tract but can be performed on other hollow organs, such as the bladder or gallbladder [3]. The gut, and in particular the stomach, are monitored above other viscera for several reasons.

In addition to being easily accessible, the GI tract is a sentinel organ in the detection of a failing circulation. Splanchnic organs are especially vulnerable, because of

M. K. Herbert et al. (Eds.), Problems of the Gastrointestinal Tract in Anesthesia...

the countercurrent flow of their microcirculation and the higher critical oxygen requirements of their cells [4]. Occult tissue hypoperfusion rapidly leads to mucosal ischemia, which may result in translocation of bacteria and endotoxin into the bloodstream, a process implicated in the pathogenesis of multiple organ dysfunction syndrome (MODS).

There are other methods available to monitor GI tract perfusion, such as Doppler flowmetry, reflectance spectrophotometry [5] and portal vein catheterization; however these are complicated to perform, time consuming and mainly confined to use in the research setting.

History of GI Tonometry

Tonometry refers to the measurement of the partial pressure of a gas in tissues. In 1964 Bergofsky tested the concept of hollow visceral tonometry by measuring the PO_2 and PCO_2 of saline instilled in the bladder and gallbladder [3]. Dawson et al. used the same principle and applied it to the gastrointestinal tract [6]. In 1973 Kivisaari and Niinikoski refined the tonometric technique for the determination of PO_2 and PCO_2 in subcutaneous tissues of the forearm by using a gas-permeable, saline-filled balloon [7]. This principle has been used in the development of the Trip NGS (gastric tonometer and sump) catheter (Datex-Engstrom, Tonometrics Division, Instrumentarium, Helsinki, Finland; see Fig. 1) used commonly in gastric saline and automated air tonometry. The catheter consists of a gas-impermeable tube connecting distally with a gas-permeable silicone balloon placed in the stomach. CO_2 freely equilibrates between regional blood vessels, the gut wall, gastric luminal and balloon contents. Catheters may also be placed in the colon and have been refined in size and shape over recent years. They are available in size 18F, 16F, and 14F for adults, with 8F and 5F sizes for use in the pediatric and neonatal population [8].

Interest in the field of GI tonometry is due primarily to the research and teaching efforts of Richard Fiddian-Green, a surgeon from the U.S. who in the early 1980s adopted the saline tonometric technique for the assessment of gut luminal PCO_2 and extended its use to the calculation of what he referred to as the GI intramucosal pH (pHi) [9].

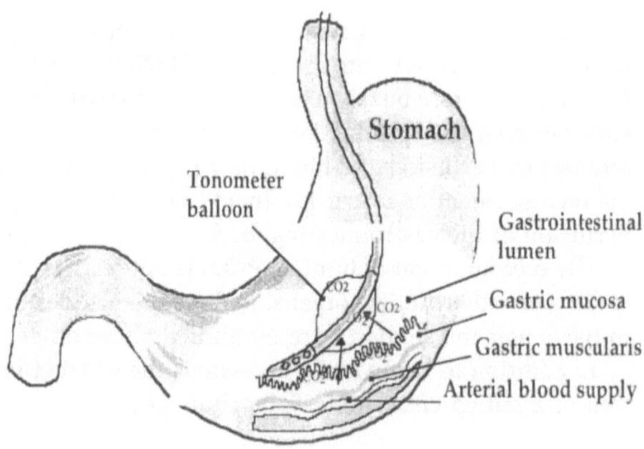

Fig. 1. TRIP NGS catheter (gastric tonometer and sump) in situ, demonstrating free equilibration of CO_2 between regional blood vessels, gastric wall, gastric luminal contents and air/saline within catheter balloon

Saline Gastric Tonometry

Principles

Gastric luminal CO_2 using saline tonometry can be measured by the installation of 2.5 ml of 0.9% saline into the balloon of a TRIP catheter placed in the stomach. The PCO_2 of the saline in the tonometer balloon following equilibration with that of the mucosa is determined with the aid of a standard blood gas analyzer. The intramucosal pH (pHi) is then calculated by substituting this value and arterial bicarbonate (HCO_3^-) (assumed to be equivalent to gastric mucosal HCO_3^-) into the following modified Henderson-Hasselbach equation:

$$\text{pHi} = 6.1 + \log_{10}\left[\text{Arterial } (HCO_3^-)/PCO_2 \text{ (tonometer)} \cdot K\right]$$

where K = time-dependent equilibration constant that corrects for the concentration gradient that exists across the tonometer membrane.

Drawbacks

The widespread acceptance of saline GI tonometry as a major monitoring tool has been impeded because of the many, mainly practical, problems associated with its use.

A laborious, meticulous technique in the handling and measurement of saline samples from the tonometer is needed to produce worthwhile and reproducible results [10]. Strict anaerobic conditions are required within the catheter, involving a time-consuming priming procedure.

One of the most important downsides of the saline tonometric technique is the need for long equilibration times between samples. Manufacturers recommend a minimum of 30–60 min before saline is aspirated and measured for CO_2 content. Consequently, results never truly reflect the patients' current condition, especially in the rapidly changing critically ill population or in acute situations such as major trauma or resuscitation. This prevents the use of saline GI tonometry to guide therapeutic interventions.

CO_2 is a highly diffusable gas, which is rapidly lost from saline because it contains no buffering systems. Studies have shown that the stability of CO_2 in the saline environment can be improved by the addition of phosphate buffers, but this lengthens equilibration times between samples because of the buffers' higher CO_2-binding capacity [11, 12].

Blood gas analyzers (BGA) exhibit errors in bias and precision because they are calibrated for the determination of PCO_2 in blood. For most commonly used machines errors are small, but certain analyzers have been shown to exhibit large and significant errors [13, 14]. Accuracy is also affected by the transit time between the sampling port and sensor of each BGA.

Research to Date

Morbidity, Mortality and Outcome

GI intramucosal pH has been shown to be a very sensitive but poorly specific indicator of outcome. On the ICU pHi has been found to be a predictor of mortality and length of stay. Doglio et al. reported a pHi of less than 7.35 to have a sensitivity of 76.5% (measured on admission and at 12 h) and a specificity of 77.5% (measured on admission only) as a predictor of mortality [15].

Studies examining the relationship between pHi and outcome following major surgery or trauma have consistently shown that a low pHi (< 7.35) is a predictor of poor outcome [16, 17] and increases postoperative complications and costs [18]. Low pHi values in the stomach and sigmoid wall during abdominal aortic reconstruction correlated with the development of ischemic colitis and visible ischemia and were highly predictive of the development of major complications [19, 20]. A prospective, randomized trial studying the effects of fluid loading in patients undergoing elective cardiac surgery with the aim of maintaining perioperative gastric mucosal perfusion showed that the incidence of a low pHi was significantly lower in the protocol group than in controls, as were the number of complications, number of days spent in hospital and subsequent cost [21].

Comparison with Other Hemodynamic Variables

In studies that have compared GI tonometry and the measurement of pHi with other routinely used monitors of cardiorespiratory function it has been found that they are more sensitive predictors of morbidity and mortality than more global measures, such as blood pressure, cardiac output and urine output [22]. The onset of a low pHi in the ICU is usually not in the setting of cardiovascular instability, highlighting the fact that conventional monitoring may not alert the practitioner to the presence of intramucosal acidosis and hypoperfusion [23]. In healthy volunteers it has been shown that early hypovolemia is associated with a deterioration of tonometrically derived variables (P_gCO_2–P_aCO_2) before overt changes in hemodynamic variables takes place (Fig. 2) [24].

Fig. 2. An observational study by Hamilton-Davies et al. [24] demonstrated the maintenance of normal cardiovascular variables but worsening tonometry variables in response to a hypovolemic insult

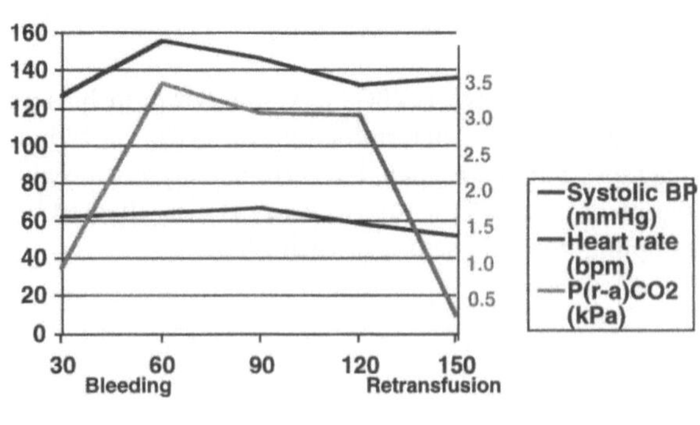

Feeding and Weaning

A low pHi has been demonstrated to predict outcome and failure of weaning from mechanical ventilation [25, 26], and further studies have shown that 28 % of attempts to wean are associated with onset of a low pHi [23]. This may suggest that withdrawal of ventilatory assistance increases blood flow to the respiratory muscles at the expense of splanchnic flow.

Enteral feeding is favored over parenteral feeding, if feasible, in critically ill patients. A low pHi is associated with GI tract dysfunction as judged by failure to acidify the gastric lumen in response to a pentagastrin test, one of the few tests available that truly reflect GI tract function [27]. A low pHi has been shown to occur temporarily at the onset of enteral nutrition, suggesting (provided any artifact has been excluded) that some form of perfusional mismatch is taking place. Although further studies are required, gastric tonometry may have the potential to identify the patient cohort more likely to be successfully enterally fed.

Catecholamine Administration

Gastric tonometry has been used to monitor the effects of various catecholamines on gut perfusion, with variable results. pHi may vary erratically in the critically ill population, because other factors apart from perfusion affect the systemic acid–base balance. These studies are difficult to compare because they vary in design, controls and randomization. Dopexamine, for instance, being an agonist at both dopaminergic and $\beta 2$-receptors with no α-agonism, is regarded by many authors as the drug of choice for reversal of low pHi [16, 28]. Several studies have suggested that dopexamine produces significant increases in pHi [29, 30] whereas a randomized placebo-controlled trial studying the effect of dopexamine (in conjunction with colloid) on low pHi failed to demonstrate an improvement in this variable [31].

Interventional Studies

Disappointingly, studies examining the outcome of pHi-guided therapy are few in number, probably because of the methodological problems in sample handling and long equilibration times mentioned above.

In a prospective, randomized, multicenter South American trial of pHi-guided therapy, over 25 % improvement in survival was reported in patients who were admitted to the ICU with a normal pHi and were treated according to a pHi-guided protocol. This study failed to show any benefit to those admitted with an already abnormal pHi, suggesting the importance of early diagnosis of GI hypoperfusion and intervention [32].

GI tonometry has proven very effective in the field of trauma. Young patients with stagnant hypoxia are common in this area, and the quick and effective restoration of circulating blood volume is paramount in their care. Splanchnic ischemia can still exist in trauma victims even when conventional resuscitation end-points have been attained [33]. Ivatury et al compared pHi and global oxygenation variables (delivery and consumption) as therapeutic indices in a prospective, randomized trial of patients in the first 24 h after major trauma. They found the mortality in the group with normalized pHi was significantly lower and the patients in the pHi-guided group tended to show improved survival, although study numbers were inadequate to confirm this. As such, tonometry variables appear superior to global oxygenation indicators of adequacy of resuscitation [34].

A prospective single-center trial with historical controls and low patient numbers has studied the impact of antioxidant and splanchnic directed therapy on persistent uncorrected pHi in a group of critically injured trauma patients. The protocol differed from controls by the administration of folate, mannitol and low-dose isoproterenol and the administration of splanchnic sparing inotropic and vasodilatory agents to optimize cardiac output. Compared with controls, the "splanchnic therapy" group had fewer organ system failures and shorter intensive care and hospital stays [35].

Automated Air Gastric Tonometry

The introduction of the Tonocap monitor (Datex-Engstrom, Tonometrics Division, Instrumentarium, Helsinki, Finland) in 1996 represents a major advance in the field of GI tonometry (Fig. 3). As an automated, semicontinuous combined air tonometer and capnograph, it overcomes many of the methodological problems presented by the saline technique. It demonstrates greater accuracy and precision with faster equilibration times and is a closed circuit, thereby limiting atmospheric contamination. A semiconstant display of the P_rCO_2 (P_gCO_2) value removes the errors resulting from frequent human sampling during the saline technique.

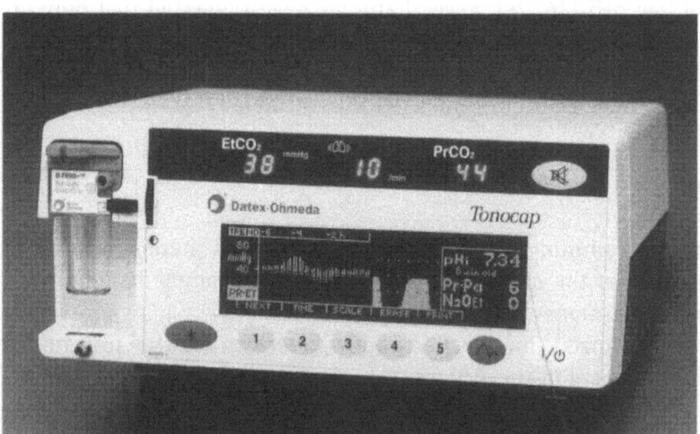

Fig. 3. The Tonocap: a monitor used for semicontinuous air gastrointestinal tonometry, introduced in 1996

Working Principle

The Tonocap monitor (Fig. 4) is attached to a standard TRIP catheter. The tonometer catheter balloon is automatically filled with 5 ml of room air, which is kept in the balloon for a preselected equilibration period to allow CO_2 diffusion from the gastric lumen. The cycle time automatically sets to 10-min intervals. The sample then empties back into an infrared measuring chamber for analysis. The air is recycled to the catheter balloon to avoid CO_2 depletion in the catheter system, thereby decreasing subsequent equilibration times.

The software of the Tonocap adjusts the measured CO_2 concentration after calculating an appropriate correction factor that allows for incomplete equilibration. If two consecutive samples are very different (as may happen at the beginning of use) the P_gCO_2 values will be corrected by 6–7 % towards the previous value. During steady state conditions there is a permanent correction factor of about 2 % to allow for catheter dead space.

Using a catheter attached to the patients endotracheal tube the Tonocap samples and analyzes airway gases for nitrous oxide (N_2O) concentration, end-tidal carbon dioxide ($EtCO_2$) and respiratory rate, which are continuously displayed.

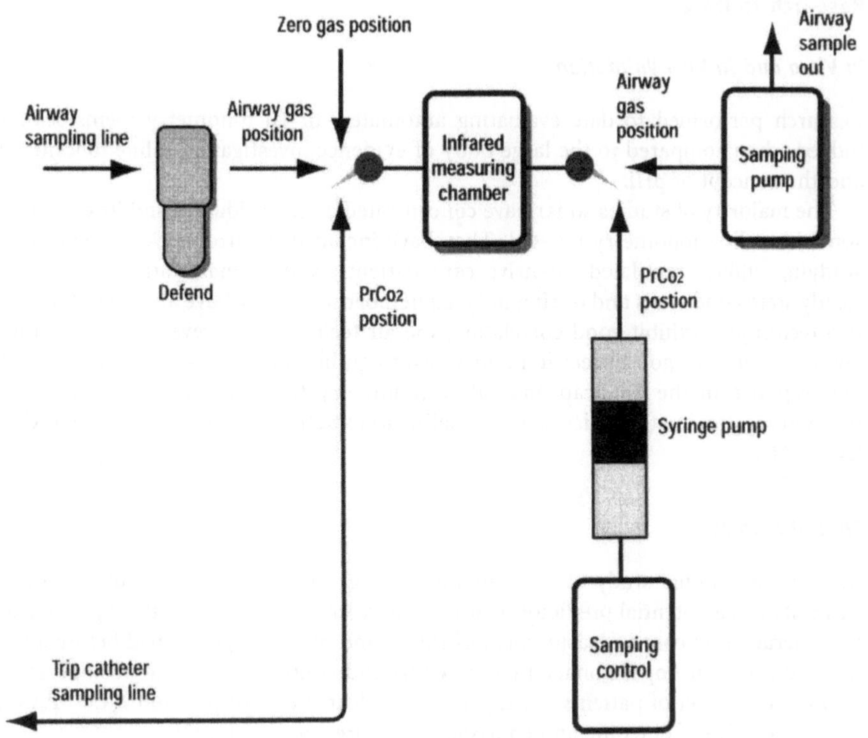

Fig. 4. Working principle of the Tonocap: the sampling control switches infrared analysis between airway gas and P_gCO_2 measurement according to desired cycling times

The infrared chamber is a CO_2 and N_2O dual-path photometer. Light is guided from the infrared source through measurement and reference chambers. Adjustment in the presence of N_2O is required because of the broad-band collision effect. Filters for CO_2 and N_2O are rotated and synchronized to measurements. Light is then reflected and focused into an infrared detector. The sensor signal pulses are then temperature compensated and amplified.

The Tonocap monitor provides an automated measurement of P_gCO_2. It can calculate the pHi from the P_aCO_2, the arterial pHa entered by the user and the measured P_gCO_2. Results of sampling may be viewed as CO_2 gaps or pHi. These may then be viewed as trends over selected time periods.

Accessories for the Tonocap monitor are:

1. Trip catheter sampling line is used to connect the TRIP catheter to the Tonocap monitor.
2. A D-fend water trap collects the mucous secretions and moisture when measuring $EtCO_2$.
3. An airway sampling line is used to measure the $EtCO_2$.
4. The Tonocap monitor can be connected to a printer or PC by cable.
5. Collect software is used for PC data acquisition.

Research to Date

In Vitro and In Vivo Validation

Research performed to date evaluating automated air GI tonometry seems scanty indeed when compared to the large body of evidence investigating saline tonometry and the concept of pHi.

The majority of studies so far have concentrated on its validation and its comparison with saline tonometry [36–40]. They have included in vitro work, in vivo work studying stable, ventilated intensive care patients, and animal work during both steady state conditions and during induced hemorrhage. They have all shown that the two techniques exhibit good correlation, the air technique, however, demonstrating low levels of bias, good precision and shorter equilibration times. A comparison of the response of the Tonocap and saline tonometry to a change in CO_2 shows it responds approximately twice as fast as saline tonometry to a stepwise change in CO_2 levels [41].

Clinical Studies

In an observational study of 100 patients undergoing cardiac surgery the Tonocap was tested as a potential predictor of adverse outcome, defined as death or prolonged postoperative outcome. Measurement of P_gCO_2 and pHi were performed before, during and after cardiopulmonary bypass (CPB) and continued into the postoperative period in a subset of patients. Postoperative measurements of pHi and P_gCO_2-P_aCO_2 were predictive of outcome and consistent with previous work [42].

Both of these sets of investigators commented that the Tonocap was easy and practical to use, especially when compared with saline tonometry.

In a European multicenter study the Tonocap was used in ASA III patients undergoing elective, noncardiac surgery expected to last more than 2 h. A functional recovery assessment at postoperative day 8 was used as the main outcome variable. The study demonstrated poorer predictive power for tonometric variables than in previous studies, but a cumulative P_g–$EtCO_2$ gap above normal (assumed to be 1.3 kPa) was the best predictor of this outcome measure (A. R. Webb, personal communication).

Parameters to Measure: pHi or P_gCO_2–P_aCO_2 Gap?

In the calculation of pHi the important assumption is made that the HCO_3^- of gastric mucosal tissue is in equilibrium with the systemic arterial HCO_3^-, which may not be correct. When gastric blood flow decreases in shock the local gastric tissue HCO_3^- may be significantly lower than systemic levels, which results in an overestimation of gastric pHi. Furthermore systemic metabolic acidosis and alkalosis, very common in the critically ill, can change systemic arterial HCO_3^- and therefore influence and confound the interpretation of gastric pHi [43, 44]. Indeed this may in part explain the predictive power of pHi seen in the critically ill, and the data suggesting that base deficit or other parameters of systemic disturbances of acid-base balance are as predictive as pHi of poor outcome in an ICU population [45].

Gastric luminal partial pressure of CO_2 (P_gCO_2) is the variable now thought to be most representative of gastrointestinal hypoperfusion. It does not assume equilibration of gastric mucosal and systemic arterial HCO_3^- values and is not directly changed by metabolic acid-base disturbances. During steady state, it reflects the balance between CO_2 production and CO_2 removal by gastric blood flow. Its value can increase to abnormal levels following a decrease in gastric blood flow alone without anaerobic generation of CO_2, suggesting that it is a more specific indicator of isolated GI mucosal hypoperfusion. The situation, however, is not as simple as it initially seems. The production of CO_2 as a by-product of anaerobic metabolism will occur when gastric oxygen delivery (DO_2) falls below a critical level tending to increase P_gCO_2 [2], however, there is an accompanying fall in CO_2 production via conventional metabolism, which also occurs below the critical level of DO_2 decreasing P_gCO_2.

P_gCO_2 is influenced by systemic arterial PCO_2 values (P_aCO_2), which in the critically ill population can vary rapidly. This can be corrected for by calculating the gastric–arterial CO_2 gap (P_gCO_2–P_aCO_2). Furthermore the Tonocap is able to measure end-tidal CO_2 ($EtCO_2$). By assuming that patients without significant ventilation/perfusion mismatch have a constant P_aCO_2–$EtCO_2$ difference this can be taken to represent P_aCO_2 which removes the need for blood gas analysis in the calculation of CO_2 gap.

There is a paucity of evidence assessing the significance of P_gCO_2–P_aCO_2 gap in the clinical setting compared with the body of research that has evaluated pHi, and we must therefore be wary of embracing it as an immediate replacement. It may be that the predictive power of pHi centers on the fact that it becomes abnormal when an index of global tissue perfusion (arterial HCO_3^-) and one of regional perfusion (P_gCO_2) each become only *mildly* deranged. This would not apply to the CO_2 gap. It may be that pHi represents a very sensitive predictor of outcome whereas the

P_gCO_2–P_aCO_2 gap is a more specific indicator of isolated gastric mucosal hypoperfusion. Some investigators have found pHi to be no more predictive of outcome than traditional measures of perfusion and oxygenation [45], whereas others have shown it to be more so [46]. Friedman et al. recently investigated the predictive power of a low pHi (< 7.32) in 35 patients with severe sepsis and found that the low specificity in predicting ICU mortality could be improved by combining low pHi with systemic lactate concentrations [47]. This may result from the combination of the predictive ability of the P_gCO_2–P_aCO_2 gap with that of the systemic acid–base balance. A recent study by Gomersall et al. [48] in 62 ICU patients who were studied within 6 h of admission showed no significant difference at 0, 12, 24 h in the pH gap and P_gCO_2–P_aCO_2 gap between survivors and nonsurvivors, although there was a statistically significant difference in pHi and pHa between the two groups. This emphasizes that we cannot simply insert P_gCO_2–P_aCO_2 gap into the slot so far occupied by pHi without support from further studies.

Potential Sources of Error in the Use of Gastric Tonometry

It is important when a monitor is used that its strengths and weaknesses are known, along with possible reasons why it may or may not be working properly. There are several sources of error inherent in the technique of GI tonometry and some specific to the Tonocap, which result from the fact that measurement of P_gCO_2 is now in the gaseous phase.

General Sources of Error

Positioning

Correct positioning of the gastrointestinal tonometer is essential for meaningful measurement. If it is too close to the pylorus, reflux from the duodenum may cause erroneous elevation of luminal CO_2 levels. Catheters have insertion length markers on them at 45, 55, 65 and 75 cm, but the manufacturer recommends confirming correct location with an X-ray.

Increased Luminal Generation of CO_2

The luminal generation of CO_2 not related to tissue perfusion, which can be caused by the reaction of gastric acid and bicarbonate, is an important potential source of error. This has been demonstrated to cause marked acute increases in tonometrically derived P_gCO_2 in normal volunteers [49]. The phenomenon can be controlled by the use of histamine (H_2) receptor blockade. This may not be such an important problem in intensive care, because the ability of the critically ill to produce gastric acid is often impaired [27, 50]. This, coupled with the idiosyncratic response to H_2 blockers exhibited by many patients, highlights the importance of measuring gastric juice pH at the start of GI tonometry. Therapy should aim to raise the pH above 4, and proton pump inhibitors should be prescribed if H_2 receptor blockade is not enough to achieve this.

Enteral Feeding

Enteral feeding also causes increased luminal CO_2 production. The presence of food in the stomach may generate sufficient amounts of CO_2 to cause an apparent increase in P_gCO_2 [51]. In practice at least 60 min should elapse between feeding and P_gCO_2 measurement for it to be reliable.

Suction

Nasogastric (NG) suction via the catheter has been suspected as a potential source of error. In healthy volunteers, NG suction has no effect on the results [52]. In case of doubt, suctioning should be discontinued 30–60 min before measurement.

Sources of Error Specific to the Tonocap

Temperature

The Tonocap's ability to measure P_gCO_2 reliably under normal conditions has been validated (see above). The studies have not, however, considered the effect of temperature on both measured and derived variables.

The solubility of a gas in a liquid depends not only on its partial pressure but also on temperature [53]. When the saline technique is used both arterial and gastric tonometer samples are in the liquid phase and are measured in a blood gas analyzer. This automatically corrects the samples for temperature by heating them to 37 °C. The Tonocap, however, compares a P_gCO_2 value measured in the gaseous phase at actual body temperature (which in many critically ill and surgical patients may be higher or lower than 37 °C) with an arterial blood gas sample corrected by the BGA to 37 °C. As the effect of temperature on the value of P_aCO_2 is not considered, the calculated P_gCO_2–P_aCO_2 gap or pHi may not be truly representative. This is important because it may mean that pathologic values for the P_gCO_2–P_aCO_2 gap and for pHi remain unrecognized or therapeutic interventions are started for nonsignificant values. The Tonocap is also more accurate at differing temperatures, with a 0.3 %/°C measurement error margin as against the 4.5 %/°C of the Corning 800 BGA (K. Blomquist, personal communication).

In consideration of P_gCO_2–$EtCO_2$ levels it must be remembered that the relationship between P_aCO_2 and $EtCO_2$ does not remain constant at varying temperatures. For this to be so P_aCO_2 values must be corrected for body temperature [54].

Similar principles underlie the well-recognized “pH stat versus alpha stat” debate on acid–base management in patients undergoing hypothermic cardiopulmonary bypass (CPB) [55].

Nitrous Oxide

The molecular weight of nitrous oxide (N_2O) is the same as that of CO_2. This may result in it being mistaken for CO_2, affecting P_gCO_2 values. The concomitant direct measurement of N_2O via the same infrared technique as CO_2 removes this potential source of error.

Pressure Effects

In contrast to saline tonometry, the Tonocap measures CO_2 in the gaseous phase. Results will therefore be affected by the pressure of surrounding anatomical compartments and atmospheric pressure. When the Tonocap is used a sensor measures absolute pressure in the balloon prior to sampling then measures the CO_2 concentration at a known sensor pressure (slightly less than atmospheric) and finally calculates and displays the partial CO_2 pressure in the balloon according to the following equation:

$$P_gCO_{2\ \text{balloon}}\ (\text{mmHg}) = P_{\text{balloon}}/P_{\text{sensor}} \cdot P_gCO_{2\ \text{sensor}}\ (\%) \cdot \text{P}_{\text{ambient}}\ (\text{mmHg})$$

Equilibration Times

During the first 2–3 cycles of P_gCO_2 measurement CO_2 depletion will occur in the gastric balloon, as the air is removed for sampling, resulting in erroneously low values. This effect still occurs despite the sample of air being recycled back to the catheter balloon in order to reduce equilibration times. Following this a steady state is reached, where removal and repletion of sampled gas will not unduly decrease P_gCO_2 levels.

P_gCO_2–$EtCO_2$ Gap

This parameter can be used instead of P_gCO_2–P_aCO_2. It is very user friendly and represents one of the major advantages of the Tonocap over saline tonometry, since no arterial blood gases are required and the monitor is able to display a continuous CO_2 gap trend. An important assumption is made however: that the P_aCO_2–$EtCO_2$ difference is constant. This may not be the case if significant ventilation/perfusion mismatching occurs because of severe pulmonary disease or circulatory problems.

Conclusion

The technique of GI tonometry and measurement of pHi using the saline method has (unlike many other monitors in everyday use) been validated by a large body of research showing it to be a sensitive predictor of outcome in the high risk surgical and critically ill population. Many of the methodological problems of saline tonometry have been overcome by the introduction of the Tonocap, which represents an exciting advance in this field.

It must be remembered, however, that the Tonocap remains simply a monitor. Outcome following its use will depend on the therapeutic interventions performed in response to and guided by its readings. We therefore await results from the further assessment of the Tonocap in the clinical setting.

References

1. McIver M (1926) Gaseous exchange between the blood and the lumen of the stomach and intestine. Am J Physiol 76:92–111
2. Schlichtig R, Bowles SA (1994) Distinguishing between aerobic and anaerobic appearance of dissolved CO_2 in intestine during low flow. J Appl Physiol 76:2443–2451
3. Bergofsky EH (1964) Determination of tissue O_2 tensions by hollow visceral tonometers: effect of breathing enriched O_2 mixtures. J Clin Invest 43:192–200
4. Nelson D, Beyer C, Samsel R, Wood L, Schumaker P (1987) Pathologic supply dependence of O_2 uptake during bacteremia in dogs. J Appl Physiol 63:1487–1492
5. Elizalde JI, Hernandez C, Llach J, Monton C, Bordas JM, Pique JM, Torres A (1998) Gastric intramucosal acidosis in mechanically ventilated patients: role of mucosal blood flow Crit Care Med 26:827–832
6. Dawson AM, Trenchard D, Guz A (1965) Small bowel tonometry: assessment of small gut mucosal oxygen tension in dog and man. Nature 206:943–944
7. Kivisaari J, Niinikoski J (1973) Use of Silastic sampling tube and capillary sampling technique in the measurement of tissue PO_2 and PCO_2. Am J Surg 125:623–627
8. Casado-Flores J, Mora E, Perez-Corral F, Martinez-Azagra A, Garcia-Teresa MA, Ruiz-Lopez MJ (1998) Prognostic value of gastric intramucosal pH in critically ill children. Crit Care Med 26:1123–1127
9. Fiddian-Green RG, McGough E, Pittenger G, Rothman E (1983) Predictive value of intramural pH and other risk factors for massive bleeding from stress ulceration. Gastroenterology 85:613–620
10. Crispin C, Jones W, Daffurn K (1995) How consistently do RNs perform the procedure of collecting specimens for measurement of gastric pHi and CO_2? Intensive Crit Care Nurs 11:123–125
11. Knichwitz G, Kuhmann M, Brodner G, Mertes N, Goeters C, Brussel T (1996) Gastric tonometry: precision and reliability are improved by a phosphate buffered solution. Crit Care Med 24:512–516
12. Kolkman JJ, Zwarekant LJ, Boshuizen K, Groeneveld AB, Steverink PJ, Meuwissen SG (1997) Type of solution and PCO2 measurement errors during tonometry. Intensive Care Med 23:658–663
13. Riddington D, Venkatesh K, Clutton-brock T, Bion J (1994) Quantification of two blood gas analyzers. Crit Care Med 22:96–100
14. Takala J, Parviainen I, Siloaho M, Ruokonen E, Hamalainen E (1994) Saline PCO_2 is an important source of error in the assessment of gastric intramucosal pH. Crit Care Med 22:1877–1880
15. Doglio GR, Pusajo JF, Egurrola MA, Bonfigli GC, Parra C, Vetere L, Fernandez MS, Fernandez S, Gutierrez G (1991) Gastric mucosal pH as a prognostic index of mortality in critically ill patients. Crit Care Med 19:1037–1040
16. Mythen MG, Webb AR (1994) The role of gut mucosal hypoperfusion in the pathogenesis of postoperative organ dysfunction. Intensive Care Med 20:203–209
17. Kirton OC, Windsor J, Wedderburn R, Hudson-Civetta J, Shatz DV, Mataragas NR, Civetta JM (1998) Failure of splanchnic resuscitation in the acutely injured trauma patient correlates with multiple organ system failure and length of stay in the ICU. Chest 113:1064–1069
18. Mythen MG, Webb AR (1994) Intraoperative gut mucosal hypoperfusion is associated with increased postoperative complications and costs. Intensive Care Med 20:99–104
19. Bjork M, Hedberg B (1994) Early detection of major complications after abdominal aortic surgery: predictive value of sigmoid and gastric intramucosal pH monitoring. Br J Surg 81:25–30
20. Soong CV, Halliday MI, Barclay GR, Hood JM, Rowlands BJ, Barros D'Sa AA (1997) Intramucosal acidosis and systemic host response in abdominal aortic aneurysm surgery. Crit Care Med 25:1472–1479
21. Mythen MG, Webb AR (1995) Peri-operative plasma volume expansion reduces the incidence of gut mucosal hypoperfusion during cardiac surgery. Arch Surg 130:423–429
22. Mythen MG, Hamilton-Davies C, Webb AR (1996) Perioperative gastrointestinal tonometry. In: Vincent JL (ed) Yearbook of intensive care and emergency medicine. Springer, Berlin Heidelberg New York, pp 227–240
23. Trinder JL, Lavery GG, Fee JPH, Lowery KG (1995) Low gastric intramucosal pH: incidence and significance in intensive care patients. Anaesth Intensive Care 23:315–321
24. Hamilton-Davies C, Mythen MG, Salmon JB, Jacobson D, Shukla A, Webb AR (1997) Comparison of commonly used clinical indicators of hypovolaemia with gastrointestinal tonometry. Intensive Care Med 23:276–281
25. Mohsenifar Z, Hay A, Hay J, Lewis MI, Koerner SK (1993) Gastric intramural pH as a predictor of success or failure in weaning patients from mechanical ventilation. Ann Intern Med 119:794–798
26. Bouachour G, Guiraud MP, Gouello JP, Roy PM, Alquier P (1996) Gastric intramucosal pH: an indicator of weaning outcome from mechanical ventilation in COPD patients. Eur Respir J 9:1868–1873

27. Higgins D, Mythen MG, Webb AR (1994) Low intramucosal pH is associated with failure to acidify the gastric lumen in response to pentagastrin. Intensive Care Med 20:105–108
28. Lokhandwala MF, Jandhyala BS (1992) Effects of dopaminergic agonists on organ blood flow and function. Clin Intensive Care 3:12–15
29. Smithies M, Yee TH, Jackson L, Beale R, Bihari D (1994) Protecting the gut and the liver in the critically ill: effects of dopexamine. Crit Care Med 22:789–795
30. Maynard N, Smithies MN, Mason B, Bihari DJ (1992) Dopexamine and gastric intramucosal pH in critically ill patients (abstract). Intensive Care Med 18:134
31. Trinder TJ, Lavery GG, Fee JPH, Lowry KG (1995) Correction of splanchnic oxygen deficit in the intensive care unit: dopexamine and colloid versus placebo. Anaesth Intensive Care 23:178–182
32. Gutierrez G, Palizas F, Doglio G, Wainsztein N, Gallesio A, Pacin J, Dublin A, Schiavi E, Jorge M, Pusajo S, Kilein F, San Roman E, Dorfman B, Shottlender J, Giniger R (1992) Gastric intramucosal pH as a therapeutic index of tissue oxygenation in critically ill patients. Lancet 339:195–199
33. Chang MC, Meredith JW (1997) Occult hypovolaemia and subsequent splanchnic ischaemia in globally resuscitated trauma patients is associated with multiple organ failure and mortality. J Trauma 42:577–584
34. Ivatury RR, Simon RJ, Havrila KD, Garcia C, Greenbarg J, Stahl WM (1995) Gastric mucosal pH and oxygen delivary and oxygen consumption indices in the assessment of adequacy of resuscitation after trauma: a prospective, randomized study. J Trauma 39:128–134
35. Barquist E, Kirton O, Windsor J, Hudson-Civetta J, Lynn M, Herman M, Civetta J (1998) The impact of antioxidant and splanchnic-directed therapy on persistent uncorrected gastric mucosal pH in the critically injured trauma patient. J Trauma 44:355–360
36. Creteur J, De Backer D, Vincent JL (1997) Monitoring gastric mucosal carbon dioxide pressure using gas tonometry: in vitro and in vivo validation studies. Anesthesiology 87:504–510
37. Temmesfeld-Wollbruck B, Szalay A, Olschewski H, Grimminger F, Seeger W (1997) Advantage of buffered solutions or automated capnometry in air-filled balloons for use in gastric tonometry. Intensive Care Med 23:423–427
38. Venkatesh B, Morgan J, Jones RD, Clague A (1998) Validation of air as an equilibration medium in gastric tonometry: an in vitro evaluation of two techniques for measuring air PCO_2. Anaesth Intensive Care 26:46–50
39. Guzman JA, Kruse JA (1997) Continuous assessment of gastric intramucosal PCO2 and pH in hemorrhagic shock using capnometric recirculating gas tonometry. Crit Care Med 25:533–537
40. Heinonen PO, Jousela IT, Blomqvist KA, Olkkola KT, Takkunen OS (1997) Validation of air tonometric measurement of gastric regional concentrations of CO_2 in critically ill septic patients. Intensive Care Med 23:524–529
41. Noone RB, Mythen MG, Vaslef SN (1997) A comparison of the response of the Tonocap and saline tonometry to a change in CO_2 (abstract). Crit Care Med 1:P88
42. Bennett-Guierro E (1997) Anesthesiology (in press)
43. Russell JA (1997) Gastric tonometry: does it work? Intensive Care Med 23:3–6
44. Brinkert W, Bakker J (1998) Is it time to abandon the pHi concept? Int J Intensive Care 5:16–21
45. Boyd O, Mackay CJ, Lamb G, Bland JM, Grounds RM, Bennett ED (1993) Comparison of clinical information gained from routine blood-gas analysis and from gastric tonometry for intramural pH Lancet 341:142–146
46. Maynard N, Bihari D, Beale R, Smithies M, Baldock G, Mason R, McColl I (1993) Assessment of splanchnic oxygenation by gastric tonometry in patients with acute circulatory failure JAMA 270:1203–1210
47. Friedman G, Berlot G, Kahn RJ, Vincent JL (1995) Combined measurement of blood lactate concentrations and gastric intramucosal pH in patients with severe sepsis. Crit Care Med 23:1184–1193
48. Gomersall CD, Joynt GM, Ho KM, Young RJ, Buckley TA, Oh TE (1997) Gastric tonometry and prediction of outcome in the critically ill. Arterial to intramucosal pH gradient and carbon dioxide gradient Anaesthesia 52:619–623
49. Kolkman J, Groeneveld A, Meuwisen S (1994) Effect of ranitidine on basal and bicarbonate enhanced intragastric PCO_2: a tonometric study. Gut 35:737–741
50. Calvet X, Baigorri F, Duarte M, Saura P, Royo C, Joseph D, Mas A, Artigas A (1998) Effect of ranitidine on gastric intramucosal pH in critically ill patients. Intensive Care Med 24:12–17
51. Marik PE, Lorenzana A (1996) Effect of tube feeding on the measurement of gastric intraluminal pH. Crit Care Med 24:1498–1500
52. Parviainen I, Vaisanen O, Roukonen E, Takala J (1996) Effect of nasogastric suction and ranitidine on the calculated gastric intramucosal pH. Intensive Care Med 22:319–323
53. Parbrook G, Davies P, Parbrook E (1993) Basic physics and measurement in anaesthesia. Butterworth-Heinemann, London

54. Sitzwohl C, Kettner SC, Reinprecht A, Dietrich W, Klimscha W, Fridich P, Sladen RN, Illievich UM (1998) The arterial to end-tidal carbon dioxide gradient increases with uncorrected but not with temperature corrected P_aCO_2 determination during mild to moderate hypothermia. Anesth Analg 86:1131–1136
55. Tallman R (1997) Acid-base regulation, alpha stat, and the Emperor's new clothes. J Cardiothorac Vasc Anesth 11:282–288

Continuous Mucosal PCO_2 Monitoring of the Gastrointestinal Tract

G. Knichwitz · T. Brüssel

Klinik und Poliklinik für Anästhesiologie und operative Intensivmedizin der Westfälischen Wilhelms-Universität Münster, 48149 Münster, Germany

Introduction

The gastrointestinal tract is especially vulnerable to ischemia and hypoxia. Therefore, monitoring of the perfusion of the gastrointestinal tract should be accepted as significant in critical illness. Under clinical conditions, the direct determination of the perfusion of the gastrointestinal tract is not feasible. However, hypoxia and ischemia can also be detected indirectly by way of metabolic parameters. In addition to a reduction in pH and lactic acidosis, an increase in the partial pressure of carbon dioxide (PCO_2) can be considered a sign of gastrointestinal malperfusion.

The following physicochemical properties of carbon dioxide (CO_2) suggest it is quite suitable for the monitoring of the gastrointestinal tract:

- The solubility of CO_2 in plasma is 21 times that of oxygen (O_2).
- CO_2 easily diffuses through various tissues and spaces (air, water).
- In hollow visceral organs (gut, bladder) an equilibrium exists for the PCO_2 of the mucosa and that of the lumen, so that the regional organ CO_2 can be determined indirectly inside their lumina.
- Even small amounts of the CO_2 produced within a certain tissue will cause a manifold increase in the monitored PCO_2 value. [1 mmol/l results in an increase in PCO_2 by 33 mmHg (= torr)].

Intramucosal PCO_2 Measurement in the Gastrointestinal Tract

The first report on the intraluminal PCO_2 determination in the gastrointestinal tract was published in 1968 by Hamilton et al. [1]. But it took until 1982 for Fiddian-Green to introduce the concept of "gastric tonometry" for the determination of the intramucosal PCO_2 (P_iCO_2) in the lumen of the stomach [2].

A gastric tonometer probe is placed transorally directly into the lumen of the stomach. The PCO_2 measured in the lumen of the stomach is in equilibrium with the intramucosal PCO_2 of the stomach and will thus provide direct information on any ischemia-induced CO_2 accumulation in the stomach mucosa with the possible loss of the gastrointestinal barrier function. The tonometer probe can also be placed in different areas of the gastrointestinal tract.

The manual and discontinuous technique of gastric tonometry was formerly the only means of detecting gastrointestinal malperfusion with moderate invasiveness. However, several authors [3–6] have shown that when a standard blood gas analyzer

M. K. Herbert et al. (Eds.), Problems of the Gastrointestinal Tract in Anesthesia ...

is used, PCO_2 determination in an unbuffered aqueous solution, as recommended in gastric tonometry, can vary by up to 57.5 %, depending on the type of blood gas analyzer used [3]. With a buffered tonometer solution, e.g. a phosphate buffer [3, 4] the precision of the determination can be increased. However, several other methodological problems – the handling of the nasogastric tonometer and the CO_2 sample, the long equilibration periods and mistakes from equilibration – remain [7]. These methodological insufficiencies have led to the development of newer techniques for the continuous and automated determination of the intramucosal PCO_2 in the lumen of the gastrointestinal tract.

New Methods of Determining P_iCO_2

The new methods for the determination of P_iCO_2 are summarized in Table 1. Salzman et al. [8] developed a "balloonless air technique" for the indirect intraluminal measurement of P_iCO_2 with a gas sample obtained from the gastrointestinal tract via a gastric probe. Similarly, Guzman and Kruse [9, 10] used air as the tonometer medium, but still used the conventional nasogastric tonometer. The introduction of air not only resulted in an improvement in precision but allowed the continuous measurement of P_iCO_2 via a closed loop recirculation system. As the P_iCO_2 is determined online by the infrared sensor of a capnograph, Guzman and Kruse called their method "capnometric recirculating gas tonometry" (CRGT) [9].

Table 1. Comparison of different methods for P_iCO_2 determination (P_iCO_2 = intramucosal PCO_2). From [15]

	Nasogastric and sigmoid tonometers	Capnographic gas tonometry	Capnographic recirculating gas tonometry	Fiberoptic CO_2 sensor
Kind of intraluminal P_iCO_2 determination	Indirect via tonometric solution and standard blood gas analyzer	Indirect via single air insufflation and capnograph	Indirect via recirculating air insufflation and capnograph	Direct via fiberoptic CO2 sensor in lumen of GI tract
Mode	Discontinuous	10 min (5 min)	Continuous	Continuous
Handling	Manual	Automatic	Automatic	Automatic
Additional requirements	(1) Blood gas analyzer, (2) tonometric solution, (3) individual, time-dependent correction factors	(1) Nasogastric tonometer, (2) system- and time-dependent correction factors	(1) Modified nasogastric tonometer, (2) system- and time-dependent correction factors	Introduction tube
Clinical availability	Tonometrics (Datex-Ohmeda) TRIP NGS tonometer, TRIP sigmoid tonometer	Tonometrics (Datex-Ohmeda) TC-200 Tonocap CO_2 monitor	Not commercially available at present	Biomedical Sensors (Diametrics Medical) modified Paratrend 7 system

The Tonocap System (Datex, Helsinki, Finland) represents a similar concept of gas tonometry. In an automated procedure, air instilled into the balloon of a nasogastric tube is aspirated after a predefined equilibration time (5–10 min) and then subjected to PCO_2 determination by capnography. Creteur et al. showed that this technique can improve the precision of P_iCO_2 determination significantly compared with conventional gastric tonometry [11].

All the above methods determine P_iCO_2 indirectly, outside the gastrointestinal tract, but there is a direct method for continuous intraluminal P_iCO_2 measurement [12, 13]. This method uses a fiberoptic CO_2 sensor, which is placed in the lumen of the gastrointestinal tract. Green light is passed down a 60 cm fiber glass to an acrylamide gel colored with Phenol Red at the fiber tip. This acrylamide gel is fixed in bicarbonate buffer and coated with an ion-resisting membrane that is permeable to CO_2. If CO_2 diffuses through the acrylamide gel, the pH and thus the absorption characteristics of the Phenol Red are changed. Depending on these pH changes, the absorption of the green light is altered. After proper calibration, this technique provides direct information on the PCO_2 in the lumen of the gastrointestinal tract.

In vitro validation showed that within 9 min the fiberoptic CO_2 sensor will continuously detect a known PCO_2 value with an error of ± 3.5 % (Fig. 1) [12]. This is a major improvement over the conventional indirect technique, which is not only discontinuous and indirect but has errors of −12.5 % even after 90 min. The complete CO_2 equilibration inside the tonometer balloon depends on time and on the tonome-

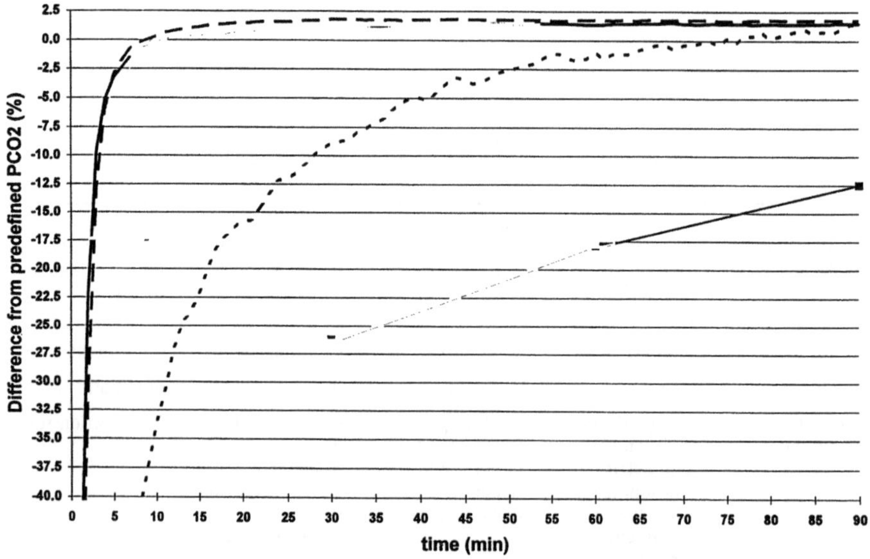

Fig. 1. PCO_2 differences (measured PCO_2 minus predefined PCO_2) in percent, (mean, n = 12). Data shown represent the continuous PCO_2-measurement with the fiberoptic CO_2-sensor in water shown by solid line (—) and in humidified air as fat plotted line (---). The closed squares (■—■) represent the measurements with the conventional nasogastric tonometer after 30, 60 and 90 minutes of equilibration time. The measurement with the fiberoptic CO_2-sensor introduced into the saline filled balloon of the conventional nasogastric tonometer was determined in a single cas (----). [Original figure from Knichwitz et al (12)]

ter medium used (air or saline). As a consequence, the CRGT or the Tonocap system must incorporate correction factors. (Table 1 shows the various techniques for the intramucosal PCO_2 determination.)

The continuous measurement of P_iCO_2 has many advantages over the discontinuous methods. Depending on the set limits of P_iCO_2 it will automatically alarm the clinician when the value is beyond the normal range. It can detect short-term changes in P_iCO_2 and can therefore be used for the early detection of gastrointestinal perfusion disturbances [9, 11–13]. Finally, it offers another possibility. It is known that intragastric CO_2 production from duodenal bicarbonate reflux interferes with the conventional measurement of intramucosal PCO_2. Continuous P_iCO_2 measurement offers the chance to differentiate between ischemia and such a reflux. With bicarbonate reflux present, the aspiration of the gastric content will rapidly alter the produced signal.

Apart from these technical variations, the evaluation of gastrointestinal malperfusion using the calculated intramucosal pH value (pHi) alone proved to be meaningless. Thus, not only was discontinuous gastric tonometry given up, but with it the conventional concept of the pHi determination [14, 15].

As a result of the improvements in monitoring techniques a new line of applications seems possible that will allow the early detection of gastrointestinal blood flow alterations. For the clinical interpretation of continuous P_iCO_2 measurement proper distinctions between "hypoxia/ischemia", "systemic/local", and "open/closed CO_2 system" are mandatory [15].

Physiologic Basis of Gastrointestinal PCO_2 Measurement

For the hypoxic or ischemic gastrointestinal PCO_2 increase, two pathophysiological mechanisms play an important part [16, 17]:

1. CO_2 accumulation. The reduced washout of CO_2 due to an impaired blood flow causes a CO_2 accumulation in the tissues. This CO_2 will be eliminated with reperfusion and will then be exhaled by the lung.
2. CO_2 production under the condition of anaerobic energy metabolism. During anaerobic energy production, hydrogen ions (H^+) are generated from two metabolic pathways: with anaerobic glycolysis, the metabolism of glucose to lactic acid forms two hydrogen ions.

$$\text{D-Glucose} \rightarrow 2\text{ATP} + 2\text{Lactate}^- + 2\text{H}^+$$

The adenylate kinase reaction transforms ATP to energy and leads to the intracellular generation of hydrogen, which is not used for the resynthesis of ATP

$$2\text{ADP} \rightarrow ATP + \text{AMP}$$
$$ATP \rightarrow \text{ADP} + \text{P}_i + \text{H}^+ + \text{Energy}$$

With hypoxia, this increased production of H^+ ions results in an increased production of CO_2

$$\text{H}^+ + \text{HCO}_3^- \leftrightarrow \text{H}_2\text{O} + \text{CO}_2$$

The CO_2 accumulation and anaerobic CO_2 production are interrelated pathways, but their relative importance differs depending on the circumstances. Only the regional CO_2 accumulation forms the basis for a regional P_iCO_2 measurement [15]. Without CO_2 accumulation, no P_iCO_2 increase can occur. This basic postulate is of the utmost importance for the interpretation of gastrointestinal P_iCO_2.

Significance of Increased Intramucosal CO_2 Production

The early detection of anaerobic energy metabolism that can result in irreversible tissue damage is of major clinical interest. The key point of the intramucosal PCO_2 measurement is the relation between blood flow reduction and CO_2 increase.

In theory, if CO_2 production is constant, any twofold increase in arteriovenous CO_2 difference in a particular region will represent a reduction of that region's perfusion by 50 %. Under these circumstances, a linear relation between blood flow and P_iCO_2 should exist. However, in the presence of ischemia or hypoxia the circumstances are less predictable and less constant, resulting in an additional CO_2 increase, as shown in Fig. 2 [13]. These results were obtained in experiments on six pigs with stepwise reduction of the superior mesenteric arterial blood flow at 10-min intervals. The resulting P_iCO_2 changes were detected with a fiberoptic CO_2 sensor placed within the ileal lumen. Following a period with only minor P_iCO_2 changes, a dramatic P_iCO_2 increase occurred, corresponding with a blood-flow reduction of approximately 60 %. This finding supports the observations published by Zhang and Vincent [18], Schlich-

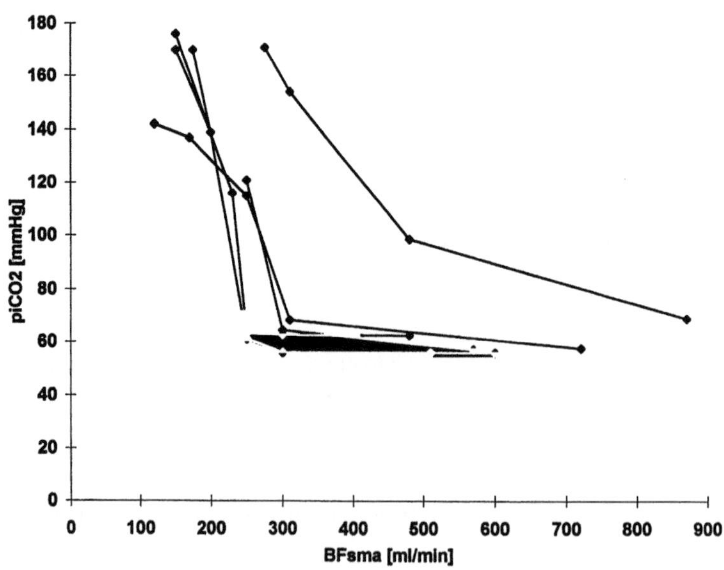

Fig. 2. Individual changes (n = 6 pigs) of the ileal intramucosal pCO_2 ($piCO_2$) measured by the fiberoptic CO_2-sensor (■—■) with stepwise reduction of the superior mesentric artery bloodflow (BF_{SMA}). [Original figure from Knichwitz et al (13)]

tig and Bowles [19] and Rozenfeld et al. [16], who demonstrated a similar critical limit of blood flow which, if surpassed, produced a sudden PCO_2 increase. This sudden CO_2 change reflects a metabolic decompensation.

The P_iCO_2 continuously measured with the fiberoptic CO_2 sensor can detect this threshold between compensated and decompensated mesenteric perfusion. Rozenfeld et al. [16] and Schlichtig and Bowles [19] postulated that this sudden CO_2 increase is caused mainly by the anaerobic energy production.

However, the differentiation between the two conditions of isolated regional mesenteric ischemia and global systemic ischemia also has an important impact on anaerobic CO_2 production and the HCO_3–CO_2 buffer system.

The Bicarbonate – Carbon Dioxide Buffer System

At first sight, the HCO_3–CO_2 buffer, with its pK of 6.1 and a blood pH of 7.40, seems to be a rather unimportant and inefficient buffering system. Its enormous effectivity is the result of the constant HCO_3^- production and CO_2 exhalation, which causes an imbalance between HCO_3^- and CO_2 with a ratio of 20:1. The Hendersen-Hasselbalch equation reads:

$$\mathrm{pH} = \mathrm{pK} + \log_{10}\frac{[\mathrm{HCO_3^-}]\ \mathrm{mmol/l}}{[\mathrm{CO_2}]\ \mathrm{mmol/l}} \rightarrow 7.40 = 6.1 + \log_{10}\frac{24.0\ \mathrm{mmol/l}}{1{,}2\ \mathrm{mmol/l}}$$

For the HCO_3–CO_2 buffer system, the undisturbed exhalation by the lungs of the CO_2 produced is of great importance. These circumstances will be called the "open CO_2 system". A condition that results in a CO_2 accumulation is defined as a "closed CO_2 system."

Under open CO_2 system conditions, the addition of 2 mmol/l H^+ will result in a pH of 7.36, as only the numerator of the Hendersen-Hasselbalch equation will be changed. In contrast, under closed CO_2 system conditions, the CO_2 produced will not be removed and thus will alter the denominator of the equation. As the HCO_3–CO_2 buffer system cannot work effectively under these conditions, there will be a theoretical decrease of the pH to 6.93 (disregarding the nonbicarbonate buffer system).

$$\mathrm{pH} = 6.1 + \log_{10}\frac{22\ \mathrm{mmol/l}}{3.2\ \mathrm{mmol/l}} = 6{,}93$$

The closed CO_2 system with CO_2 accumulation has a lower bicarbonate buffer capacity because the product of the chemical balance is not removed. A new balance is found between CO_2 and HCO_3^- with reduced consumption of HCO_3^-. With this closed CO_2 system the nonbicarbonate buffer system (hemoglobin, phosphate buffer, plasma protein) plays an important part as it neutralizes the hydrogen ions. The closed CO_2 system is characterized by smaller HCO_3^- shifts than the open CO_2 system [15].

P_iCO_2 Alterations in the Open and the Closed Systems

The described difference between open and closed CO_2 systems is of major importance for P_iCO_2 measurement. We conducted a number of animal experiments to explain this influence on the intramucosal PCO_2 [13].

Figure 3a and b shows the P_iCO_2 determined by a fiberoptic CO_2 sensor in the ileal lumen of a pig. After baseline measurements (0 min) were obtained, gastrointestinal ischemia was induced by a 70 % reduction of the blood flow in the superior mesenteric artery for 180 min [13], after which the gut was reperfused for 120 min. This model represented a closed CO_2 system, because the reduced perfusion did not allow adequate washout of the produced CO_2. While the arterial PCO_2 (Fig. 3a) remained constant at around 40 mmHg, a sudden significant P_iCO_2 increase occurred in the intestinal mucosa (Fig. 3a). This P_iCO_2 increase was most probably caused by CO_2 accumulation with an additional CO_2 production from anaerobic energy metabolism. The lactate concentration in the mesenteric venous blood was 6.5 mmol/l. If the PCO_2 was determined in a large vein outside the gut mucosa, i.e. the superior mesenteric vein, a parallel, but smaller, PCO_2 increase was noted (Fig. 3a).

Another interesting finding was observed during the 120 min of reperfusion. While the PCO_2 in the superior mesenteric vein reached its baseline value immediately after the onset of reperfusion, the intramucosal PCO_2 remained elevated at 80 mmHg (Fig. 3a). This can be explained by the various locations of the PCO_2 determinations, which represent different tissue areas. Owing to its intraluminal location, the P_iCO_2 measurement can detect alterations in the villus, which is highly vulnerable to ischemia. In this area, reperfusion and thus CO_2 washout are blocked by shunts and capillary destruction. In contrast, the superior mesenteric venous PCO_2 represented only unimpaired CO_2 washout, and as such areas that allowed proper reperfusion. Histological examination of the ileum showed signs of typical ischemic destruction.

The specific vascular anatomy of the gastrointestinal tract plays an important part in the explanation of the observed ischemic destruction of the villus. The artery of the villus runs centrally to the tip of the villus and then spreads into a dense capillary network to allow nutritive perfusion. The central artery runs very close to the countercurrent vein. The vessels are only 20 μm apart and so oxygen exchange can occur along the concentration gradient of both vessels [20]. As a result, oxygen can bypass the tip of the villus and reach the vein. Depending on the degree of blood flow reduction and the duration of the ischemic episode, an increasing tissue swelling occurs that causes destruction of the villus and results in an even further reduced CO_2 washout with CO_2 accumulation. To detect these pathophysiological changes the P_iCO_2 should be measured.

The matching pHi value (Fig. 3b) calculated using P_iCO_2 and mesenteric venous $cHCO_3^-$ (Fig. 3b) represented severe acidosis with a pHi of 6.75. However, as significant mesenteric venous $cHCO_3^-$ changes could not be seen under such closed CO_2 system conditions, this observed pHi decrease must have originated solely from the local intestinal P_iCO_2 increase.

The alterations are completely different under open CO_2 system conditions, a situation that we introduced with cardiopulmonary bypass. The results are shown in detail in Fig. 4a and b. A pig was placed on cardiopulmonary bypass for 180 min,

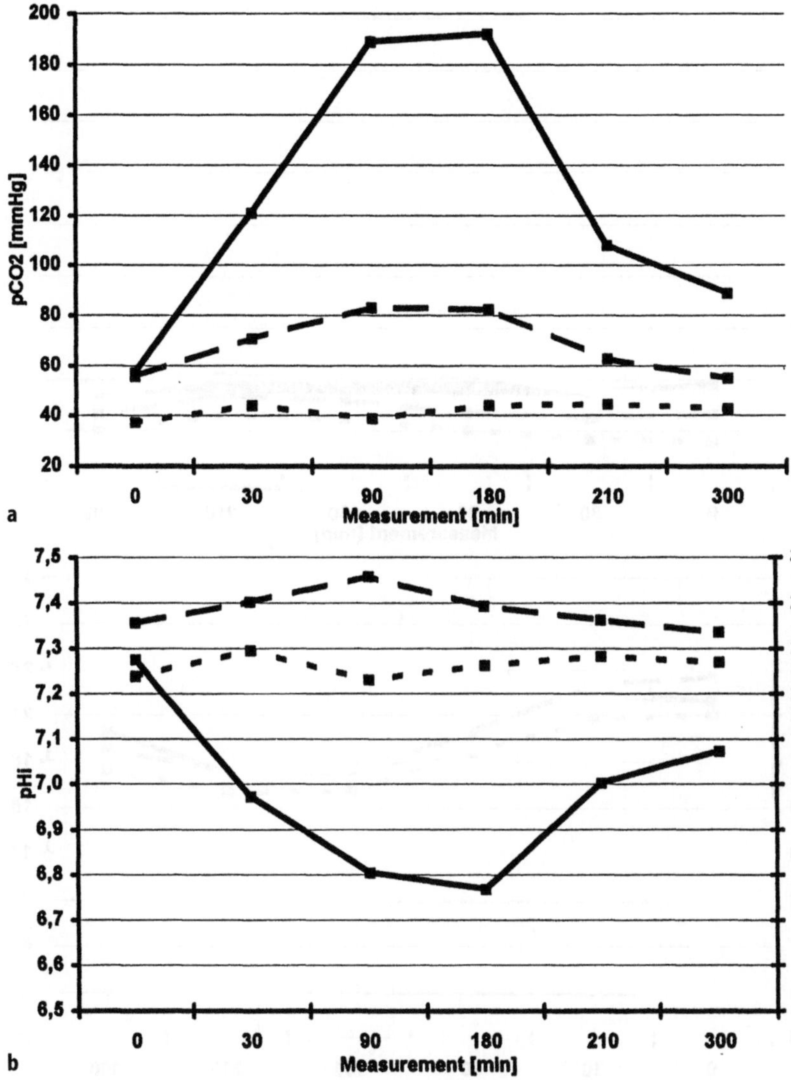

Fig. 3 a, b. "Closed system" condition: Systemic and local changes under mesentric ischemia induced by a 70% reduction of the superior mesenteric artery blood flow for 180 minutes. Single measurement of a pig. Measurement: 0 min = baseline; 30, 90, 180 min = mesenteric ischemia; 210, 300 min = mesenteric reperfusion.

a Changes in intramucosal pCO_2 ($piCO_2$ = —■—), mesenteric venous pCO_2 (--■--) and arterial pCO_2 (---■---).

b Changes in intramucosal pH (pHi = —■—), mesenteric venous (--■--) and arterial (---■---) bicarbonate concentration ($cHCO_3^-$). [single observation from Knichwitz et al (13)]

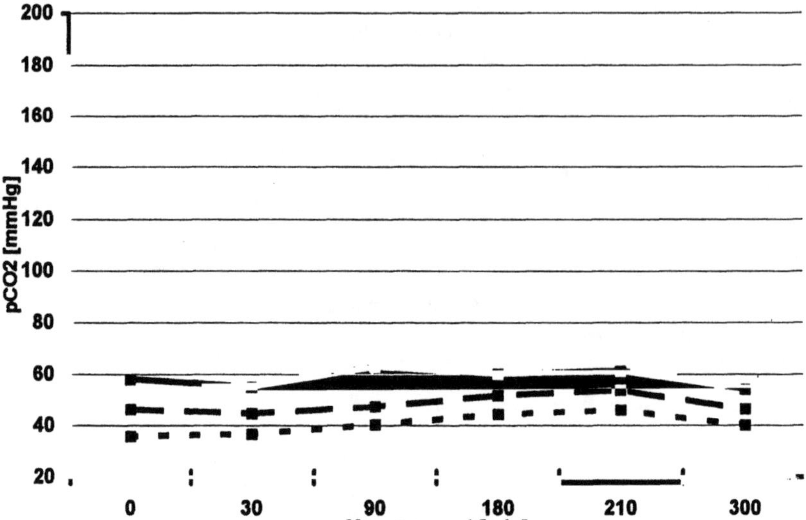

a

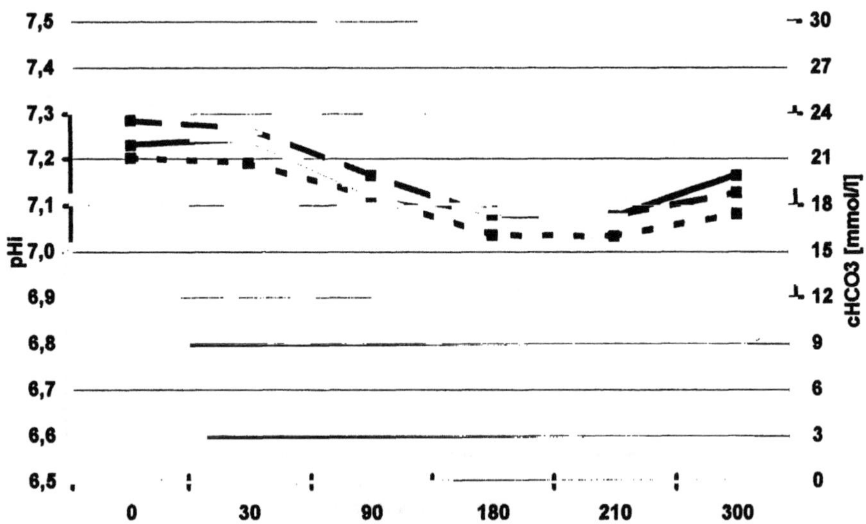

b

Fig. 4a, b. "Open system" condition: Systemic and local changes under cardiopulmonary bypass for 180 minutes. Single measurement of a pig. Measurement: 0 min = baseline; 30, 90, 180 min = cardiopulmonary bypass; 210, 300 min = after cardiopulmonary bypass.
a Changes in intramucosal pCO_2 ($piCO_2$ = —■—), mesenteric venous pCO_2 (--■--) and arterial pCO_2 (---■---).
b Changes in intramucosal pH (pHi = —■—), mesenteric venous (--■--) and arterial (---■---) bicarbonate concentration ($cHCO_3^-$). [Original figure from Knichwitz et al (15)]

followed by an additional observation period of 120 min. During normothermic bypass a lactic acidosis with a serum lactate concentration of 10 mmol/l and an arterial pH of 7.20 was noted. The blood flow in the superior mesenteric artery was not changed from baseline. Under these open system conditions, the CO_2 produced as a result of anaerobic metabolism was washed out and eliminated by the membrane oxygenator. As a consequence, there was no significant change in intramucosal, mesenteric venous or arterial PCO_2 (Fig. 4a). CO_2 was eliminated from the system and bicarbonate was spent by buffering of hydrogen ions. As a consequence, a significant arterial (Fig. 4b) and mesenteric venous reduction in $cHCO_3^-$ (Fig. 4b) from 24 mmol/l to 17 mmol/l) was noted. As the P_iCO_2 did not change, the calculated pHi decrease (Fig. 4b) originated from the $cHCO_3^-$ reduction. Histological examination of ileal tissues from this experiment showed no pathologic destruction of the gastrointestinal villi. The cardiopulmonary bypass led to a systemic acidosis that was associated with a local intestinal acidosis. This acidosis was less severe than that under closed CO_2 system conditions, did not cause irreversible mucosal swelling or capillary destruction and thus did not inhibit the CO_2 washout. The continuous measurement of P_iCO_2 under open system conditions showed no pathologic P_iCO_2 increase.

From these observations, it is quite clear that evaluation of the gastrointestinal perfusion by means of pHi alone is obsolete.

The interpretation of the P_iCO_2 data not only asks for an assessment between CO_2 accumulation and anaerobic CO_2 production but also, importantly, needs the distinction between "hypoxia/ischemia", "systemic/local", and open/closed CO_2 system [15].

A pure regional blood flow reduction (ischemia) primarily causes CO_2 accumulation, as the locally generated CO_2 cannot be washed out. Under these conditions of a closed CO_2 system an additional secondary hypoxia induced CO_2 production will develop.

Under closed CO_2 system conditions any impending organ damage from CO_2 accumulation can easily be detected very early by the locally measured PCO_2 increase.

On the other hand, hypoxia without disturbed organ blood flow will result primarily in an increased anaerobic CO_2 production. If this additionally generated CO_2 can be washed out and exhaled the condition is called open CO_2 system.

Under these conditions the CO_2 equilibrium is determined mainly by the following three determinants: tissue CO_2 production (e.g. gut), CO_2 transport capacity of the circulation and CO_2 exhalation by the lung (see Table 2).

An increase in hypoxic CO_2 production of intestinal tissues will not result in a PCO_2 increase in the intestine as long as blood flow and ventilation are increasing.

Table 2. Relation between CO_2 production, transport, and exhalation and the expected measured intramucosal PCO_2 (P_iCO_2) value in the lumen of the gut

Gastrointestinal tract CO_2 production	Circulation CO_2 transport	Lung CO_2 exhalation	Expected P_iCO_2 value in the gut
Increased	Increased	Increased	Normal
Increased	Decreased	Normal	High
Increased	Decreased	Decreased	High
Normal	Normal	Increased	Low
Normal	Normal	Decreased	High

Only when the CO_2 transport capacity is significantly lower than the hypoxic CO_2 production will a CO_2 accumulation in the tissue occur.

As long as the anaerobically produced CO_2 is washed out under open CO_2 system conditions a PCO_2 increase will not occur. Only if hypoxia has induced edema formation will tissue destruction or shunts lead to a secondary impairment of the perfusion. As a consequence the CO_2 will accumulate and cause a regionally detectable PCO_2 increase that can be monitored clinically.

Under open CO_2 system condition the pending organ damage can only be detected after secondary CO_2 accumulation resulting from the transformation of "open" to "closed system" conditions.

In everyday clinical practice it is often difficult to differentiate between open and closed CO_2 system, as both conditions may occur within a single patient. Independent of the disease, a gastrointestinal perfusion disorder normally starts under open system conditions. Depending on the illness, closed system conditions are introduced additionally when CO_2 washout is inhibited by shunting and/or impaired capillary function. The detection of this time-point must be the most important purpose of any intramucosal PCO_2 measurement.

Only continuous PCO_2 measurement will allow the determination of the exact time point when CO_2 accumulation in the mucosa starts. This time-point corresponds to the time at which a certain area is excluded from perfusion and thus represents a closed system. This is the time point where severe tissue damage is likely to become inevitable unless adequate perfusion is restored.

Independently of local ischemia and CO_2 accumulation, the calculated pHi can decrease as a result of a systemic bicarbonate reduction. Thus, only the P_iCO_2 can provide the information necessary to allow detection of the change from open CO_2 system to closed CO_2 system conditions.

Optimum Placement of the P_iCO_2 Measurement Probe in the Gastrointestinal Tract

To date nasogastric placement of the P_iCO_2 measurement device is most commonly used. It is assumed that ischemic alterations of the stomach can give a timely indication of possible blood flow alterations in the residual intestine. However, this assumption is not always correct. The important distinction between "hypoxia/ischemia", "systemic/local alterations" and "open/closed CO_2 system" must also be considered when the P_iCO_2 measurement probe is placed in the gastrointestinal tract (see Table 3).

Not detectable is a generally or locally caused hypoxia of the gastrointestinal tract despite anaerobic CO_2 production as long as the CO_2 elimination remains intact.

Gastrointestinal ischemia with consecutive CO_2 accumulation would be detectable if the CO_2 sensor were placed in the affected segment of the intestine. This, however, is difficult to achieve if the ischemia is not global but affects a certain, unknown, segment of the gastrointestinal tract.

Determination in the stomach is adequate if the insult is of systemic proportions and as such affects the whole gastrointestinal tract – a scenario typical for septicemia or catecholamine therapy. In those cases with systemic alterations of the circulation nasogastric placement of the P_iCO_2 probe can be recommended.

Table 3. Intraluminal placement of continuous P_iCO_2 monitoring in the gastrointestinal tract

Type of event	Ischemia: closed CO_2 system	Hypoxia: open CO_2 system	Hypoxia/ischemia: closed CO_2 system
Local event	Site of occurrence	Not detectable	Site of occurrence
Global event	Anywhere in the GIT	Not detectable	Anywhere in the GIT

Table 4. Automated air tonometry with the Tonocap system

Location	Gastric, using a special nasogastric tonometer
Technique	Automated insufflation of air into the gastric balloon of the probe 10 min of equilibration Aspiration of air and CO_2 determination by infrared capnography
Interval	10 min
Influencing factors	Nutrition: stop enteral feeding for 30 min Gastric acidosis with duodenal reflux: antacids, lavage Gastric lavage: stop for 30 min Hyper-/hypoventilation Intravenous bicarbonate administrations
Parameter	Intramucosal PCO_2 (P_iCO_2) of the stomach Purpose: evaluation of gastric blood flow alterations
P_iCO_2 normal value	<50 mmHg
$aiDCO_2$	Partial pressure difference in arterio-intramucosal CO_2 $aiDCO_2 = P_aCO_2 - P_iCO_2$ (mmHg) - Normal value: <10 mmHg - Exclusion of PCO_2 alterations from ventilatory changes

Clinical Applicability

The Tonocap automated air tonometry system (Datex-Ohmeda) is the only commercial system available on the market. It offers the profile shown in Table 4.

No studies are available that involved determination of normal values or gave a therapeutic algorithm for the new continuous method of P_iCO_2 measurement. Rather, the stated normal values are the result of limited experience. Thus, in the assessment of the obtained values their variation over time is more important than any single value.

P_iCO_2-related Therapy

Over the last 10 years, several studies have examined the influence of various therapeutic regimens on pHi but not on P_iCO_2. As mentioned above, the pHi is a mathematical construct derived from the combination of systemic $cHCO_3^-$ and local P_iCO_2. Combining these two parameters has led to an increase in sensitivity regarding the outcome of critical illness. However, as discussed in the previous paragraphs, it does not yield any information on a possible gastrointestinal perfusion disorder. Yet many studies have been published in which the pHi was used as an indicator of impaired gastrointestinal perfusion. The only parameter that can provide such information on gastrointestinal blood flow is P_iCO_2. It must, however, be kept in mind that P_iCO_2 is a qualitative value and can only distinguish an impaired capillary perfusion from a normal perfusion by a P_iCO_2 increase.

With impaired gastrointestinal perfusion and elevated P_iCO_2 levels, the efficacy of any therapy can only be judged by a decrease in P_iCO_2 due to CO_2 washout with capillary reperfusion. There are a few studies that provide data on P_iCO_2, $cHCO_3^-$ and pHi, and give some insight into related therapeutic concepts [21–25].

Mythen et al. [21] demonstrated that early preoperative plasma volume expansion with colloid during cardiac surgery prevented intramucosal CO_2 accumulation and therefore was able to reduce the incidence of gut mucosal hypoperfusion. Gutierrez et al. [22] found a dose-related effect of dobutamine abolished intestinal CO_2 accumulation in septic patients independently of cardiac index. In addition, Neviere et al. [23] agreed with these findings by Gutierrez and were also able to exclude such an effect for dopamine. Levy et al. [24] demonstrated that the administration of epinephrine instead of a combined therapy with dobutamine/norepinephrine increased the intramucosal CO_2 production. As a consequence the author could not recommend epinephrine for the support of gastrointestinal perfusion in septic patients. Finally, the new specific drug dopexamine, thought to increase gastrointestinal perfusion, was unable to wash out accumulated CO_2 in the gastric mucosa [25]. This finding led Temmesfeld-Wollbrück et al. [25] to conclude that the impact of dopexamine on gastrointestinal perfusion needs further elucidation.

Terminology and Conclusion

Since a common terminology is lacking for the monitoring of gastrointestinal perfusion, a number of terms are used synonymously: gastric tonometry, pHi measurement or P_iCO_2 measurement. This has led to confusion that could be eliminated if the method were named after the primary parameter that it actually intends to measure: "intramucosal PCO_2 measurement" [15].

Intramucosal PCO_2 measurement can be summarized as follows:

1. The P_iCO_2 is the primary parameter of this gastrointestinal monitoring technique and allows an evaluation only for the hollow visceral organ in which it is placed. An increase in P_iCO_2 suggests a local malperfusion with CO_2 accumulation in the respective region of the gastrointestinal tract.
2. P_iCO_2 measurement does not allow numerical conclusions on the gastrointestinal blood flow. It gives qualitative information on normal or impaired perfusion.
3. Data from animal experiments suggest that a threshold of impaired perfusion exists at approximately 40 % of the gastrointestinal blood flow. Any further reduction in blood flow causes a sudden severe increase in P_iCO_2 with additional CO_2 production.
4. Any interpretation of P_iCO_2 alterations demands consideration of metabolic changes (acidosis of acute renal failure, alkalosis of hepatic insufficiency) and respiratory PCO_2 changes. Within minutes hypercarbia causes a P_iCO_2 increase [12].
5. Adequate interpretation of any P_iCO_2 value obtained essentially requires the additional information on the difference between intramucosal and arterial PCO_2 (PCO_2 gap).

6. Any consideration regarding open and closed systems will necessitate the simultaneous measurement of P_iCO_2 and the arterial HCO_3^- concentration.
7. The calculated pHi can serve as a sensitive outcome parameter. It will not, however, allow conclusions regarding regional perfusion alterations.

With few exceptions, all studies on gastrointestinal perfusion derangement over the last decade have used conventional discontinuous nasogastric tonometry. As this technique can only provide information on the average pHi over a certain period, many short-term alterations will remain undetected. Only the introduction of automatic continuous devices such as the fiberoptic CO_2 sensor will allow accurate online detection of important P_iCO_2 changes. Since 1996, several research groups have performed clinical studies with a continuous technique. Before this technique can be recommended for routine clinical application, additional studies are needed. These should try to establish a normal range and therapeutic concepts that might lead to an improvement of gastrointestinal perfusion derangement.

References

1. Hamilton JD, Dawson AM, Webb PW (1968) Observation upon small gut "mucosal" pO_2 and pCO_2 in anaesthetized dogs. Gastroenterology 55:52–60
2. Fiddian-Green RG, Pittenger BS, Whitehouse WM (1982) Back diffusion of CO_2 and its influence on the intramural pH in gastric mucosa. J Surg Res 33:39–48
3. Knichwitz G, Mertes N, Kuhmann M (1995) Improved PCO_2-measurement of six standard blood gas analysers with a phophate-buffered solution for gastric tonometry. Anaesthesia 50:532–534
4. Knichwitz G, Kuhmann M, Brodner G, Mertes N, Goeters C, Brüssel T (1996) Gastric tonometry: precision and reliability are improved by a phosphate buffered solution. Crit Care Med 24:512–516
5. Riddington D, Venkatesh B, Clutton-Brock T, Bion J (1992) Potential hazards in estimation of gastric intramucosal pH (letter). Lancet 340:547
6. Takala J, Parviainen I, Siloaho M, Ruokonen E, Hämäläinen E (1994) Saline PCO_2 is an important source of error in the assessment of gastric intramucosal pH. Crit Care Med 22:1877–1879
7. Knichwitz G, Brüssel T (1996) Use of phosphate buffered solution in gastric tonometry: reply. Crit Care Med 24:1932–1933
8. Salzmann AL, Strong KE, Wang H, Wollert S, Vandermeer TJ, Fink MP (1994) Intraluminal "balloonless" air tonometry: a new method for determination of gastrointestinal mucosal carbon dioxide tension. Crit Care Med 22:126–134
9. Guzman JA, Kruse JA (1996) Development and validation of a technique for continuous monitoring of gastric intramucosal pH. Am J Respir Crit Care Med 153:694–700
10. Guzman JA, Kruse JA (1997) Continuous assessment of gastric intramucosal pCO2 and pH in hemorrhagic shock using capnometric recirculating gas tonometry. Crit Care Med 25:533–537
11. Creteur J, De Backer D, Vincent J-L (1997) Monitoring gastric mucosal carbon dioxide pressure using gas tonometry. Anaesthesiology 87:504–510
12. Knichwitz G, Rötker J, Brüssel T, Kuhmann M, Mertes N, Möllhoff T (1996) A new method for continuous intramucosal pCO_2-measurement in the gastrointestinal tract. Anesth Analg 83:6–11
13. Knichwitz G, Rötker J, Möllhoff T, Richter KD, Brüssel T (1998) Continuous intramucosal pCO_2-measurement allows the early detection of intestinal malperfusion. Crit Care Med 26:550–557
14. Schlichtig R, Mehta N, Gayowski TJP (1996) Tissue-arterial pCO_2 difference is a better marker of ischemia than intramural pH (pHi) or arterial pH–pHi difference. J Crit Care 11:51–56
15. Knichwitz G, Van Aken H, Brüssel T (1998) Gastrointestinal monitoring using the intramucosal pCO_2 measurement. Anesth Analg 86: 134–142
16. Rozenfeld RA, Dishart MK, Tonnessen I, Schlichtig R (1996) Methods for detecting local intestinal ischemic anaerobic metabolic acidosis by pCO_2. J Appl Physiol 81:1834–1842
17. Gutierrez G (1991) Cellular energy metabolism during hypoxia. Crit Care Med 19:619–626
18. Zhang H, Vincent JL (1993) Arteriovenous differences in PCO_2 and pH are good indicators of critical hypoperfusion. Am Rev Respir Dis 148:867–871

19. Schlichtig R, Bowles S (1994) Distinguishing between aerobic and anaerobic appearance of dissolved CO_2 in intestine during low flow. J Appl Physiol 76:2443–2451
20. Lundgren O, Haglund U (1978) The pathophysiology of the intestinal countercurrent exchanger. Life Sci 23:1411–1422
21. Mythen MG, Webb AR (1995) Perioperative plasma volume expansion reduces the incidence of gut mucosal hypoperfusion during cardiac surgery. Arch Surg 130:423–429
22. Gutierrez G, Clark C, Brown SD, Price K, Ortiz L, Nelson C (1994) Effect of dobutamine on oxygen consumption and gastric mucosal pH in septic patients. Am J Respir Crit Care Med 150:324–329
23. Neviere R, Mathieu D, Chagnon J-L, Lebleu N, Wattel F (1996) The contrasting effect of dobutamine and dopamine on gastric mucosal perfusion in septic patients. Am J Resp Crit Care Med 154:1684–1688
24. Levy B, Bollaert P-E, Charpentier C, Nace L, Audibert G, Bauer P, Nabet P, Larcan A (1997) Comparison of norepinephrine and dobutamine to epinephrine for hemodynamics, lactate metabolism, and gastric tonometric variables in septic shock: a prospective, randomized study. Intensive Care Med 23:282–287
25. Temmesfeld-Wollbrück B, Szalay A, Mayer K, Olschewski H, Seeger W, Grimminger F (1998) Abnormalities of gastric mucosal oxygenation in septic shock. Partial responsiveness to dopexamine. Am J Resp Crit Care Med 157:1586–1592

The Potential of Tissue Lightguide Spectrophotometry for Monitoring Gastric Mucosal Oxygenation During Mechanical Ventilation

A. Fournell · L. A. Schwarte · T. W. L. Scheeren

Zentrum für Anaesthesiologie, Heinrich-Heine-Universität, Moorenstrasse 5, 40225 Düsseldorf, Germany

Introduction

In pathologic conditions such as sepsis, assessment of global parameters of circulation and oxygenation can show quite normal results contrasting with values in microcirculatory regions, where hypoxia may still prevail. One of the areas of special interest in this context is the splanchnic region. But the significance of the gastrointestinal tract (GI) as the "canary" of the body [1] is at odds with the tools we have available to monitor splanchnic circulation, and especially oxygenation, which are very limited. Gastric tonometry may provide us with some useful information about flow in the GI, but in no way does it measure oxygen [2]. This obvious lack of suitable methods prompted us to look for alternatives, and tissue lightguide spectrophotometry [3] seems to be an appropriate way of achieving genuine measurements of oxygen in tissue.

Spectroscopy to Assess Tissue Oxygenation

Spectroscopic techniques are based on the law of Beer-Lambert, which describes the relation between the amount of absorbed/reflected light and the concentration of the material absorbing the light. Spectrophotometry used to assess tissue oxygen saturation (HbO_2) exploits the fact that oxygenated and deoxygenated hemoglobin have different absorption spectra. Oxyhemoglobin has a two-peaked spectrum, whereas deoxyhemoglobin has only one peak in its spectrum. Every unknown hemoglobin spectrum must lie somewhere between these two spectra, and it can be imagined easily that its "shape" and hence the actual oxygen saturation can be derived by a procedure of iteration and comparison. This algorithm has been published by Frank et al. [3].

The Erlangen microlightguide spectrophotometer "EMPHO" (Bodensee Gerätetechnik, D-88641 Überlingen, Germany) provides the hardware for determination of HbO_2. It consists of four functional modules: the light source, the micro-lightguide cable, the detection device, and a computing system. The light from a xenon arc lamp is transmitted by a highly flexible micro-lightguide (250 μm diameter) to the tissue. The light reflected from the tissue is transferred by a hexagon of six lightguides (250 μm diameter) surrounding the illuminating lightguide to a rotating interference band-pass filter disk, where it is monochromatized in a range of 502–603 nm. The photons are detected by a photomultiplier. The electrical signals are converted from

M. K. Herbert et al. (Eds.), Problems of the Gastrointestinal Tract in Anesthesia...

analog to digital and then processed and stored by a personal computer. All lightguides are encased in a flexible rubber tube with an outer diameter of approximately 2.0 mm.

Animal Studies

We have used this method in an experimental study in chronically instrumented dogs during general anesthesia [4]. The objective of this study was to evaluate the ability of tissue lightguide spectrophotometry to monitor the effects of positive end-expiratory pressure (PEEP) during intermittent positive pressure ventilation (IPPV) on local intracapillary hemoglobin saturation (HbO_2) of gastric mucosa. This seems to be an important issue, because inadequate oxygen delivery to the gut is commonly regarded as the initial event in the development of multiple organ dysfunction syndrome (MODS), a clinical syndrome that usually includes the lungs as one organ system affected in the first line [5]. The developing acute respiratory failure (ARF) makes mechanical ventilation necessary. Besides all modifications regarding the appropriate level, the addition of PEEP remains one of the mainstays in this crucial situation [6].

In this study the micro-lightguide was introduced through a flexible orogastric tube into the stomach of the dog after induction of anesthesia. The correct position of the lightguide (facing the greater curvature of the stomach) was identified by means of gastroscopy. The flexible gastroscope was afterwards removed to avoid trauma to the gastric mucosa and to achieve a competent closure of the cardiac orifice of the stomach.

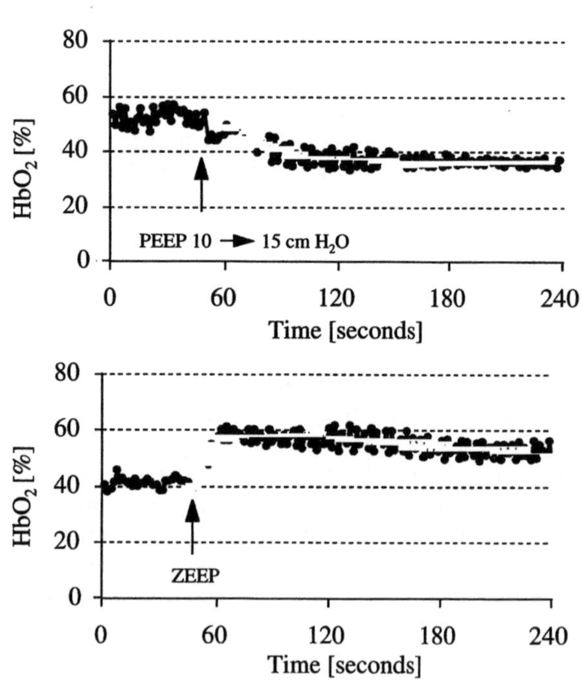

Fig. 1. The implementation of positive end-expiratory pressure (PEEP) during intermittent positive pressure ventilation (IPPV) reversibly depresses HbO_2 of gastric mucosa: when PEEP is increased from 10 cm to 15 cm H_2O (*upper registration*, indicated by *arrow*) HbO_2 decreases, whereas it is improved (*lower registration*) when PEEP is turned off. Modified from [4]

Fig. 2. Incremental levels of PEEP initiate a dose-related reduction in HbO_2 of gastric mucosa. Values are mean ± SEM. *$P < 0.05$ for PEEP 10 cm H_2O and PEEP 15 cm H_2O vs ZEEP (zero end-expiratory pressure; Wilcoxon signed rank test); 10 experiments in 6 dogs. Modified from [4]

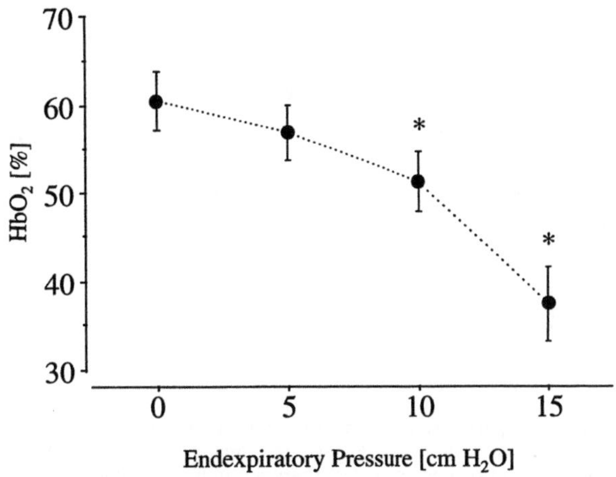

As shown in Fig. 1, oxygen saturation of gastric mucosa, already diminished as a result of PEEP to 10 cmH_2O less than normal baseline values, dropped further when PEEP was increased from 10 to 15 cm H_2O and improved after end-expiratory pressure was switched to zero (ZEEP).

The same pattern was observed in every experiment (Fig. 2): PEEP decreased the HbO_2 level in the gastric mucosa in a dose-dependent manner despite unaltered systemic arterial oxygenation (98.1 ± 0.6 %, 98.0 ± 0.6 %, 97.8 ± 0.7 %, and 97.3 ± 0.6 % during ventilation with ZEEP and PEEP levels 5, 10, and 15 cm H_2O, respectively; values are mean ± SEM). At the highest level of PEEP (15 cm H_2O) HbO_2 was reduced from 60.6 ± 3.3 % during ZEEP to 37.5 ± 4.3 % (mean ± SEM).

PEEP decreases cardiac output (CO) by diminishing ventricular preload. As ventricular contractility is not compromised in normal ventricular function by PEEP [7, 8], restoration of ventricular preload should normalize CO. But it is questionable whether normalization of CO during ventilation with PEEP also normalizes HbO_2 of the gastric mucosa.

We addressed this problem in a second study in dogs. The animals were chronically instrumented with carotid loops and an ultrasonic flowprobe implanted around the pulmonary artery to allow continuous measurement of systemic mean arterial pressure (MAP) and CO.

Simultaneously with the attenuation of CO and MAP (Fig. 3), HbO_2 in the gastric mucosa decreased from 59.7 ± 2.4 % during IPPV with ZEEP to 44.4 ± 3.1 % during IPPV with PEEP 15 cm H_2O (Fig. 4). But in contrast to CO and MAP, which both returned completely to baseline values after intravascular volume was expanded by an infusion of HES (hydroxyethyl starch, 5–10 ml kg^{-1}) to restore preload, the HbO_2 level in the gastric mucosa remained statistically significantly below baseline values, although it also improved, to 51.2 ± 2.8 %.

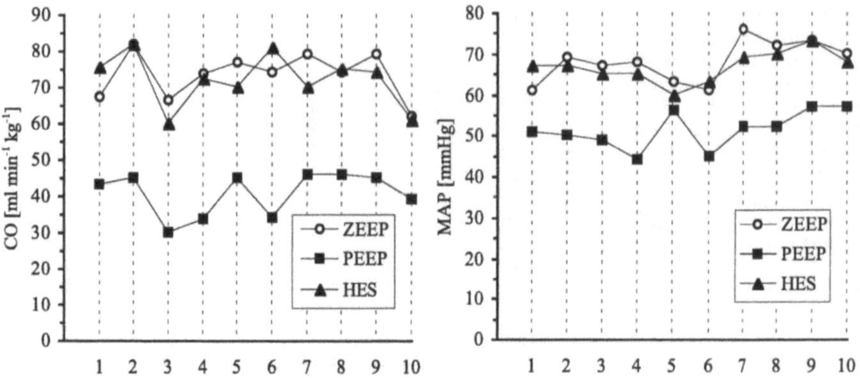

Fig. 3. Compared with baseline values during ventilation with ZEEP (*open circles*) both CO and MAP decline in each individual experiment during IPPV with PEEP (*closed squares*). After preload has been restored (*closed triangles*) there are only negligible differences from baseline values. *Numbers 1–10* indicate 10 consecutive experiments in 5 dogs

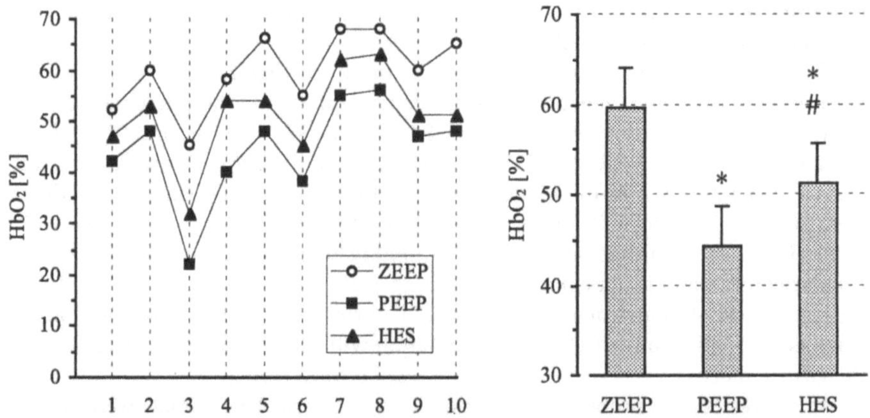

Fig. 4. Although HbO_2 of gastric mucosa is improved after volume expansion and hence normalization of cardiac output (CO) and mean arterial pressure (MAP) in each experiment, it remains well below baseline values (10 experiments in 5 dogs). *ZEEP vs PEEP, *ZEEP vs HES, #PEEP vs HES, $P < 0.0001$ (Wilcoxon signed rank test)

Study in Volunteers

Patterns of reaction to exposure to PEEP similar to those in the animal studies have also been observed in an ongoing study during spontaneous breathing with PEEP (continuous positive airway pressure, CPAP) in volunteers (Fig. 5).

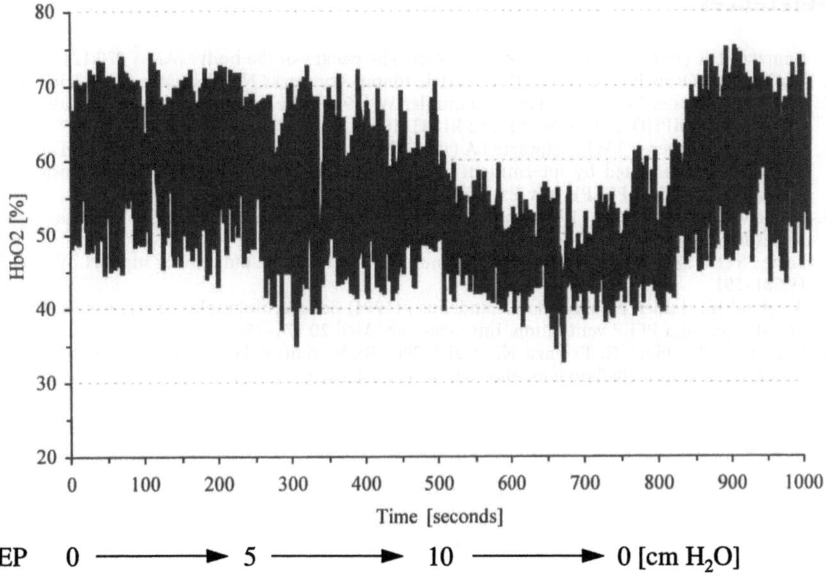

Fig. 5. Increasing levels of end-expiratory pressure during spontaneous breathing per face mask (continuous positive airway pressure; CPAP) progressively depress HbO_2 of gastric mucosa in a volunteer without sedation. After end-expiratory pressure is switched to zero, HbO_2 returns to baseline values

Conclusions

Our studies show that lightguide spectrophotometry can be used to monitor tissue oxygenation reliably in the splanchnic region, an area that is particularly sensitive to impaired oxygen supply in impending MODS. Because any further attenuation in tissue oxygen availability in this crucial situation could possibly enhance the development of organ failure, it is of the utmost importance that any detrimental effects are recognized as soon as possible. As in our studies, measurements of global variables in systemic circulation do not necessarily reflect regional abnormalities, so that the need for a continuous supply of information about changes in particular organ systems such as the gut is obvious. Tissue lightguide spectrophotometry fulfills this task in an ideal way. The method is only slightly invasive, so that possible complications are negligible and it can be applied continuously to ensure online information about any changes in the actual oxygen status of the bowel. This may be of great importance when it comes to deciding what therapeutic interventions are appropriate in specific situations and monitoring their effects.

References

1. Dantzker DR (1993) The gastrointestinal tract. The canary of the body? JAMA 270:1247–1248
2. Benjamin E, Oropello JM (1996) Does gastric tonometry work? No. Crit Care Clin 12:587–601
3. Frank KH, Kessler M, Appelbaum K, Dümmler W (1989) The Erlangen micro-lightguide spectrophotometer EMPHO I. Phys Med Biol 34:1883–1900
4. Fournell A, Scheeren TWL, Schwarte LA (1997) Oxygenation of the intestinal mucosa in anaesthetized dogs is attenuated by intermittent positive pressure ventilation (IPPV) with positive end-expiratory pressure (PEEP). Adv Exp Med Biol 428:385–389
5. Landow L, Andersen LW (1994) Splanchnic ischaemia and its role in multiple organ failure. Acta Anaesthesiol Scand 38:626–639
6. Barie PS (1995) Organ-specific support in multiple organ failure: pulmonary support. World J Surg 19:581–591
7. Berglund JE, Halden E, Jakobson S, Landelius J (1994) Echocardiographic analysis of cardiac function during high PEEP ventilation. Intensive Care Med 20:174–180
8. Dambrosio M, Fiore G, Brienza N, et al (1996) Right ventricular myocardial function in ARF patients. PEEP as a challenge for the right heart. Intensive Care Med 22:772–780

PART III

Nutritional Aspects

INVITED ARTICLE

The Colon as a Metabolically Active Organ: Implications for the Composition of Enteral Formula Diets

W. M. Scheppach

Department of Medicine, University of Würzburg, Josef-Schneider-Str. 2, 97080 Würzburg, Germany

Introduction

Dietary fiber is widely accepted as an important part of healthy human nutrition. There is, however, controversy over the use of fiber in artificial enteral nutrition, although fiber-enriched formula diets are marketed in the United States and in Europe [1, 2]. The term dietary fiber comprises a heterogeneous group of polysaccharides (non-starch polysaccharides, NSPs) and lignin (a polyphenol) with varying physicochemical properties. An important feature of NSPs is their fermentability by colonic anaerobic bacteria [3, 4]. The principal end products of bacterial fiber degradation are short-chain fatty acids (SCFAs), of which acetate, propionate, and n-butyrate are most important quantitatively. SCFAs are the predominant anions in the colonic lumen and are thought to have a major impact on luminal and mucosal metabolism. If the addition of fiber to liquid formula diets is beneficial to the patient, it is probably by offering fermentable substrates to the colonic microflora, resulting in SCFA production. Two topics are discussed below:

1. What is the experimental evidence that may form a basis for the use of dietary fiber in artificial enteral nutrition?
2. Have clinical studies shown an advantage of fiber-enriched diets over fiber-free formulas?

Experimental Evidence for Use of Fiber in Formula Diets

Colonic SCFAs and Sodium Absorption

SCFAs are rapidly absorbed from the colonic lumen by a concentration-dependent transcellular process, probably by coupled anion exchange (SCFA anion against bicarbonate) [5, 6]. In contrast, the transport of SCFA anions via the paracellular route seems less effective, as shown in the guinea pig large intestine [7]. In the healthy human colon, 80 g lactulose can be metabolized without the occurrence of osmotic diarrhea [8]. SCFA absorption is coupled with sodium absorption; although there are open questions regarding the exact mechanism [9, 10] it is clear that the net effect of bacterial fermentation is the removal of sugars, water, and sodium from the colonic lumen. Butyrate also reverses the effect of cholera toxin on the rat colon by converting net water secretion into net water absorption and by significantly reducing the net secretion of Na^+ [11]. This antidiarrheal effect should be considered in artificial enteral nutrition where osmotic diarrhea is a frequent problem in clinical practice.

M. K. Herbert et al. (Eds.), Problems of the Gastrointestinal Tract in Anesthesia...

SCFAs and Mucosal Energy Metabolism

After absorption from the colonic lumen, SCFAs are handled in different ways by the colonocytes. The 2- and 3-carbon acids are released into portal blood to reach the liver [12], where propionate is taken up quantitatively by hepatocytes. Gut-derived acetate, however, is recovered in peripheral blood to serve as a systemic fuel [13]. Little butyrate is detected in the portal vein [12]; this fatty acid is metabolized by the colonic epithelium to β-OH-butyrate and CO_2. From Roediger's fundamental studies in isolated colonocytes of humans [14] and rats [15], it is known that luminal butyrate is used as a nutrient in preference to glucose, glutamine, and ketone bodies. The distal colon, in particular, relies on butyrate as a metabolic fuel. When glucose and butyrate were available as substrates, n-butyrate accounted for 59 % of the oxygen consumption in the ascending colon and 72 % in the descending colon [14]. In chronically malnourished and acutely fasted rats, butyrate oxidation is substantially reduced, which shows the vulnerability of the colonic mucosa to luminal energy deprivation [16]. Roediger [17] discussed a link between energy metabolism and sodium absorption: epithelia lacking their preferred nutrient may be rendered incapable of absorbing sodium and water at normal rates ("starvation diarrhea").

A starving colonic epithelium is at risk of developing chronic colitis [18]. This is particularly evident in diversion colitis, where complete diversion of the fecal stream deprives the distal colon of its preferred nutrients (SCFAs) [19]. SCFA irrigation can ameliorate mucosal inflammation in diversion colitis [20] and in distal ulcerative colitis [21, 22]; in the latter condition, diminished SCFA concentrations have been reported [23].

SCFAs and Epithelial Proliferation

Dietary fibers (especially highly fermentable components) are trophic to the colonic epithelium of rats, as shown by an increase in mucosal DNA, RNA, and protein content [24]. The same effect occurs when starch is malabsorbed and serves as a fermentable substrate to the microflora [25]. Inert bulk (kaolin), however, does not affect the crypt cell production rate of mouse colonic mucosa [26]. The proliferative effect of fiber on rat colonocytes is seen in conventional but not in germ-free animals. It can be concluded from this finding that products of fiber breakdown and not fiber per se stimulate cell proliferation [27]. Infusion of SCFAs (the main end products of fiber degradation) into the colon of rats stimulates epithelial growth [28]. The SCFA solution (70 mM acetate, 35 mM propionate, 20 mM butyrate) and the butyrate solution (20 mM) raised mucosal parameters of cellularity to the same extent.

These findings in experimental animals were confirmed in humans [29]. Biopsies from healthy cecal mucosa were incubated in vitro with a SCFA combination (60 mM acetate, 25 mM propionate, 10 mM butyrate, sodium salts) or with sodium butyrate (10 mM) alone. Butyrate stimulated DNA synthesis (measured by incorporation of [^{3}H]thymidine; labeling index = number of labeled crypt cells divided by the total number of crypt cells) in a way similar to the SCFA combination. This finding emphasizes the importance of n-butyrate for the colonic mucosa.

The stimulation of colonic mucosal proliferation is physiologically important if it improves large intestine function under certain stress conditions. This issue was addressed in a series of rat studies. Colonic infusion of SCFAs accelerated wound healing after colonic transection and reanastomosis. Spontaneous anastomotic dehiscence was significantly less in the SCFAs than in the control group; the anastomotic suture line burst in fewer colons from the SCFA group when tension was applied to the bowel wall [30]. After 80 % small-bowel resection (i.e., in a model of the short-bowel syndrome) pectin (a highly fermentable dietary fiber) enhanced intestinal adaptation by increasing colonic mucosal DNA, RNA, and protein contents [31]; this resulted in a less pronounced postoperative weight loss than under control conditions. Under the same experimental conditions, intravenous SCFAs added to total parenteral nutrition (TPN) raised jejunal and ileal mucosal parameters. With regard to the colon, there was a trend toward greater mucosal parameters ($P = 0.06$) [32]. Summarizing these data from animal studies, there is evidence that the trophic effect of SCFAs may enhance intestinal adaptation to surgical stress.

Fiber and Gut Barrier

A complex system with interrelated factors prevents the penetration of the small and, more importantly, the large intestinal wall by bacteria: the gut barrier. Little is known about the effect of fiber or its degradation products on the gut-associated immune system. There is a preliminary report showing stimulated DNA synthesis by lymphocytes in vitro in the presence of sodium butyrate [33]. Similarly, glutamine (a non-fiber nutrient for enterocytes) affects the metabolism and function of lymphocytes, which may add to host defenses against bacterial invasion [34].

Unspecific epithelial defenses may also add to the gut barrier function. Colonic crypt proliferation with desquamation of mature cells may present an obstacle to bacterial surface adhesion [35], which precedes colonization and possibly invasion. In the rat model, the effect of fiber on bacterial translocation from the gut to mesenteric lymph nodes, liver, and spleen has been tested. The addition of cellulose to an orally administered TPN solution diminished ileal protein loss and reduced the incidence of bacterial translocation (compared with TPN alone); supplementation with citrus pectin had no effect in this experimental setting [36]. The addition of corncobs, but not soy fiber, to a defined fiber-free formula diet reduced the translocation rate significantly [37]. Both glutamine and fiber (psyllium), when added to a fiber-free formula diet, prevented loss of bowel mass, but neither substance protected effectively against spontaneous or endotoxin-induced bacterial translocation [38], a phenomenon primarily noted in experimental animals. Which fiber component is the most effective in supporting epithelial defenses must be evaluated.

The ecology of the resident microflora may be disturbed by a lack of fermentable substrate or by concomitant antibiotic treatment of patients on TPN or artificial enteral feeding. The activity of bacterial carbohydrate fermentation is depressed by oral ampicillin [39], penicillin, and metronidazole [40], as measured by the hydrogen breath technique. This may result in antibiotic-associated diarrhea – one third of cases exhibited overgrowth of toxin-forming *Clostridium difficile*. Products of fermentation may inhibit the growth of pathogens. Butyrate (25 mM) suppresses the in vitro multiplication of *C. difficile* and may thus play a role in the development of colonization resistance [41]. Conversely, cecectomy (i.e., the removal of the fermentative organ) makes mice more susceptible to peroral challenge by *Salmonella enteritidis*

[42]. Theoretically, impairment of fermentation induces calorie loss. By SCFA absorption, ~ 100–200 kcal/day is salvaged from a Western diet in the absence of diarrhea [43]. Because only 5 %–10 % of human energy requirements may come from SCFA absorption, the effects of antibiotics on water and electrolyte losses may be more important than on energy losses.

Components of nutrition (fiber, glutamine) may interact with host factors and strengthen the gut barrier. More information from animal and human studies is needed until recommendations can be given.

Clinical Studies with Fiber Supplements in Liquid Formulas

With regard to the supplementation of liquid formula diets with dietary fiber, fiber extracts are used that have little in common with the physically intact fiber in plant cell walls. The source of fiber most often added to formulas is soy polysaccharide, consisting of cellulose (20 %) and hemicelluloses (80 %), with traces of lignin; it is highly (~ 70 %) fermentable in the human colon. Soy fiber has only a moderate effect on viscosity, therefore, delivery of fiber-containing diets through 9–15 French feeding tubes (gastrostomy or nasogastric/ nasoduodenal tube) is not accompanied by a higher incidence of blockage (compared with fiber-free formulas). When the effects of fiber supplements to enteral feeding are reviewed, the underlying clinical setting is found to be of major significance.

Healthy Volunteers

Slavin et al. [44] conducted a trial in 16 healthy young men consuming either a self-selected diet or liquid formulas with the addition of 0, 30, or 60 g/day of soy fiber for 10-day periods. Stool weights on the self-selected (144.6 ± 52.5 g/day, means ± SD) and the 60-g/day soy fiber (150.3 ± 78.4 g/day) diets were significantly greater than stool weights on the fiber-free (67.3 ± 20.8 g/day) and 30-g/day soy fiber (100.2 ± 40.7 g/day) diets. Stool weights on the 30-g/day soy fiber diet were also greater than on the fiber-free diet. Matzkies and Webs [45] fed a fiber-free formula to eight volunteers for 3 weeks. In week 2 and 3, soy fiber (30 g/day) was added. Stool weight rose from 57 ± 15 g/day (end of week 1) to 86 ± 4 g/day (end of week 3). The difference was not statistically significant; a control group was not included in this study.

Zimmaro et al. [46] studied 13 healthy adults consuming a regular diet for 3 days and then an isotonic tube-feeding formula for 9 days. Afterwards, the subjects were randomly assigned to tube feeding with pectin (range 14.5–31.5 g/day) or continuation of the fiber-free tube feeding. Fiber-free tube feeding resulted in liquid stools in 60 % of subjects, whereas diarrhea was not seen in those with a regular diet. The addition of pectin completely reversed the high percentage of liquid stools seen during fiber-free tube feeding.

Raimundo et al. [47] reported that the addition of soy polysaccharide to a fiber-free enteral diet had no effect on the parameters of bowel function (stool weight, stool frequency, whole-gut transit time) in seven volunteers (7-day periods). However, SCFA production was increased in vitro (fecal incubation of stool samples from the soy fiber period).

In summary, the results from these publications are conflicting, probably because of inadequately short study periods and time-treatment interactions. It is estimated that at least 4-week periods would be appropriate to allow adaptation to dietary changes and to avoid overlapping effects in crossover designs.

The possibility of mineral depletion with fiber-containing enteral feedings has been a concern. Taper et al. [48] investigated Cu, Zn, Fe, Mg, K, and PO_4 retention in 22 healthy men. The addition of 40 g/day soy fiber to a fiber-free liquid formula resulted in significantly lower Cu, Zn, Fe, and Mg retentions than did the 20-g/day supplement; the 30-g/day fiber supplement had an intermediate effect. Except for slightly negative Cu and Fe retentions with the 40-g/day fiber diet, retentions of all minerals remained positive throughout the study. Shinnick et al. [49] reported a decreased absorption of folate and Zn when 10–15 g/day soy polysaccharide was added to a fiber-free formula. Because elemental diets often deliver minerals in excess of the recommended daily allowance, it is unlikely that fiber supplementation leads to a clinically significant mineral deficit [50].

Stable Medical Patients

Two controlled studies have been performed in stable patients. Patil et al. [51] studied five patients who were admitted to the hospital for investigation of abdominal pain and/ or frequency of bowel action; there was no evidence of organic disease. During two 15-day periods they were given either a polymeric fiber-free diet or the same diet supplemented with 24 g/day carrot fiber (8 g cellulose, 16 g pectin) by continuous nasogastric infusion. Frequency of bowel action and wet stool weights were not significantly different between study periods. Heymsfield et al. [50] studied eight patients with various diagnoses (e.g., postmyocardial infarction, diabetes, chronic lung disease, depression, muscular dystrophy). They evaluated the effects of soy polysaccharide (12.4 and 38.5 g/day) added to a fiber-free liquid formula. After 1–2 weeks, stool wet and dry weights were similar with the fiber-free and fiber-augmented formulas.

These studies suggest that, in clinical practice, fiber-containing enteral diets have no advantage over low-residue diets. However, it must still be argued that additional large-scale investigations in well-defined patient groups over longer treatment periods are needed to verify these results.

Patients with Psychiatric or Neurological Disorders

Fischer et al. [52] published results of a prospective crossover study in 28 mentally retarded young individuals suffering from chronic constipation. Subjects received a fiber-free formula for 4 weeks and, subsequently, a feeding supplemented with soy polysaccharide (15.6–17.4 g/day) for 2 weeks. In this short-term trial, addition of soy fiber did not change stool weight, stool frequency, or transit time. More recently, investigators from the same institution reported a 1-year trial in 11 mentally retarded youths. [53]. The patients were suffering from constipation and were fed formula diets with or without soy fiber, by gastrostomy. With fiber-free enteral feeding, wet stool weight was 30 ± 13 g/day. This figure increased significantly to 87 ± 45 g/day with supplementation with 18–25 g/day soy fiber. Similarly, mean daily stool frequencies rose significantly, from 0.6 ± 0.2 to 1.1 ± 0.5. During the soy fiber period, N, Mg, Ca, and PO_4 remained in positive balance, whereas one third of Zn balances were negative. [54].

Shankardass et al. [55] studied 28 patients with neurological disorders (e.g., cerebrovascular accidents, head injury, epilepsy, Guillain-Barre syndrome, multiple sclerosis) who were on long-term tube feeding (21 gastrostomy, 7 nasogastric tube) for coma ($n = 21$) or inability to swallow. Patients received, at random, a fiber-free or a fiber-augmented formula (12.8 g/1000 ml soy fiber) in two consecutive 6-week periods. Whereas fecal weight and stool frequency were not different between study periods, the requirement of laxatives was significantly reduced during the fiber period.

The study populations of Liebl et al. [53] and Shankardass et al. [55] are not comparable because constipation was not a clinical problem (mean fecal wet weights: 156.5 g/day fiber, 142.6 g/day no fiber) in the latter. These studies show that fiber supplementation may be beneficial in enteral nutrition of selected patients with a tendency toward constipation. In particular, the trial by Liebl et al. [53] demonstrates that long observation periods may be required in order to show fiber effects on bowel function that are missed in 1- to 2-week periods.

Intensive Care Patients

Guenter et al. [56] studied 100 acutely ill patients, who received tube feeding for an average of 15.8 days. Patients were randomly assigned to either a fiber-free or a soy fiber (14.4 g/1000 ml)-supplemented formula. The incidence of diarrhea was most strongly associated with the use of antibiotics, when the percentage of days with diarrhea and the presence of *C. difficile* in patients with diarrhea was not different between groups. Hart and Dobb [57] reported a trial in which 68 critically ill patients received a fiber-free formula with or without addition of ispaghula husk (7 g/day). The duration of enteral feeding was 8–9 days on average. The addition of fiber to enteral feeds did not affect diarrhea. Again, there was a correlation between diarrhea and the administration of antibiotics. In another study from the same intensive care unit, the feeding of a soy fiber-containing formula (14.4 g/1000 ml) had no advantage over a fiber-free diet with regard to a diarrhea score (calculated from the frequency, volume, and consistency of stools) [58]. Frankenfield and Beyer [59] studied nine head-injury patients who were on ventilators in an intensive care unit. During 4- to 6-day periods, patients received either a fiber-free or a fiber-augmented (14 g/1000 ml soy fiber) formula (crossover design). The incidence of diarrhea between treatments was not significantly different. The study was criticized for time-treatment interactions because of short intervention periods without a washout phase. Heimbach et al. [60] compared a fiber-free formula with a fiber-supplemented diet (21.1 g/1000 ml soy polysaccharide) in 30 burn patients for 16-day periods. Stool weight and frequency were not different between groups. However, patients fed the fiber-containing formula were able to ingest a significantly greater number of calories without developing diarrhea than patients given the fiber-free diet. Homann et al. [61] fed a formula containing partially hydrolyzed guar to 50 postoperative patients; in the control group ($n = 50$) a fiber-free standard diet was administered. The patients on the fiber-supplemented diet experienced significantly less diarrhea than those on the standard diet.

In conclusion, data obtained in patients under intensive care are controversial. The negative effects of drugs (e.g., antibiotics) and physiological stress interfere with the potential benefit of a fiber-containing formula. Moreover, patients usually remain under intensive care for relatively short time periods; thus intestinal adaptation to fiber-containing enteral feeding may not yet have occurred at the end of the feeding period.

Conclusion

There is good experimental evidence that fiber, an integral part of normal human nutrition, may play a role as a supplement to artificial enteral feedings. SCFAs, as bacterial breakdown products of fiber, stimulate colonic sodium and water absorption and should thus have an antidiarrheal effect. Butyrate is the preferred metabolic fuel of colonocytes. SCFAs stimulate colonic epithelial proliferation and prevent mucosal atrophy associated with fiber-free tube feeding. They may also strengthen the gut barrier and reduce bacterial translocation. Good hypotheses have evolved from experimental settings that are worth testing in clinical trials.

However, the results obtained in clinical studies (of healthy volunteers and patient groups) have been inconsistent. This may be due to short study periods, time-treatment interactions, small sample sizes, lack of stratification according to disease acuity, and semiquantitative measurements [62]. From the available data, it can cautiously be concluded that fiber supplementation may be beneficial in long-term tube feeding of constipated patients and in intensive-care units, but drugs and stress however, are powerful confounding variables in studies evaluating the effects of a fiber supplement on bowel function.

All the studies outlined above were performed on subjects with intact bowel function. It would be interesting to learn whether specific intestinal disorders could be ameliorated by fiber-augmented tube feeding, including investigating: Intestinal adaptation to massive small-bowel resection, if normal food is inadequate to maximize epithelial response; prevention of colonic anastomotic leakage; intestinal atrophy after long-term parenteral nutrition, as a step toward normal food intake; and response of chronically inflamed mucosa to butyrate arising from fiber fermentation. In addition, different types of fiber yielding different proportions of SCFAs could be tested [63]. It may also be possible to introduce modified starches that reach the colon and release high amounts of butyrate in vivo [64] and in vitro [65]. Until this work has been done, the rationale to add fiber to artificial enteral nutrition remains open for debate.

References

1. Silk DBA (1989) Progress report: fibre and enteral nutrition. Gut 30:246–264
2. Scheppach W, Burghardt W, Bartram P, et al (1990) Addition of dietary fiber to liquid formula diets: the pros and cons. JPEN 14:204–209
3. Cummings JH, Macfarlane GT (1991) The control and consequences of bacterial fermentation in the human colon. J Appl Bacteriol 70:443–459
4. Macfarlane GT, Cummings JH (1991) The colonic flora, fermentation, and large bowel digestive function. In: Phillips, SF, Pemberton JH, Shorter RG (eds) The large intestine: physiology, pathophysiology and disease. Raven, New York, pp 51–92

5. Ruppin H, Bar-Meir S, Soergel KH, et al (1980) Absorption of short-chain fatty acids by the colon. Gastroenterology 78:1500–1507
6. Cummings JH (1984) Colonic absorption: the importance of short-chain fatty acids in man. Scand J Gastroenterol Suppl 93:S 89- S 99
7. Von Engelhardt W, Busche R, Gros G, et al (1991) Absorption of short-chain fatty acids: mechanisms and regional differences in the large intestine. In: Roche AF (ed) Short-chain fatty acids: metabolism and clinical importance. Ross Laboratories, Columbus, pp 60–62
8. Hammer HF, Santa Ana C, Schiller LR, et al (1989) Studies of osmotic diarrhea induced in normal subjects by ingestion of polyethylene glycol and lactulose. J Clin Invest 84:1056–1062
9. Roediger WEW, Rigol G (1984) Sodium absorption with bacterial fatty acids and bile salts in the proximal and distal colon as a guide to colonic resection. Dis Colon Rectum 27:1–5
10. Binder HJ, Mehta P (1989) Short-chain fatty acids stimulate active sodium and chloride absorption in vitro in the rat distal colon. Gastroenterology 96:989–996
11. Ramakrishna BS, Nance SH, Roberts-Thomson IC, et al (1990) The effects of enterotoxins and short-chain fatty acids on water and electrolyte fluxes in ileal and colonic loops in vivo in the rat. Digestion 45:93–101
12. Cummings JH, Pomare EW, Branch WJ, et al (1987) Short chain fatty acids in human large intestine, portal, hepatic and venous blood. Gut 28:1221–1227
13. Scheppach W, Pomare EW, Elia M, et al (1991) The contribution of the large intestine to blood acetate in man. Clin Sci 80:177–182
14. Roediger WEW (1980) Role of anaerobic bacteria in the metabolic welfare of the colonic mucosa in man. Gut 21:793–798
15. Roediger WEW (1982) Utilization of nutrients by isolated epithelial cells of the rat colon. Gastroenterology 83:424–429
16. Firmansyah A, Penn D, and Lebenthal E (1989) Isolated colonocyte metabolism of glucose, glutamine, n-butyrate, and b-hydroxybutyrate in malnutrition. Gastroenterology 97:622–627
17. Roediger WEW (1986) Metabolic basis of starvation diarrhoea: implications for treatment. Lancet 1:1082–1084
18. Roediger WEW (1990) The starved colon – diminished mucosal nutrition, diminished absorption, and colitis. Dis Colon Rectum 33:858–862
19. Glotzer DJ, Glick ME, Goldman H (1981) Proctitis and colitis following diversion of the faecal steam. Gastroenterology 80:438–441
20. Harig JM, Soergel KH, Komorowski RA, et al (1989) Treatment of diversion colitis with short-chain-fatty acid irrigation. N Engl J Med 320:23–28
21. Breuer RI, Buto SK, Christ ML, et al (1991) Rectal irrigation with short-chain fatty acids for distal ulcerative colitis: preliminary report. Dig Dis Sci 36:185–187
22. Scheppach W, Sommer H, Kirchner T, et al (1992) Effect of butyrate enemas on the colonic mucosa in distal ulcerative colitis. Gastroenterology 103:51–56
23. Vernia P, Gnaedinger MS, Hauck W, et al (1988) Organic anions and the diarrhea of inflammatory bowel disease. Dig Dis Sci 33:1353–1358
24. Jacobs LR, Lupton JR (1984) Effect of dietary fibers on rat large bowel mucosal growth and cell proliferation. Am J Physiol 246:G 378- G 385
25. Calvert RJ, Otsuka M, Satchithanandam S (1989) Consumption of raw potato starch alters intestinal function and colonic cell proliferation in the rat. J Nutr 119:1610–1616
26. Goodlad RA, Wright NA (1983) Effects of addition of kaolin or cellulose to an elemental diet in intestinal cell proliferation in the mouse. Br J Nutr 50:91–98
27. Goodlad RA, Ratcliffe B, Fordham JP, et al (1989) Does dietary fibre stimulate intestinal epithelial cell proliferation in germ free rats? Gut 30:820–825
28. Kripke SA, Fox AD, Berman JM, et al (1989) Stimulation of intestinal mucosal growth with intracolonic infusion of short-chain fatty acids. JPEN 12:109–116
29. Scheppach W, Bartram P, Richter A, et al (1992) The effect of short-chain fatty acids on the human colonic mucosa in vitro. JPEN 16:43–48
30. Rolandelli RH, Koruda MJ, Settle RG, et al (1986) Effects of intraluminal infusion of short-chain acids on the healing of colonic anastomosis in the rat. Surgery 100:198–203
31. Koruda MJ, Rolandelli RH, Settle RG, et al (1986) The effect of a pectin supplemented elemental diet on intestinal adaptation to massive small bowel resection. JPEN 10:343–350
32. Koruda MJ, Rolandelli RH, Settle RG, et al (1988) Effect of parenteral nutrition supplemented with short-chain fatty acids on adaptation to massive small bowel resection. Gastroenterology 95:715–720
33. Carpaneto EM, Mariani MR, Ferrini S, et al (1991) Stimulation of DNA synthesis in primary culture of human lymphocytes by sodium butyrate. Proc Am Assoc Cancer Res 32:331–336
34. Newsholme EA, Crabtree B, Ardawi MSM (1985) Glutamine metabolism in lymphocytes: its biochemical, physiological and clinical importance. Q J Exp Physiol 70:473–489

35. Sherman P, Soni R, Karmali M (1988) Attaching and effacing adherence of vero cytotoxin-producing *Escherichia coli* to rabbit intestinal epithelium in vivo. Infect Immunol 56:756–761
36. Spaeth G, Specian RD, Berg RD, et al (1990) Bulk prevents bacterial translocation induced by the oral administration of total parenteral nutrition solution. JPEN 14:442–447
37. Alverdy JC, Aoys E, Moss GS (1990) Effect of commercially available chemically defined liquid diets on the intestinal microflora and bacterial translocation from the gut. JPEN 14:1–5
38. Barber AE, Jones WG, Minei JP, et al (1990) Glutamine or fiber supplementation of a defined formula diet: impact on bacterial translocation, tissue composition, and response to endotoxin. JPEN 14:335–343
39. Rao SSC, Edwards CA, Austen CJ, et al (1988) Impaired colonic fermentation of carbohydrate after ampicillin. Gastroenterology 94:928–934
40. Bjorneklett A, Midtvedt T (1981) Influence of three antimicrobial agents – penicillin, metronidazole, and doxycyclin – on the intestinal microflora of healthy humans. Scand J Gastroenterol 16:473–478
41. Rolfe RD (1984) Role of volatile fatty acids in colonization resistance to *Clostridium difficile*. Infect Immunol 54:185–191
42. Voravuthikunchai SP, Lee A (1987) Cecectomy causes long-term reduction of colonization resistance in the mouse gastrointestinal tract. Infect Immunol 55:995–1000
43. McNeil NI (1984) The contribution of the large intestine to energy supplies in man. Am J Clin Nutr 39:338–342
44. Slavin JL, Nelson NL, McNamara EA, et al (1985) Bowel function of healthy men consuming liquid diets with and without dietary fiber. JPEN 9:317–321
45. Matzkies F, Webs B (1985) Wirkung einer neuen Sondennahrung auf den Stoffwechsel, die Urinelektrolyte und den Gastrointestinaltrakt beim gesunden Erwachsenen mit und ohne Zulage eines Ballaststoffes aus Sojakleie. Z Ernährungswiss 24:105–112
46. Zimmaro DM, Rolandelli RH, Koruda MJ, et al (1989) Isotonic tube feeding formula induces liquid stools in normal subjects: reversal by pectin. JPEN 13:117–123
47. Raimundo AH, Kapadia S, Terry DL, et al (1992) The effect of fibre-free enteral diets and the addition of soy polysaccharide on human bowel function and short chain fatty acid (SCFA) production. JPEN 16:298–303
48. Taper LJ, Milam RS, McCallister MS, et al (1988) Mineral retention in young men consuming soy-fiber-augmented liquid-formula diets. Am J Clin Nutr 48:305–311
49. Shinnick FL, Hess RL, Fischer MH, et al (1989) Apparent nutrient absorption and upper gastrointestinal transit with fiber-containing enteral feedings. Am J Clin Nutr 49:471–475
50. Heymsfield SB, Roongspisuthipong C, Evert M, et al (1988) Fiber supplementation of enteral formulas: effects on the bioavailability of major nutrients and gastrointestinal tolerance. JPEN 12:265–273
51. Patil DH, Grimble GK, Keohane P, et al (1985) Do fibre containing enteral diets have advantages over existing low residue diets? Clin Nutr 4:67–71
52. Fischer M, Adkins W, Hall L, et al (1985) The effect of dietary fibre in a liquid diet on bowel function of mentally retarded individuals. J Ment Defic Res 29:373–381
53. Liebl BH, Fischer MH, Van Calcar SC, et al (1990) Dietary fiber and long term large bowel response in enterally nourished nonambulatory profoundly retarded youths. JPEN 14:371–375
54. Van Calcar SC, Liebl BH, Fischer MH, et al (1989) Long-term nutritional status of an enterally nourished institutionalized population. Am J Clin Nutr 50:381–390
55. Shankardass K, Chuchmach S, Chelswick K, et al (1990) Bowel function of long-term tube-fed patients consuming formulae with and without dietary fiber. JPEN 14:508–512
56. Guenter PA, Settle RG, Perlmutter S, et al (1991) Tube-feeding related diarrhea in acutely ill patients. JPEN 15:277–280
57. Hart GK, Dobb GJ (1988) Effect of a fecal bulking agent on diarrhea during enteral feeding in the critically ill. JPEN 12:465–468
58. Dobb GJ, Towler SC (1990) Diarrhoea during enteral feeding in the critically ill: a comparison of feeds with and without fibre. Intensive Care Med 16:252–255
59. Frankenfield DC, Beyer PL (1989) Soy-polysaccharide fiber: effect on diarrhea in tube-fed, head-injured patients. Am J Clin Nutr 50:533–538
60. Heimbach DM, Williamson J, Marvin J (1985) The gastrointestinal tolerance of a fibre-supplemented tube feeding formula in burn patients. In: The clinical role of fibre. MES Medical Education Services, Toronto, S 67–72
61. Homann HH, Kemen M, Fuessenich C, et al (1994) Reduction in diarrhea incidence by soluble fiber in patients receiving total or supplemented enteral nutrition. JPEN 18:486–490
62. Frankenfield DC, Beyer PL (1991) Dietary fiber and bowel function in tube-fed patients. J Am Diet Assoc 91:590–596

63. McBurney MI, Thompson LU (1991) Dietary fiber and total enteral nutrition: fermentative assessment of five fiber supplements. JPEN 15:267–270
64. Scheppach W, Fabian C, Sachs M, et al (1988) The effect of starch malabsorption on fecal short-chain fatty acid excretion in man. Scand J Gastroenterol 23:755–759
65. Macfarlane GT, Englyst HN (1986) Starch utilization by the human large intestinal microflora. J Appl Bacteriol 60:195–201

Early Enteral Nutrition Influences Immunological Response of Lymphocyte Subsets After Polytrauma

J. M. Engel · T. Menges · G. Hempelmann

Department of Anaesthesiology and Intensive Care Medicine, Justus-Liebig-University Giessen, 35390 Giessen, Germany

Introduction

Severely injured trauma patients have a high blood loss resulting in a centralised circulation with hypoperfusion of organs. After volume replacement and reconstitution of the microcirculation, the ischemic damage to the epithelial layer and the intestinal tissues is aggravated due to "reperfusion-syndrome" from a primary functional to a structural organ failure. The gut is one of the most vulnerable organs, as the intestinal mucosa has a high oxygen demand. Because of the high number of α-receptors, the circulation of the gut is dramatically reduced in cases of shock, and the terminal vascular bed suffers from an inadequate oxygen delivery. This unfavourable combination results in mucosal acidosis. The consequences are disintegration of the epithelium and the breakdown of the intestinal mucosal barrier with the risk of bacterial translocation. Translocation is defined as the passage of bacteria or toxins from the endoluminal space of the gastrointestinal tract to extraintestinal sites such as mesenteric lymph nodes, liver, spleen, peritoneum, and blood. The host immune response is able to destroy bacteria or clear toxins prior to their systemic spread. In the case of an intestinal barrier breakdown and an overwhelming host defence, the number of bacteria and toxins increases dramatically in the interstitial space and the systemic circulation, resulting in systemic bacteremia. This might be an explanation for the occurrence of septic-toxic complications, sepsis, and multiple organ dysfunctions.

The exposure of cellular elements to humoral immune systems triggers the release of inflammatory mediators. The Systemic Inflammatory Response Syndrome (SIRS) is the result of an uncontrolled, generalised inflammatory response and a concurrent overwhelming host defence. Sepsis and SIRS promote the manifestation of a subsequent Multi Organ Dysfunction Syndrome (MODS). The gut therefore, is often called the motor of MODS.

Other factors contributing to an increased translocation rate in polytraumatised patients are suppression of the immune system, alterations of the normal bowel flora, and a lack of intraluminal nutrients. Enteral nutrition stimulates mesenteric blood flow and enhances perfusion of the gut. The increased blood flow improves the oxygen supply to the intestinal systems. Several studies confirmed the importance of intraluminal nutrients in reducing the rate of mucosal cell atrophy and in maintaining mucosal barrier integrity.

In contrast to parenteral nutrition, enteral nutrition includes substrates of importance for the physiological balance of digestive processes and intraluminal gut conditions. Firstly, nutritive substrates such as glutamine, cysteine, complex carbohydrates

M. K. Herbert et al. (Eds.), Problems of the Gastrointestinal Tract in Anesthesia...

such as fiber, and medium chain- and long chain omega-3-lipids are important to stabilize the physiological gut conditions [12]. Secondly, these substrates stimulate gut hormones such as gastrin and enteroglucagon. A physiological function of gastrin is to stimulate cell proliferation, and to increase levels of DNA, RNA and protein synthesis in duodenal, ileal and proximal colonic mucosa [2, 6]. Moreover, increased enteroglucagon levels are correlated with an increased intestinal mucosal growth [5].

Enteral nutritional support seems to be favourable for critically ill patients. Clinical studies describe the importance of enteral nutrition, due to an increase in the synthesis of structural proteins resulting in reduced septic complications, in comparison to parenteral nutrition [7, 9, 10, 11]. The liberation of tumour necrosis factor-α (TNF-α) into the hepatic and systemic circulation is less extensive [4]. The number of all T lymphocytes, especially CD4+ (helper) lymphocytes, is greater [3] when enteral nutrients are given. Moore et al. [8] investigated the clinical consequences of early enteral nutritional support in patients with abdominal trauma. Group 1 patients were enterally nourished within 12–18 h postoperatively, whereas group 2 patients were fed enterally after 5 days. Of the group 2 patients, 29 % suffered infectious complications whereas only 9 % of group 1 patients revealed septic-toxic complications. Bower et al. [1] found a lower mortality rate in critically ill patients with early enteral nutrition as predicted by the Therapeutic Intervention Scoring System (TISS).

In critically ill patients, initial feeding by tube into the stomach often does not work sufficiently because of functional gastroparesis and pylorospasm. X-ray or endoscopic guidance may be necessary for insertion of a transpyloric tube. Because of difficult and time-consuming techniques, early tube feeding is often not applied. To evaluate its significance, we investigated the effects on lymphocyte subsets, of early enteral nutrition in trauma patients.

Methods

Institution approval was obtained, and 20 trauma patients with an Injury Severity Score > 30 points were included in the study. They received enteral nutritional support (standard diet) for 7 days. The patients were randomly grouped after administration on the intensive care ward. Group 1 patients were fed within the first 36 h via duodenal tubes, starting with an infusion rate of 25 ml/h and increasing by 25 ml/h amounts until the final dose, as measured by indirect calorimetry, was reached. Group 2 patients, after normalisation of gastric peristalsis, were fed isocaloric and isonitrogen diets via gastric tubes, starting on day four after trauma. In the first four days they were fed the isocaloric diet parenterally. Exclusion criteria were high-grade intestinal stenosis, decompensated insufficiency of liver and kidneys, necrotising pancreatitis, high dose of catecholamine requirement, and immunosuppressive therapy including the administration of glucocorticoids.

All patients received a standard infusion and transfusion therapy; antibiotics were given according to microbiological testing. The patients were on controlled mechanical ventilation and continuous sedation (fentanyl 5 μg/kg/h and midazolam 0.25 mg/kg/h). On days 1, 3, 5, 7 and 9, CD3+, CD19+, CD4+, CD8+ and CD3 HLA-DR+ lymphocyte subsets and natural killer (NK) cells were measured by flow cytometry.

Results

Both groups were comparable in their demographic data. The Injury Severity Score was 41 ± 4 in group 1 compared to 39 ± 5 in group 2. The number of CD3+ cells (see Fig. 1) was slightly elevated in group 1 compared to group 2 throughout the study period. CD4+ cell numbers (see Fig. 2) were higher in the early enterally fed group, and reached 49.2 ± 2.5 % on day 7 (group 2: 43.8 ± 3.4 %), and 51.2 ± 1.2 % on day 9 (group 2: 49.4 ± 2.1 %). The numbers of CD8+-, CD3-HLA-DR+-, and CD19+-lymphocyte subsets, and NK-cells showed no differences.

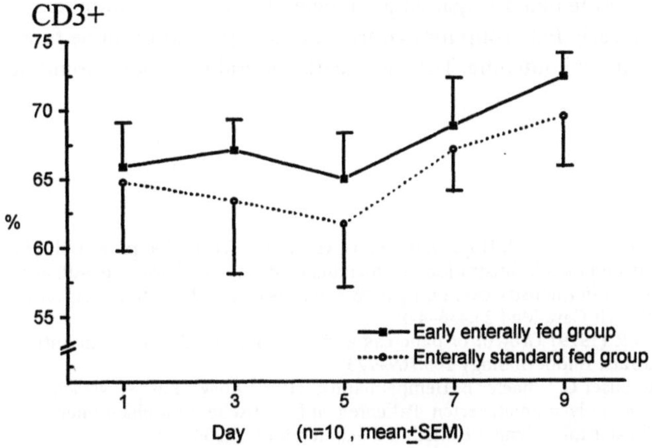

Fig. 1. Course of CD3+ (T) cells throughout the study period. The cells in group 1 were slightly elevated compared to group 2

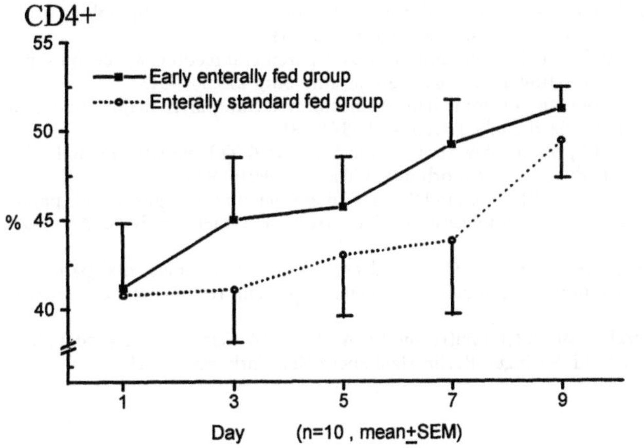

Fig. 2. Course of CD4+ (helper) cells throughout the study period. The cells in the early enterally fed group were higher than in the control group

Conclusion

In polytraumatised patients fed early by the enteral route, a tendency toward increased numbers of CD4+ cells and unchanged CD8+-levels was observed. This result is important because lymphocytes are cross wires of the humoral and cellular host immune response. CD3+ (T) lymphocytes are connected with cytokines to other immunologically active cells. In this way they can regulate the immune response. They can amplify this response in the form of CD4+ (helper) cells. For example, activated CD4+ (helper) cells induce the production and liberation of antibodies in B-cells. These functions characterise CD4+ (helper) cells as crucial elements of the immune system. Dysfunction of CD4+ (helper) cells can have deleterious consequences for the organism in the defence against pathogens. The increased numbers of CD4+ (helper) cells in the early fed group may contribute to improved immune function, suggesting a better clinical outcome. Therefore early enteral nutrition should be applied in trauma patients.

References

1. Bower R, Cerra F, Bershadsky B, Licari J, Hoyt D, Jensen G, van Buren CT, Rothkopf M, Daly JM, Adelsberger B (1995) Early enteral administration of a formula (Impact) supplemented with arginine, nucleotides, and fish oil in intensive care unit patients: results of a multicenter, prospective, randomized, clinical trial. Crit Care Med 23:436–449
2. Dembinski AB, Johnson LR (1979) Growth of pancreas and gastrointestinal mucosa in antrectoma and gastrin treated rats. Endocrinology 105:769–773
3. Engel JM, Menges T, Neuhäuser C, Schaefer B, Hempelmann G (1997) Auswirkungen verschiedener Ernährungsregime bei polytraumatisierten Patienten auf septische Komplikationen und Immunparameter. Anästhesiol Intensivmed Notfallmed Schmerzther 32:234–239
4. Fong Y, Marano MA, Barber A, He W, Moldawer LL, Bushman D, Coyle SM, Shires GT, Lowry SF (1989) Total parenteral nutrition and bowel rest modify the metabolic response to endotoxin in humans. Ann Surg 210:449–456
5. Goodlad RA, Al Mukhtar MYT, Ghatei MA, Bloom SR, Wright NA (1983) Cell proliferation plasma enteroglucagon and plasma gastrin levels in starved and refed rats. Virchows Arch Cell Path 43:55–62
6. Johnson LR (1987) Regulation of gastrointestinal growth. In: Johnson LR (ed) Physiology of the gastrointestinal tract. 2nd edn. Raven Press, New York, pp 301–333
7. Kudsk KA, Croce MA, Fabian TC et al. (1992) Enteral versus parenteral feeding: effects on septic morbidity after blunt and penetrating abdominal trauma. Ann Surg 215:503–513
8. Moore EE, Jones TN (1986) Benefits of immediate jejunostomy feeding after major abdominal trauma – A prospective, randomized study. J Trauma 26:874–881
9. Moore FA, Moore EE, Jones TN, McCroskey BL, Peterson VM (1989) TEN versus TPN following major abdominal trauma – Reduced septic morbidity. J Trauma 29:916–923
10. Moore FA, Feliciano DV, Andrassy RJ et al. (1992) Early enteral feeding, compared with parenteral, reduces postoperative septic complications. The result of a meta-analysis. Ann Surg 216:172–183
11. Peterson VM, Moore EE, Jones TN et al. (1988) Total enteral nutrition versus total parenteral nutrition after major torso injury: attenuation of hepatic protein reprioritization. Surgery 104:199–207
12. Zaloga GP (1993) Parenteral versus enteral nutrition. In: Wilmore DW, Carpentier YA (eds) Metabolic support of the critically ill. Springer, Berlin Heidelberg New York, pp 267–293

INVITED ARTICLE

Glutamine-supplemented Parenteral Nutrition

R. D. Griffiths · C. Esanu-Varnav

Department of Medicine, University of Liverpool, U.C.D. Duncan Building, Liverpool L69 3GA, UK

Abstract. Glutamine, a non-essential amino acid, is widely abundant in the body and in the food we eat. In times of stress it is released from skeletal muscle and acts as an interorgan nitrogen and carbon transporter. It is an important energy source directly to many cells and indirectly through glycogen metabolism. It is fundamental for protein synthesis, where it donates nitrogen for the synthesis of purines, pyrimidines, nucleotides and amino sugars, and is a precursor for the synthesis of the major antioxidant, glutathione. The kidney, liver, small intestine and cells of the immune system all use glutamine. Over the long term, the liver and immune systems predominate and use glutamine for synthetic processes and immune modulation.

L-Glutamine is absent from traditional parenteral amino acid solutions. Through a wealth of clinical studies, parenteral glutamine administration in the less severely ill has shown benefits to intestinal integrity and immune function, and can counteract the fall in muscle glutamine and protein synthesis following surgery. In the critically ill patient glutamine is depleted in plasma and skeletal muscle consistent with an excessive demand greater than can be met by endogenous supply. Exogenous glutamine, by promoting tissue integrity and enhancing the immune system, should improve outcome where supply is limited. In patients dependent on parenteral nutrition (PN), the benefit of its replacement would be seen by the prevention of late deaths, after the mortality risk of the initial illness has been overtaken by the other risks of a sustained ICU stay.

This hypothesis was examined in ICU patients unable to receive enteral feed. A prospective block-randomised, double-blind study compared a glutamine-PN with an isonitrogenous, isoenergetic control-PN, with the primary endpoint of mortality at six months post intervention and secondary endpoints of organ failure and cost (Griffiths RD et al., Nutrition 1997: 13:295–302). Survival at six months was significantly improved in those receiving glutamine parenteral nutrition (24/42 v 14/42; $P = 0.049$). More deaths occurred in the patients requiring control-PN for more than 10 days ($P = 0.03$). Control-PN deaths occurred later with a greater use of ICU and significantly longer total hospital post-intervention stay ($P = 0.012$). In the glutamine recipients, the total ICU and hospital cost *per survivor* was reduced by 50 %.

Introduction

Within the concept of nutrient provision, glutamine is traditionally considered to be a non-essential amino acid in the well, normal adult, because it can be synthesized within the body. However, over the last half-century, the importance and essential

M. K. Herbert et al. (Eds.), Problems of the Gastrointestinal Tract in Anesthesia...

nature of glutamine in human metabolism have been well documented. Furthermore, it is recognized that it becomes an essential nutrient for optimal tissue metabolism [1] during catabolic processes following injury, inflammation or infection, because demand may outstrip endogenous supply. Work in recent years has suggested that in the critically ill a deficiency state develops, and that supplementation with additional glutamine can correct this deficiency and improve outcome.

Physiology of Glutamine

Cell and Tissue Metabolism

Glutamine is the most prevalent free amino acid, and in skeletal muscle is about 60 % of the free amino acid pool[2]. Glutamine constitutes about 25 % of the total circulating free amino acids and is the most abundant amino acid in protein structures [3]. Glutamine is synthesised by the cytosolic glutamine synthetase in most tissues, and is degraded in the mitochondria by glutaminase. It is almost fifty years since glutamine was first shown to be a required nutrient for cell growth and proliferation in tissue culture, and in the early fifties Eagles tissue culture medium was developed, containing 2 mmol/l glutamine. Glutamine has been shown to be critical for the integrity and function of high turnover or metabolically active tissues [4] (immune system, small intestine and kidney). This is most strikingly illustrated by the cells of the immune system which show wide functional regulation within the physiological range of plasma glutamine levels experienced in health and disease [5]. Glutamine is the principle interorgan donor of carbon and nitrogen, for instance regulating purine, pyrimidine and nucleotide synthesis. Its very abundance, with large interorgan fluxes combined with a diverse participation in transamination reactions means that glutamine is a regulator of amino acid homeostasis [6].

The Immune System

Glutamine is metabolised by lymphocytes and macrophages at a rate which can be higher than that for glucose [7]. Only 5 %–25 % of glutamine carbons are oxidized completely, the rest being converted to glutamate, aspartate, alanine and carbon dioxide. This allows rapid clonal expansion and protein synthesis in lymphocytes, the repair of DNA and RNA damaged by reactive oxidative species in the phagocytic cells, mRNA synthesis and the release of cytokines in macrophages and lymphocytes. A rapid response to an immune challenge requires permanently high glutamine utilisation [8], known as branch-point sensitivity in control mechanisms. Both animal and ex-vivo studies on lymphocytes demonstrate a striking dose response relationship at physiological plasma glutamine concentrations that is critical for T lymphocyte function [9]. In patients with severe burns the rate of proliferation of lymphocytes and of phagocytosis by macrophages was impaired at the reduced plasma glutamine levels found in these patients [10]. Treatment of neutrophils ex-vivo with glutamine restored normal phagocytic function against *Staphylococcus aureus* in paediatric burn patients [11]. Recent work [12] suggests that glutamine enhances preferentially the Th1 lymphocyte response characterised by IL-2 production, macrophage activation and improved cell mediated immunity towards bacteria, fungi, viruses and tumour cells. Apoptosis occurs in lymphoid and parenchymal cells during sepsis [13]. In cell culture systems glutamine is protective against apoptosis in immune [14] and endothelial [15] cell lines. In promonocytic cell cultures, glutamine in the medium protected against heat induced apoptosis by enhancing the expression of heat shock proteins [16]. Whether this is a direct effect, or is mediated via increasing glutathione and protection of oxidative stress induced mechanisms, is unresolved. Most dietary glutamine is utilised primarily by the enterocytes and gut associated lymphoid tissue (GALT) [17], so the high glutamine requirement of immune cells outside the gastrointestinal (GI) tract must be met from the systemic circulation, and are as a consequence influenced by circulating levels. The migration of lymphocytes through the GALT means that secretory IgA function at all mucosal sites is influenced by GALT activity. Glutamine enterally could improve the primary immune defences against infections that have been shown in mice [18]. Infections are common following marathon races which are a major stress with a marked cytokine response. There is a 21 % decline in plasma glutamine and a marked leukocytosis and lymphopenia seen at 2 h following the race. In a randomised double-blind study of 151 subjects given a glutamine or a control drink immediately after, and 2 h following the race, the incidence of infections in the subsequent week was reduced from 52 % in the control to 19 % in the glutamine recipients [19].

Muscle Metabolism

Although most cells of the body possess glutamine synthetase only a few tissues produce glutamine for export to other organs. Both the lung and the brain produce glutamine, however it is skeletal muscle by virtue of its size that is the most important glutamine store, and this, together with its ability to synthesize glutamine de novo, makes it the most important source of glutamine for the bloodstream. Glutamine transport capacity across the sarcolemma is the main controlling factor in releasing glutamine into the bloodstream and in regulating its level [20]. The synthesis, storage and rapid release of glutamine makes the skeletal muscle an important participant in the immune response [21]. One of the initial responses to trauma or surgical stress [22], and in particular corticosteroids [23], is to export glutamine to the splanchnic bed from the free amino acid pool in muscle, leading to protein breakdown and de novo synthesis of glutamine. Skeletal muscle accounts for more than two thirds of the postabsorptive glutamine turnover. The contribution from protein breakdown or de novo synthesis has been reappraised, using improved analytical methods for the amount of protein-bound glutamine in the muscle. It had been thought that de novo synthesis contributed to 60 % of the turnover rate, but it is now recognised that this may be as much as 85 % [24]. The release of amino acids during catabolic stress can be modified by glucose and insulin, but while this attenuates alanine and other non-essential amino acid release, the efflux of glutamine continues [25].

Intestinal Metabolism

The gastrointestinal tract, particularly the enterocyte, is a net consumer of glutamine in part as a respiratory fuel. The uptake of glutamine is concentration- and therefore supply-dependent. The concentrations and distribution of the key enzymes involved in glutamine synthesis (glutamine synthetase) and breakdown (glutaminase) have been mapped along the human gastrointestinal tract [26]. The small and to some extent the large bowel have the greatest ability to utilize glutamine, but have little synthesizing capacity. In contrast neither the oesophagus nor stomach have much glutaminase and therefore probably use little glutamine. The stomach, uniquely, has substantial capacity to synthesize glutamine. The lowest glutamine and highest glutamate concentrations are found in the duodenum, consistent with the small bowel as the greatest consumer of glutamine, which it must derive from the lumen or from the circulation. Glutamine utilisation in the small intestine may be more important for cellular respiration than glucose [27]. In the small intestine, glutamine carbon atoms can be metabolised via two main routes. The Krebs cycle represents the first route (75 % of the carbon atoms) with more than 50 % of carbon atoms being oxidized to CO_2, and the remainder forming citrate, lactate, other intermediate compounds, and glucose [28]. The second route will lead to the incorporation of glutamine in protein structures (10 %–15 %). The last 10 % of the glutamine carbon atoms will result in the formation of proline, ornithine and citrulline, which are then exported by the circulation to be utilised in other organs [29]. Enterocytes have a dual source of glutamine: the arterial blood and the intestinal lumen. Evidence suggests that the enterocyte can utilise other substrates such as glutamate when presented on the luminal side [17] but in the absence of feeding, arterial glutamine supply may become critical for glutamine dependent metabolism. As has been discussed above for immune cells, in a cell line of rat small intestine, the presence of glutamine induced the expression of heat shock proteins (HSP70) and conferred protection against lethal heat stress [30].

Liver Metabolism

Glutamine plays a very important role in ammonia and urea metabolism in the liver. In the splanchnic bed, the majority of glutamine is only partially metabolised to intermediate products of metabolism, with the nitrogen released as ammonia and alanine in the portal vein. In the liver, ammonia is transformed by the periportal, glutaminase-rich hepatocytes into urea, consuming bicarbonate ions in molar proportions. A smaller population of perivenous hepatocytes, devoid of urea-synthesizing enzymes but rich in glutamine synthetase, takes up the ammonia which escapes detoxification by urea synthesis, together with glutamate, aspartate and α-oxoglutarate and synthesizes glutamine [31]. In normal conditions, the end result of this process of cycling of glutamine is the metabolisation of ammonia, with synthesis of urea and no significant glutamine flux in the liver [32]. In a state of metabolic acidosis, there is a decrease in the synthesis of urea, with an increase in perivenous glutamine synthesis. Urea synthesis is a major pathway for bicarbonate elimination, the reduction in urea synthesis representing a homeostatic response to acidosis and bicarbonate conservation [33].

Glutamine is an important substrate for the synthesis of glutathione, which is predominantly synthesized in the liver but also in many other tissues. Glutathione is abundant in many mammalian tissues and acts as an endogenous scavenger with the ability to counteract oxidative injury from oxygen free radicals. In animal models glutamine-enriched total parenteral nutrition has been shown to enhance plasma glutathione [34] and to protect the liver against paracetamol toxicity [35]. Glutamine availability may determine the size and distribution of the glutathione stores in the body and, ultimately, the organism's capacity to oppose an oxidative insult.

Kidney Metabolism

During normal acid-base balance little glutamine will be taken and metabolized by the kidney. There is an increased utilisation of glutamine in acidosis. In an acute episode certain enzymes will be activated by the low pH, while in chronic acidosis enzyme induction is the main mechanism. The extracted glutamine is deaminated and deamidated, generating two ammonia ions. This will provide a cation for excretion, with preservation of the sodium and potassium and the generation of bicarbonate ions [36]. The kidney also participates in the glutamine metabolism, by utilising the citrulline produced from glutamine metabolism in the gut, as the sole precursor for the synthesis of arginine [37]. Arginine, a conditionally essential amino acid, participates in the urea cycle and in the citric acid cycle, is a nitrogen source for the nitric oxide synthesis and stimulates the secretion of anabolic hormones (growth hormone, insulin). Whilst glutamine increases arginine production, it has been shown to paradoxically reduce NO production, playing, as yet, a poorly explored role in endothelial metabolism and vascular control [38].

Lung Metabolism

The lung has capacity to synthesize glutamine, and in normal circumstances it is an organ of net release of glutamine in the systemic circulation [39], as shown by measurements using cardiac catheters. In surgical patients, very early in a septic episode there is a significant release of glutamine from the lung [40]. Development of a lung injury will lead to an inability of the lung to release glutamine, followed by a net utilisation of glutamine [41].

Parenteral Glutamine

Safety and Tolerance of Intravenous Glutamine in Humans

Products

The dialyzed enzymatic casein hydrolysates used in the 1940s and 1950s for intravenous nutrition were comprised of amino acids and low molecular weight peptides with significant amount of glutamine in the original protein. With the development of amino acid solutions in the 1970s glutamine was not included in the formulations. It

Table 1. Randomised clinical studies using parenteral glutamine

Patient group	Outcome	Comment
Elective abdominal or hip surgery	Improves nitrogen balance Prevents decline in muscle glutamine Prevents fall in protein synthesis in muscle	Stehle P et al.(1989) Lancet 1:231–233 Hammarqvist F et al. (1989) Ann. Surg 209:455–461 Blomqvist BI et al. (1995) Metabolism 44:1215–22
Bone marrow transplants	Reduces infectious complications Shorter hospital stay Prevents decline in protein C levels from liver	Ziegler TR et al. (1992) Ann Intern Med 116:821 Schloerb PR et al. JPEN 1993: 17:407–413 Brown SA et al. (1998) Bone Marrow Transplantation 22:281–284
Colorectal surgery	Increases immune cell proliferation and function Increases immune cell proliferation and function Shorter hospital stay	O'Riordain MG et al. (1994) Ann Surg 220:212–221 Morlion BJ et al. (1998) Ann Surg 227:302–308
TPN pre-operative bowel surgery	Counteracts increased gut permeability, preserves intestinal morphology, restores mucosal glutamine, and modifies intraepithelial immune cell responses	van der Hulst RRWJ et al. (1993)Lancet 334:1363–1365 van der Hulst RRWJ et al. (1996) Surg Res 62:30–34 van der Hulst RRWJ et al. (1997) JPEN 21:310–315
Pre-term infants	Fewer septic episodes Earlier onset of feeding	Lacey JM et al. (1996) JPEN 20:74–80
ICU patients	Enhances D-xylose absorption in small bowel	Tremel B et al. Gastroenterology 1994: 107:1595–1601
ICU patients with MOF	Improved 6-month survival	Griffiths RD et al. (1997) Nutrition 13:295–303

was considered impracticable to include glutamine, since to have a good shelf life the solutions required heat sterilization, and glutamine would thus be converted to the cyclic compound pyroglutamic acid, with the quantitative elimination of ammonia [42]. Recently, to overcome this problem commercially, heat-stable, synthetic glutamine-containing dipeptides are now incorporated into some parenteral formulations [43]. Alternatively, solutions of L-glutamine can be prepared under aseptic conditions and sterilised by filtration [44] but solubility of L-glutamine generally means that only a 2.5 % solution can be safely made to avoid precipitation. The general stability of L-glutamine solutions in practice is good and whether there is any real clinical risk of toxicity from pyroglutamate has been well argued against [45]. In humans there is a wide expression of 5-oxoprolinase, the enzyme responsible for the conversion back to glutamic acid as an integral part of the glutathione pathway [46]. Furthermore the early protein hydrolysates had much of the glutamine probably converted to pyroglutamic acid, and were used successfully without apparent ill effect [47]. The clinical studies discussed below (and in Table1) have used either L-glutamine solutions, on their own and as part of all-in-one mixtures, or have used the dipeptides L-alanyl-L-glutamine (Ala-Gln) or glycyl-L-glutamine (Gly-Gln), the former having almost a four-fold better solubility.

Human Studies

Human volunteer studies using L-glutamine infusions showed that it was rapidly distributed into the extracellular space. Elevations in normal plasma levels of glutamine could be achieved with doses of between 0.285 g Gln/kg/day and 0.570 g Gln/Kg/day, which for a 70 kg male would require between 20 and 42 g of glutamine per day [48]. There was no apparent toxicity without any significant increase in circulating glutamate or ammonia. Giving the dipeptides to human volunteers [49] has shown that the dipeptide is rapidly hydrolyzed to the amino acids intra- and extra-cellularly with no tissue accumulation of the dipeptide or transfer across the normal blood brain barrier [50]. Infusion studies of Ala-Gln [51] and Gly-Gln [52] in the post-absorptive and starved human suggest an important role for the kidney in dipeptide clearance. This was associated with increased plasma concentrations and enhanced splanchnic uptake of their respective amino acids. Ala-Gln has a faster clearance than Gly-Gln but there is no physiological evidence to suggest an advantage of one over the other [53] as a method of delivering glutamine. Glutamine has been administered for up to four weeks at about 20 g/day in stable patients on home parenteral nutrition. The addition of glutamine was discontinued because there was an increase in liver enzyme activity, but no change in ammonia metabolism, and in those few patients it was resolved when glutamine administration was ceased [54]. There is no theoretical evidence to suggest that healthy subjects would require glutamine, and these patients had short bowels and possibly even had reduced glutamine requirements. The excess glutamine would then have had to be metabolized by the liver.

The Mechanism for the Glutamine Clinical Effects

Skeletal Muscle and Nitrogen Balance

The first clinical studies to examine physiological effects were performed on patients undergoing elective operations where the surgical stress was predictable and standardized, and the decline of free glutamine in muscle well documented.

Following trauma or surgery there is a consistent and similar pattern of amino acid changes in skeletal muscle, that occurs promptly and takes many days to recover [55]. There is a marked depletion of non-essential amino acids, notably glutamine, with an increase in essential amino acids. The most distinct rise is in the branched chain amino acids (precursors of glutamine), phenylalanine, tyrosine and methionine. Studies using isonitrogenous, isoenergetic controls have indicated that the administration of parenteral nutrition supplemented with glutamine [56], ornithine-alpha-ketoglutarate [57], or dipeptide alanyl-glutamine, reduces nitrogen loss [58] and the depletion of intracellular glutamine following the stress of elective abdominal surgery. In patients undergoing hip replacement, glutamine as the sole nitrogen source has been shown to acutely attenuate the intracellular glutamine loss and reduction in protein synthesis as measured by polyribosome concentration [59]. The changes in muscle glutamine over one month have been followed in elective cholecystectomy patients receiving parenteral Gly-Gln (25 g) for 3 days post-operatively, before returning to a normal diet [60]. The presence of glutamine prevented the initial decline in plasma and muscle glutamine, but this fell once oral diet started so that by 10 days there was no difference between the control and glutamine recipients. The acute association between a fall in intracellular free glutamine and a decline in protein synthesis first seen in animal models was similarly observed in these studies [56, 59] but a direct relationship may not apply and is probably unlikely over several days. These studies had examined whether providing extra glutamine could prevent an acute fall in muscle glutamine. A more recent study has examined whether glutamine could replete the intracellular muscle glutamine pool and stimulate protein synthesis. Elective colon surgery patients were studied for 2 to 3 days post-operatively following an acute infusion of 0.285 g/kg body weight (about 20 g) glutamine over 5.5 h [61]. Despite a doubling in plasma glutamine there was no increase in the low intramuscular free glutamine and no stimulation of the depressed protein synthesis rates as measured by the flooding-dose stable isotope method and on ribosomal analysis. The clinical extreme is the critically ill patient with an intramuscular glutamine pool depleted by some 70 % to 80 % prior to commencing nutrition [62, 63] and where 20 g of glutamine per day for 5 days could not return this to normal. Furthermore even if it proved possible to replete the intramuscular free glutamine pool it has yet to be proved whether this could have an effect on muscle protein synthesis. At this dose in ICU patients, although there was an initial rise in plasma glutamine, a sustained statistical elevation in plasma glutamine could not be demonstrated, perhaps not unexpectedly when given as an infusion over 24 h [63]. A sustained elevation in plasma glutamine has been shown in multiple trauma patients in ICU, only when given as a larger dose, equivalent to 28 g Gln (as 40 g dipeptide Gly-Gln) [64]. This dosage was well tolerated without adverse effects. The effect on the muscle glutamine pool in critically ill patients at this dose has not been tested. A 7 g dose however, infused at three times this rate over two hours in normal subjects, doubles plasma levels and elevates muscle glutamine [65]. Compared with an infusion of alanine and glycine, glutamine alone significantly increased muscle glycogen re-accumulation post-exercise, independent of any changes in circulatory glucose or insulin. The reverse is also true in that glycogen is a precursor of tricarboxylic acid (TCA) cycle intermediates and subsequently of glutamine. As mentioned earlier the majority of glutamine is made by de novo synthesis particularly from the branched chain amino acids that are increased during protein breakdown [66]. With trauma and sepsis, the metabolism of branched chain amino acids is accelerated in muscle, and through the aminotransferase reaction uses 2-oxoglutarate in the formation of glutamate on its way to form glutamine through glutamine synthetase. Such a drain on the intermediates of the TCA cycle could compromise glutamine production [67]. However wasting of muscle means that there is also depletion in the overall production of glutamine. The wasting of muscle can be extreme. Detailed whole body composition analysis is now possible in the very sick. Recent work [68] shows that over a 21 day period, patients who were critically ill after trauma or sepsis had staggering losses of lean body mass (whole body water and protein) of almost 1 % loss *per day of illness*, far greater than can be accounted for by bed rest alone. The majority is lost from skeletal muscle, confirming biopsy studies in the very sick, that show an average loss of fibre area of more than 2 % per day [69], and protein loss to the same extent [70].

Gastrointestinal Tract and Liver

With glutamine utilisation carried out principally by the small bowel and colon it is not surprising, therefore, that studies using glutamine therapeutically to influence disorders of the mouth, oesophagus and stomach have proved unsuccessful [71]. An intraoperative study of patients with gastrointestinal cancer measured arterio-venous differences in different regions of the bowel [72]. Glutamine consumption was highest in the jejunum, three times higher than in the ileum or colon. Uptake was related to arterial glutamine concentration, suggesting reduced uptake when plasma levels fall. Small intestinal glutamine content is reduced in those patients with the reduced body mass associated with nutritional depletion secondary to cancer [73]. Arterial levels of glutamine are lower relative to the reduction below ideal body weight [72]. A glutamine-containing parenteral nutrition (about 15 g/day) for 10 days was shown to be able to return the plasma glutamine level to normal, and to increase the mucosal glutamine content in those patients who were depleted [74]. It made no difference to those who had normal glutamine content. Unlike these features of starvation the features seen in sepsis are different. The glutamine content of the duodenal mucosa in the critically ill patients that have been studied during periods of sepsis show an elevation, while it is unaltered in the colon and depressed in the rectal mucosa [75] although the plasma glutamine level was significantly depressed. This may be due to a depression in the activity of glutaminase that has been described in the mucosa in sepsis [76]. Glutamine-supplemented total parenteral nutrition (TPN) has been shown to prevent the changes in gut morphology and the increased permeability that occur with 10 days of parenteral nutrition [77] and to improve the absorptive capacity in those given glutamine [78]. A hypothesis has been developed that suggests that glutamine has a role in preserving the integrity of the intestinal tract and in supporting the barrier function against the translocation of bacteria and toxins to the portal and systemic circulation [79]. Although translocation has been described in humans it is not reflected by the changes in permeation as measured by absorbable sugars [80]. It is perhaps the immune barrier which is significant, and parenteral glutamine has been shown to decrease the intestinal immune cell activation that occurs in the absence of enteral feeding [81]. The most dramatic clinical demonstration of the protective effect of glutamine against infection comes from a recently published study of enteral nutrition given early to patients with multiple trauma. Multiple trauma patients, whilst initially uninfected, are at increased risk of infection particularly from gram-negative organisms. In a carefully structured, randomised, masked study of 60 trauma patients [82], enteral glutamine-enriched nutrition given naso-duodenally within 48 h of the trauma, significantly reduced the incidence of pneumonia and bacteremia by more than 50 %, possibly mediated by the immunoprotective mechanisms discussed earlier.

Hepatic veno-occlusive disease of the liver is a complication that can follow high-dose cytotoxic chemotherapy for bone marrow transplantation (BMT). The maintenance of adequate tissue glutathione levels may be critical for the prevention of this complication. Falling protein C levels have been shown to be predictive of severe veno-occlusive disease. In 34 patients undergoing BMT, parenteral glycyl-L-glutamine given in a randomised study was shown to prevent the fall in protein C levels suggesting a degree of hepatic protection [83].

Immune Function

The first randomised, double-blind controlled study of glutamine-supplemented parenteral nutrition was in allogenic bone marrow transplant patients [84]. Isonitrogenous infusions were continued until 50 % of oral intake was achieved. Fewer glutamine recipients developed clinical infection, and hospital stay was significantly shorter, with cost savings. This was confirmed in a similar study that also showed an improved nitrogen balance, a reduction in the number of bacterial infections, less extracellular fluid expansion and a significantly shorter hospital stay [85]. Glutamine treated patients had a greater percentage of lymphocytes after engraftment, with improvement seen in the T lymphocyte population [86]. Premature infants receiving glutamine have fewer septic episodes and an earlier onset of enteral feeding [87]. Following colorectal surgery, patients given glutamine for 5 days showed an increase in T cell DNA synthesis, compared with an isonitrogenous control [88]. The same group have also shown that glutamine reduces mononuclear cell interleukin-8 release in severe acute pancreatitis [89]. There was also some evidence of improved lymphocyte proliferation and this may account for the immune modulation of the cytokine release. In another randomised post-operative study, patients given glutamine following bowel surgery showed improved nitrogen balances, shorter lengths of stay and improved recovery of lymphocyte counts. As a measure of improved immune status, they demonstrated an improved generation of cysteinyl-leukotrienes from polymorphonuclear neutrophil granulocytes [90].

Glutamine and Critical Illness

In the critically ill, glutamine requirement can significantly outstrip the endogenous supply from muscle [91]. The alterations in the amino acid profile in critical illness are well characterized in the plasma, with an increase in the branched chain amino acids (muscle protein catabolism and lack of utilisation) and a reduction in glutamine and arginine (increased utilisation and/or decreased synthesis). A constant finding is a reduction of at least 50 % in intracellular free glutamine levels [92] in ICU patients, with intramuscular glutamine reduced by some 75 % [93, 94]. Plasma levels of arginine and glutathione are lowered, the immune function is affected and the integrity of the gut barrier is compromised. Plasma and intramuscular glutathione levels fall in critical illness [95] in parallel with the depletion of glutamine, in distinct contrast to the absence of change in the sulphur amino acid precursor, cysteine. Such reduction in the antioxidant defences of the organism comes at a time when free radicals are being produced in large numbers.

Intensive Care Glutamine Study

If a deficiency exists and glutamine supply is a limiting factor in the critically ill, the benefit of its exogenous replacement would be seen by the prevention of *late deaths*, often due to sepsis, after the mortality risk of the initial illness has been overtaken by the other risks of a sustained ICU stay. This hypothesis was examined using a prospective block-randomised, double-blind design to test whether "all in one" glutamine-PN compared with isonitrogenous, isoenergetic control-PN would influence outcome, with the endpoints of morbidity, mortality and cost at six months post intervention [96], (also see editorial reviews [97, 98]).

Eighty-four critically ill adult patients, median age 65 years, with APACHE II score >10, were started on PN if enteral nutrition was contraindicated or unsuccessful, i.e., had gastrointestinal failure. Randomisation produced well-matched groups. Plasma glutamine was reduced similarly in both groups from a normal value of 0.64 (95 % C.I. 0.55 to 0.72) mmol/l to a mean of 0.34 (95 % C.I. 0.26 to 0.43) mmol/l. In a representative sample of these patients, muscle glutamine was depleted by 75 % or more to a mean of 3.1 (95 % C.I. 2.2 to 4.0) mmol/kg wet weight. Over three-quarters of the patients had major sepsis with intra-abdominal causes being the most common. Survival at 6 months was significantly better with glutamine-PN 57 % v control-PN 33 %, $P = 0.049$. The mortality in the control group was similar to an age and illness severity matched group receiving a conventional feed in the year preceding the study. In patients who received PN for more than 10 days, there was significantly greater mortality in those dependent on the control (glutamine deficient) formulation compared with those receiving a glutamine-containing feed ($P = 0.03$). Differences in mortality increased with time in patients on PN, and were related only to the presence or absence of glutamine, and not to age, illness severity or total amount of nutrition received. (Fig. 1)

Despite the greater survival rate in the glutamine group, total hospital costs did not increase as might be expected, since the excess control-PN deaths occurred later, and the patients had a significantly longer (and therefore costlier) post-intervention stay ($P = 0.013$) and use of ICU. As a consequence, the use of glutamine-PN led to a 50 % reduction in the total ICU and hospital cost when expressed *per survivor*. A low body mass index is an independent predictor of an excess mortality rate in multiple organ failure, and this becomes evident at about 25 days into the illness [99]. Multiple organ failure (MOF) was the principal cause of death in ICU and strikingly, the deaths in the control-PN group occurred after 21 days in ICU, consistent with the time scales

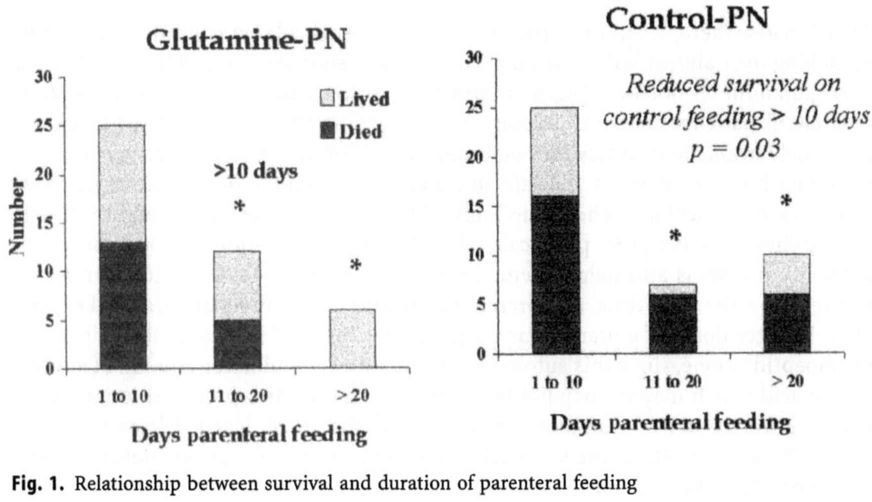

Fig. 1. Relationship between survival and duration of parenteral feeding

expected with muscle wasting, the majority of these deaths from MOF. This suggests that endogenous glutamine supply had become critical to survival, probably as a result of progressive skeletal muscle loss. Is this excess mortality rate due to a deficiency of glutamine depriving the gut, liver and immune system? Interestingly, when glutamine was replaced parenterally, the survival rate became comparable to patients with similar illness severity, fed enterally. These results do not imply a precise mechanism but suggest that instead of preserving functional muscle mass, the exogenous glutamine may confer a survival advantage by ameliorating some of the immediate consequences of the lack of endogenous glutamine supply from a reducing skeletal muscle pool.

What is the Required Dose?

There are few data to give firm advice. Most studies have used fixed proportions delivering from 15 to 30 g/day. A post-operative patient with less glutamine demand may require a figure at the lower end while a severely injured patient with multiple trauma or burns may require 25 to 35 g/day. Whether the ability to raise plasma glutamine is a sufficient indicator of appropriate dose is not clear, but the proposed benefits to the immune system would suggest that this is a reasonable approach. Clinical evidence for showing that enteral supplements significantly raise plasma or tissue glutamine levels for a sustained period is poor. Indeed, there is contrary evidence which suggests that plasma glutamine levels are slower to recover when the same dose of glutamine is given enterally rather than parenterally [100]. The enteral route may be sufficient when given early to the non-infected patient (e.g., trauma) to improve GALT function and the immune defence against infection [82], however, for the already severely stressed or infected ICU patient, enteral supplements alone may be inadequate, and parallel parenteral support is likely to be required.

Conclusion

There are few therapies in the critically ill that have such a large scientific background stretching over almost half a century. There is now sufficient evidence for one to ask why glutamine is not being used routinely as a constituent of parenteral feeds in severely ill patients unable to tolerate enteral feeding [98]. In the United Kingdom, the widely available facilities for combining sterile products in pharmacies found in nearly all hospitals permits the safe addition of L-glutamine to parenteral nutrition solutions for clinical use. The limited solubility of L-glutamine entails larger volumes, so elsewhere this is not so practicable, but the newer dipeptide solutions overcome solubility problems and help provide longer shelf lives for storage. However, we do not yet know the right dose, and present formulations merely reflect practical expedience. If larger doses of glutamine are required this may not be practicable with a single dipeptide alone, since this automatically supplies an equimolar amount of another amino acid which may or may not be necessary. The sceptics prepared to ignore the evidence for the use of glutamine could examine the lesson learned from the use of growth hormone in the acutely critically ill patient. Despite the good intention of trying to preserve the skeletal muscle mass, the consequence of this expensive therapy may have been to suppress the release of glutamine and, therefore, its availability to the immune system [101]. This may well have accounted for the excess mortality rate seen in two recent multi-centre studies. Perhaps this could have been avoided by giving exogenous glutamine?

Acknowledgements. I would like to thank the Sir Jules Thorn Charitable Trust, Oxford Nutrition, and the staff, colleagues and patients on the Intensive Care Unit at Whiston Hospital, Merseyside, for without them this work would not have been possible.

References

1. Lacey JM, Wilmore DW (1990) Is glutamine a conditionally essential amino acid? Nutr Rev 48:297–309
2. Bergström J, Fürst P, Noree L-O, Vinnars E (1974) Intracellular free amino acid concentration in human muscle tissue. J Appl Physiol 36:693–697
3. Souba WW (1991) Glutamine: a key substrate for the splanchnic bed. Annu Rev Nutr 11:285–308
4. Roth E, Karner J, Ollenshlager G. (1990) Glutamine: an anabolic effect? JPEN 14:130S-136S
5. Newsholme EA, Calder PC. (1997) The proposed role of glutamine in some cells of the immune system and speculative consequences for the whole animal. Nutrition 13:728–730
6. Meister A (1956) Metabolism of glutamine. Physiol Rev 36:103–127
7. Newsholme EA, Crabtree B, Ardawi MSM (1985) Glutamine metabolism in lymphocytes: its biochemical, physiological and clinical importance. Q J Exp Physiol 70:473–489
8. Calder PC (1995) Glutamine action in cells of the immune system. In: Cynober L, Furst P, Lawin P (ed) Pharmacological Nutrition Immune Nutrition (International Symposium) W. Zuckschwerdt Verlag, Munchen, 10–20
9. Yaqoob P, Calder PC (1997) Glutamine requirements of proliferating T lymphocytes. Nutrition 13: 646–651
10. Parry-Billings M, Evans J, Calder PC, Newsholme EA (1990) Does glutamine contribute to immunosuppression after major burns? Lancet 336:523–525
11. Ogle CK, Ogle JD, Mao J-X, Simon J, Noel JG, Li B-G, Alexander JW (1994) Effect of glutamine on phagocytosis and bacterial killing by normal and pediatric burn patient neutrophils. JPEN 18:128–133
12. Yaqoob P, Kew S, Wallace FA, Miles EA, Calder PC (1998) Dietary glutamine enhances Th1 lymphocyte responses. Clin Nutr 17 (suppl 1): 33-P.17
13. Kotchkiss RS, Swanson PE, Cobb JP, Jacobson A, Buchman TG, Karl IE (1997) Apoptosis in lymphoid and parenchymal cells during sepsis: findings in normal and T and B cell-deficient mice. Crit Care Med 25(8): 1298–1307
14. Petronini PG, Urbani S, Alfieri R, Borghetti AF, Guidotti GG (1996) Cell susceptibility to apoptosis by glutamine deprivation and rescue: survival and apoptotic death in cultured lymphoma-leukemia cell line. J Cell Physiol 169(1): 175–185
15. Parolari A, Sala R, Antona C, Bussolatti O, Alamanni F, Mezzadri P, Dall'Asta V, Gazzola GC, Biglioli P (1997) Hypertonicity induces injury to cultured human endothelium: attenuation by glutamine. Ann Thorac Surg 64(6): 1770–1775
16. Weingartmann G, Brabec M, Oehler R, Spittler A, Roth E (1998) Glutamine protects U937 cells against heat induced apoptosis in association with high expression of hsp70. Clin Nutr 17(Suppl 1): 34-P.18
17. Matthews DE, Marano MA, Campbell RG (1993) Splanchnic bed utilisation of glutamine and glutamic acid in humans. Am J Physiol 264:E848-E854
18. Li J, King BK, Janu PG, Renegar KB, Kudsk KA (1998) Glycyl-L-glutamine-enriched total parenteral nutrition maintains small intestine gut-associated lymphoid tissue and upper respiratory tract immunity. JPEN 22:31–36
19. Castell LM, Newsholme EA (1997) The effects of oral glutamine-supplementation on athletes after prolonged, exhaustive exercise. Nutrition 13:738–742
20. Rennie MJ, MacLennan PA, Hundal HS, Weryk B, Smith K, Taylor PM, Egan C, Watt PW (1989) Skeletal muscle glutamine transport, intramuscular glutamine concentration, and muscle protein turnover. Metabolism 38:47–51

21. Newsholme EA, Parry-Billings M (1990) Properties of glutamine release from muscle and its importance for the immune system. JPEN 14:63S-67S
22. Deutz NEP, Reijven PLM, Athanasas G, Soeters PB (1992) Post-operative changes in hepatic, intestinal, splenic and muscle fluxes of amino acids and ammonia in pigs. Clin Sci 83:607–614
23. Tamarappoo BK, Nam M, Kilberg MS, Welbourne TC (1993) Glucocorticoid regulation of splanchnic glutamine, alanine, glutamate, ammonia, and glutathione fluxes. Am J Physiol 264 (Endocrinol. Metab. 27): E526-E533
24. Kuhn KS, Schuhman K, Stehle P, Fürst P (1998) De novo synthesis represents a greater proportion of muscle glutamine turnover than previously assumed. Clin Nutr 17 (Suppl 1): 10–O.33
25. Brooks D, Bessey PQ, Black PR, Aoki TT, Wilmore DW (1986) Insulin stimulates branched chain amino acid uptake and diminishes nitrogen flux from skeletal muscle in injured patients. J Surg Res 40:395–405
26. James LA, Lunn PG, Middleton S, Elia M (1998) Distribution of glutaminase and glutamine synthetase activities in the human gastrointestinal tract. Clin Sci 94:313–319
27. Hartmann F, Plauth M (1989) Intestinal glutamine metabolism. Metabolism Suppl 1 38:18–24
28. Windmueller HG (1982) Glutamine utilisation by the small intestine. Adv Enzymol 53:201–237
29. Souba WW, Herskowitz K, Salloum RM, Chen MK, Austgen TR (1990) Gut glutamine metabolism. JPEN (Suppl 4) 14:45S-49S
30. Wischmeyer PE, Musch MW, Madonna MB, Thisted R, Chang EB (1997) Glutamine protects intestinal epithelial cells: role of inducible HSP70. Am J Physiol 272 (Gastrointest Liver Physiol 35): G879-G884
31. Haussinger D, Gerok W (1983) Hepatocyte heterogeneity in glutamate uptake by isolated perfused rat liver. Eur J Biochem 136:421–425
32. Haussinger D (1990) Liver glutamine metabolism. JPEN 14 (Suppl 4):56S-62S
33. Welbourne TC, Joshi S (1990) Intraorgan glutamine metabolism during acidosis. JPEN 14 Suppl 4:77S-85S
34. Denno R, Rounds JD, Faris R, Holejko LB, Wilmore DW (1996) Glutamine-enriched total parenteral nutrition enhances plasma glutathione in the resting state. J Surg Res 61:35–38
35. Hong RW, Rounds JD, Helton WS, Robinson MK, Wilmore DW (1992) Glutamine preserves liver glutathione after lethal hepatic injury. Ann Surg: 215:114–119
36. Sies H, Haussinger D (1984) Hepatic glutamine and ammonia metabolism. In: Haussinger D, Sies H. (ed) Glutamine metabolism in mammalian tissues. Springer, Berlin Heidelberg New York, pp 78–97
37. Houdjik APJ, Van Leeuwen PAM, Teerlink T et al. (1994) Glutamine-enriched enteral diet increases renal arginine synthesis. JPEN 18:422–426
38. Roth E (1998) L-Arginine-nitric oxide metabolism. Glutamine: a new player in this metabolic game. Editorial. Clin Nutr 17:1–2
39. Plumley DA, Austgen TR, Salloum RM, Souba WW (1990) Role of the lungs in maintaining amino acid homeostasis. JPEN 14:569–573
40. Plumley DA, Souba WW, Hautamaki RD, Martin TD, Flynn TC, Rout WR, Copeland EM (1990) Accelerated lung amino acid release in hyperdynamic septic surgical patients. Arch Surg 125:57–61
41. Souba WW, Herskowitz K, Plumley DA (1990) Lung glutamine metabolism. JPEN 14 Suppl 4:68S-70S
42. Grimble G (1993) Glutamine, glutamate and pyroglutamate – facts and fantasies. Clin Nutr 12:66–69
43. Fürst P, Pogan K, Stehle P (1997) Glutamine dipeptides in clinical nutrition. Nutrition 13:731–737
44. Khan K, Hardy G, McElroy B, Elia M (1991) The stability of L-glutamine in total parenteral nutrition solutions. Clin Nutr 10:193–198
45. Grimble GK, McElroy B, Aimer P, Hardy G, Silk DBA (1997) The stability of glutamine added to TPN regimens for critically ill patients. Br J Intensive Care 7:126–136
46. Szewczuk A, Kwiatkowska J (1970) Pyrolidonyl peptidase in animal, plant and human tissues: occurrence and some properties of the enzyme. Eur J Biochem 15:92–96
47. Aqvist S, Wretlind A (1957) Pyrolidone carboxylic acid in enzymatic casein hydrolysates. Acta Physiol Scand 39:147–157
48. Ziegler TR, Benfell K, Smith RJ, Young LS, Brown E, Ferrari-Baliviera E, Lowe DK, Wilmore DW (1990) Safety and metabolic effects of L-Glutamine administration in humans. JPEN 14:137S-146S
49. Lochs H, Hubl W (1990) Metabolic basis for selecting glutamine-containing substrates for parenteral nutrition. JPEN 14:114S-117S

50. Himmelseher S, Pfenninger E, Herrman P (1996) Cerebrospinal and plasma amino acid concentrations after administration of IV glycyl-glutamine and glycyl-tyrosine containing amino acid solutions in humans. JPEN 20:281–286
51. Lochs H, Roth E, Gasic S, Hubl W, Morse EL, Adibi SA (1990) Splanchnic, renal, and muscle clearance of alanylglutamine in man and organ fluxes of alanine and glutamine when infused in free and peptide forms. Metabolism 39:833–836
52. Lochs H, Hubl W, Gasic S, Roth E, Morse EL, Adibi SA (1992) Glycylglutamine: metabolism and effects on organ balances of amino acids in postabsorptive and starved subjects. Am J Physiol Endocrinol Metab 262:E155-E160
53. Fürst P, Albers S, Stehle P (1990) Glutamine-containing dipeptides in parenteral nutrition. JPEN 14:118S-124S
54. Hornsby-Lewis L, Shike M, Brown P, Klang M, Pearlstone D, Brennan MF (1994) L-Glutamine supplementation in home total parenteral nutrition patients: stability, safety, and effects on intestinal absorption. JPEN 18:268–273
55. Askanazi J, Carpentier YA, Michelsen CB, Elwyn DH, Furst P, Kantrowitz LR, Gump FE, Kinney JM (1980) Muscle and plasma amino acids following injury: influence of intercurrent infection. Ann Surg 192:78–85
56. Hammarqvist F, Wernerman J, Ali R, von der Decken A, Vinnars E (1989) Addition of glutamine to total parenteral nutrition after elective abdominal surgery spares free glutamine in muscle, counteracts the fall in muscle protein synthesis, and improves nitrogen balance. Ann Surg 209:455–461
57. Wernerman J, Hammarqvist F, Ali MR, Vinnars E (1989) Glutamine and ornithine-alpha-ketoglutarate but not branched-chain amino acids reduce the loss of muscle glutamine after surgical trauma. Metabolism 38 (8 suppl 1): 63–6
58. Stehle P, Zander J, Mertes N, Albers S, Puchstein C, Lawin P, Furst P (1989) Effect of parenteral glutamine peptide supplements on muscle glutamine loss and nitrogen balance after major surgery. Lancet 1 (8632): 231–3
59. Blomqvist BI, Hammarqvist F, von der Decken A, Wernerman J (1995) Glutamine and α-ketoglutarate prevent the decrease in muscle free glutamine concentration and influence protein synthesis after total hip replacement. Metabolism 44:1215–1222
60. Petersson B, Waller S-O Vinnars E, Wernerman J (1994) Long-term effect of glycyl-glutamine after elective surgery on free amino acids in muscle. JPEN 18:320–325
61. Januszkiewicz A, Essen P, McNurlan MA, Calder GA, Andersson K, Wernerman J, Garlick PJ (1996) Effect of a short-term infusion of glutamine on muscle protein metabolism postoperatively. Clin Nutr 15:267–273
62. Roth E, Funovics J, Muhlbacher F et al. (1982) Metabolic disorders in severe abdominal sepsis: glutamine deficiency in skeletal muscle. Clin Nutr 1:25–41
63. Palmer TEA, Griffiths RD, Jones C (1996) Effect of parenteral L-glutamine on muscle in the very severely ill. Nutrition 12 (5): 316–320
64. Weingartmann G, Fridrich P, Mauritz W, Götzinger P, Mittlböck M, Germann P, Karner J, Roth E (1996) Safety and efficacy of increasing dosages of glycyl-glutamine for total parenteral nutrition in polytrauma patients. Wien Klin Wochenschr 108/21:683–688
65. Varnier M, Leese GP, Thompson J, Rennie MJ (1995) Stimulatory effect of glutamine on glycogen accumulation in human skeletal muscle. Am J Physiol 269 (Endocrinol Metab 32): E309-E315
66. Darmaun D, Déchelotte P (1991) Role of leucine as a precursor of glutamine a-amino nitrogen in vivo in humans. Am J Physiol 260:E326-E329
67. Wagenmakers AJM (1992) Amino acid metabolism, muscular fatigue and muscle wasting. Speculations on adaptations at high-altitude. Int J Sports Med 13:S110-S113
68. Finn PJ, Plank LD, Clark MA, Connolly AB, Hill GL (1996) Progressive cellular dehydration and proteolysis in critically-ill patients. Lancet 347:654–56
69. Griffiths RD, Palmer TEA, Helliwell T, Maclennan P, Macmillan RR (1995) Effect of passive stretching on the wasting of muscle in the critically ill. Nutrition 11:428–432
70. Gamrin L, Essen P, Forsberg AM, Hultman E, Wernerman J (1996) A descriptive study of skeletal muscle metabolism in critically ill patients: free amino acids, energy rich phosphates, protein, nucleic acids, fat, water, and electrolytes. Crit Care Med 24:575–583
71. Elia M, Lunn PG (1997) The use of glutamine in the treatment of gastrointestinal disorders in man. Nutrition 13:743–747
72. Van der Hulst RRWJ, von Meyenfeldt MF, Deutz NEP, Soeters PB (1997) Glutamine extraction by the gut is reduced in patients with depleted gastrointestinal cancer. Ann Surg 225:112–121
73. Van der Hulst RRWJ, Deutz NEP, von Meyenfeldt MF, Elbers JMH, Stockbrügger RW, Soeters PB (1994) Decrease of mucosal glutamine concentration in the nutritionally depleted patient. Clin Nutr 13:228–233

74. Van der Hulst RRWJ, Deutz NEP, von Meyenfeldt MF, Stockbrügger RW, Soeters PB (1996) The effect of glutamine administration on intestinal glutamine content. J Surgical Res 61:30–34
75. Ahlman B, Ljungqvist O, Persson B, Bindslev L, Wernerman J (1995) Intestinal amino acid content in critically ill patients. JPEN 19:272–278
76. Salloum RM, Copeland EM, Souba WW (1991) Brush border transport of glutamine and other substrates during sepsis and endotoxaemia. Ann Surg 213:401–410
77. Van der Hulst RR, van Kreel BK, Von Meyenfeldt MF, Brummer RJ, Arends JW, Deutz NE, Soeters PB (1993) Glutamine and the preservation of gut integrity. Lancet 341:1363–1365
78. Tremel H, Kienle B, Weilemann LS, Stehle P, Fürst P (1994) Glutamine dipeptide-supplemented parenteral nutrition maintains intestinal function in the critically ill. Gastroenterology 107:1595–1601
79. Wilmore DW, Smith RJ, O'Dwyer ST, Jacobs DO, Ziegler TR, Wang XD (1988) The gut: a central organ after surgical stress. Surgery 104:917–923
80. O'Boyle, J Macfie (1998) Alterations in intestinal barrier function do not predispose to translocation of enteric bacteria in gastroenterological patients. Nutrition 14:358–362
81. Van der Hulst RRWJ, von Meyenfeldt MF, Tiebosch A, Buurman WA, Soeters PB (1997) Glutamine and intestinal immune cells in humans. JPEN 21:310–315
82. Houdijk APJ, Rijnsburger ER, Jansen J, Wesdorp RIC, Weiss JK, McCamish MA, Teerlink T, Meuwissen SGM, Haarman HJThM, Thijs LG, van Leeuwen PAM (1998) Randomised trial of glutamine-enriched enteral nutrition on infectious morbidity in patients with multiple trauma. Lancet 352:772–776
83. Brown SA, Goringe A, Fegan C, Davies SV, Giddings J, Whittaker JA, Burnett AK, Poynton CH (1998) Parenteral glutamine protects hepatic function during bone marrow transplantation. Bone Marrow Transplant 22 (3): 281–284
84. Ziegler TR, Young LS, Benfell K, Scheltinga M, Hortos K, Bye R, Morrow FD, Jacobs DO, Smith RJ, Antin JH, Wilmore DW. (1992) Clinical and metabolic efficacy of glutamine-supplemented parenteral nutrition after bone marrow transplantation. Ann Intern Med 116:821–828
85. Schloerb PR, Amare M (1993) Total parenteral nutrition with glutamine in bone marrow transplantation and other clinical applications (a randomised, double-blind study) JPEN 17:407–413
86. Ziegler TR, Bye RL, Persinger RL, Young LS, Antin JH, Wilmore DW (1998) Effect of glutamine supplementation on circulating lymphocytes after bone marrow transplantation: a pilot study. Am J Med Sci 315:4–10
87. Lacey JM, Crouch JB, Benfell K, et al. (1996) The effects of glutamine-supplemented parenteral nutrition in premature infants. JPEN 20:74–80
88. O'Riordain MG, Fearon KCH, Ross JA, Rogers P, Falconer JS, Bartolo DCC, Garden OJ, Carter DC (1994) Glutamine-supplemented total parenteral nutrition enhances T-lymphocyte response in surgical patients undergoing colorectal resection. Ann Surg 220:212–221
89. De Beaux AC, O'Riordan MG, Ross JA, Jodozi L, Carter DC, Fearon KCH (1998) Glutamine-supplemented total parenteral nutrition reduces blood mononuclear cell interleukin-8 release in severe acute pancreatitis. Nutrition 14:261–265
90. Morlion BJ, Stehle P, Wachter P, Siedhoff HP, Koller M, Konig W, Fürst P, Puchstein C (1998) Total parenteral nutrition with glutamine dipeptide after major abdominal surgery – a randomized, double-blind, controlled study. Ann Surg 227:302–308
91. Gore DC, Jahoor F (1994) Glutamine kinetics in burn patients. Comparison with hormonally induced stress in volunteers. Arch Surg 129:1318
92. Roth E, Funovics J, Muhlbacher F, et al. (1982) Metabolic disorders in severe abdominal sepsis: glutamine deficiency in skeletal muscle. Clin Nutr 1:25–41
93. Gamrin L, Andersson K, Hultman E, Nilsson E, Essen P, Wernerman J (1997) Longitudinal changes of biochemical parameters in muscle during critical illness. Metabolism 46:756–762
94. Palmer TEA, Griffiths RD, Jones C (1996) Effect of parenteral L-glutamine on muscle in the very severely ill. Nutrition 12(5): 316–320
95. Hammarqvist F, Luo J-L, Cotgreave IA, Andersson K, Wernerman J (1997) Skeletal muscle glutathione is depleted in critically ill patients. Crit Care Med 25:78–84
96. Griffiths RD, Jones C, Palmer TEA (1997) Six-month outcome of critically ill patients given glutamine supplemented parenteral nutrition. Nutrition 13:295–302
97. Wilmore DW (1997) Glutamine saves lives! What does it mean? Nutrition 13:375–376 (editorial)
98. Wernerman J (1998) Glutamine-containing TPN: a question of life and death for intensive care unit-patients? Clin Nutr 17:3–6
99. Galanos AN, Pieper CF, Kussin PS, Winchell MT, Fulkerson WJ, Harrell FE, Teno JM, Layde P, Connors AF, Phillips RS, Wenger NS: for the SUPPORT investigators (1997) Relationship of Body Mass Index to subsequent mortality among seriously ill hospitalised patients. Crit Care Med 25: 1962–1968

100. Fish J, Sporay G, Beyer K, Jones J, Kihara T, Kennedy A, Apovian C, Jensen GL (1997) A prospective randomized study of glutamine-enriched parenteral compared with enteral feeding in postoperative patients. Am J Clin Nutr 65:977–983
101. Biolo G, Iscra F, Toigo G, Ciocchi B, Situlin R, Gullo A, Guarnieri G (1997) Effects of growth hormone administration on skeletal muscle glutamine metabolism in severely traumatised patients: preliminary report. Clin Nutr 16:89–91

PART IV

Perioperative Dysfunction of the Gastrointestinal Tract

Perioperative Motility of the Foregut

K. H. Fuchs · J. Maroske · H. Tigges · J. Heimbucher · S. M. Freys · A. Thiede

Chirurgische Universitätsklinik und Poliklinik, Josef-Schneider-Strasse 2,
97080 Würzburg, Germany

Introduction

Abdominal surgery usually causes changes in gastrointestinal motility, and the nature of these changes can vary tremendously [1, 3, 4, 5, 15, 18, 19]. The changes can be differentiated into early postoperative motility disturbances and late postoperative disorders of the motor activity of the stomach and small bowel. This overview is focused on several aspects regarding perioperative motility changes of the foregut. First, an important feature is the technology currently available to assess foregut function. Second, data are available to describe physiological motility and the intraluminal environment of the different foregut compartments [2, 7, 10, 11, 14, 18]. A third important subject is the early postoperative motility changes which are usually reversible after a few days [16, 17, 18]. It can be important to assess postoperative foregut motility changes as a reason for postoperative ileus and disturbances of fluid and food passage through the intestine. A fourth subject of interest is the late postoperative persisting functional disorders which are usually caused by surgery to the foregut [9, 12, 13, 20]. The latter can cause troublesome symptoms for the patient, or even damaging exposure to toxic agents in some compartments that leads to additional disease and the need to be corrected.

Possible clinical problems caused by perioperative motility disorders are swallowing discomfort, gastroesophageal reflux, duodenogastric reflux, delayed gastric emptying and gastric dilatation as well as ileus. Other problems are possible but of minor clinical relevance. This paper will address the assessment technology, physiological data in the normal situation, and early and late postoperative changes. Objective assessment is very important since symptoms are not a reliable guide to abnormalities in esophageal and gastric function.

Assessment Technology

Several diagnostic procedures are available to assess, directly or indirectly, foregut function. Intraluminal pressure measurements are a traditional direct assessment method to evaluate esophageal, gastric, and small bowel motility [11, 16, 18]. A conventional tool is the intraluminal perfusion manometry system, which allows for continuous recording of luminal contractions. Non-occlusive contractions in an organ with a rather wide lumen can create an accuracy problem. An alternative to the perfusion system is a solid state catheter with several points of measurement, that has been

M. K. Herbert et al. (Eds.), Problems of the
Gastrointestinal Tract in Anesthesia...

introduced in the recent decades and has become a reliable tool during the past years. This system can be used for esophageal motility recordings as well as for antroduodenal and jejunal recordings [11]. The catheter must be placed transnasally, sometimes under fluoroscopic or endoscopic guidance, into the gastric lumen and small bowel. It is connected to a portable or stationary computer assisted data logger which allows for a 24 h or even a 48 h recording time. An example of antroduodenal recordings of the interdigestive motor complex in a normal healthy volunteer is shown in Fig. 1.

All potentially interfering drugs need to be discontinued at least 48 h prior to the examination. The patient is fasted overnight, and the motility catheter is passed either into the stomach or possibly under fluoroscopic guidance, to the final position down through the pylorus and into the duodenum and jejunum. For an antroduodenal recording to be produced it must be made sure that the catheter is correctly positioned, with three pressure sensors in the antral area and at least two pressure sensors in the duodenal and/or jejunal environment. Healthy volunteers and patients should perform their normal daily activity during the investigation. They should be instructed to eat at set meal times, such as lunch, dinner and breakfast as indicated in a given diary. This protocol provides adequate information of both fasting and fed

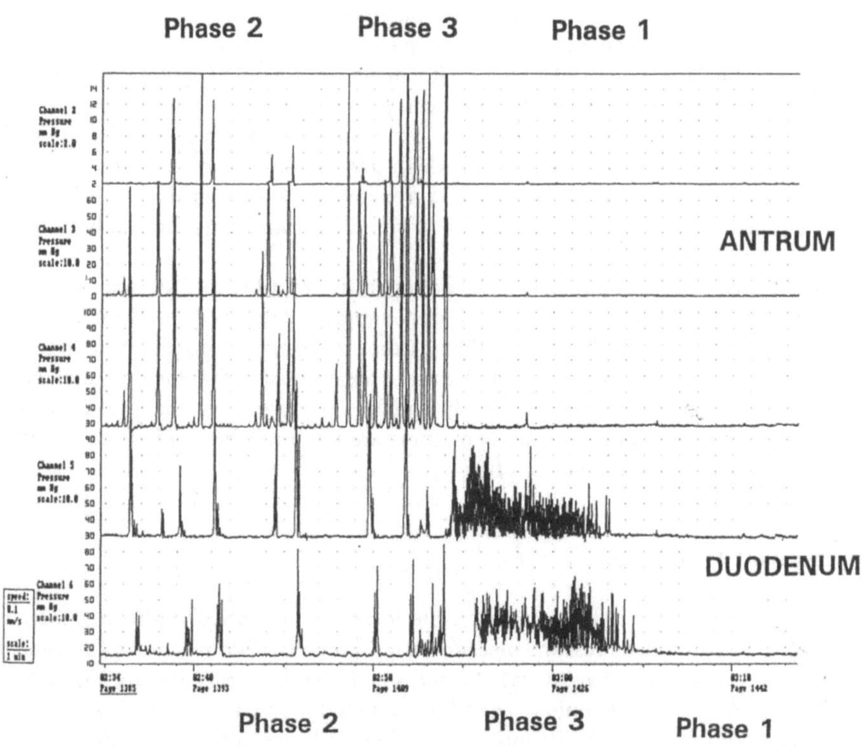

Fig. 1. Examples of normal migrating motor complex. The upper three channels represent the antral motility and the lower two channels represent the duodenal motor activity. There is an increase in amplitude and frequency of contractions from Phase 1 to Phases 2 and 3. Phase 3 lasts for 5 min in the antrum and 8 min in the duodenum

state motility patterns. The patient or the volunteer should record all symptoms during the study period in the diary to allow for a correlation of symptoms with motility features.

Indirect measurements of foregut motility provide long-term assessment of esophageal, gastric and duodenal pH environments as well as the presence of bile in these compartments [2, 6, 7, 8, 9]. An additional parameter to assess these compartments is the detection of pancreatic enzymes by aspiration of fluids. Simultaneous pH measurements are performed with glass electrodes connected to a portable data recorder (Medtronic, Düsseldorf, Germany). The pH probes are calibrated in buffer solutions of pH 1 and pH 7, before and after the measurements. A commercially available software program is utilized for data transfer and analysis (Esophagram, Medtronic, Düsseldorf, Germany).

Bilirubin is monitored by a fiberoptic probe (Bilitec 2000, Medtronic, Düsseldorf, Germany). This device displays the absorbance of bilirubin in relative units. In vitro, the absorbance of bilirubin correlates with the bile acid concentration [2, 6]. In vivo comparison of bilirubin monitoring with scintigraphy also shows significant concordance with regard to the presence or absence of reflux, and the mucosa reflux contact time [6]. This assessment gives a semiquantitative estimate of the amount of bile refluxing from the duodenum into the stomach and further up into the esophagus, thus reflecting the antroduodenal motility, which causes a reflux. Bilitec tracings are analyzed, and the percentage time with an absorbance higher than a given threshold

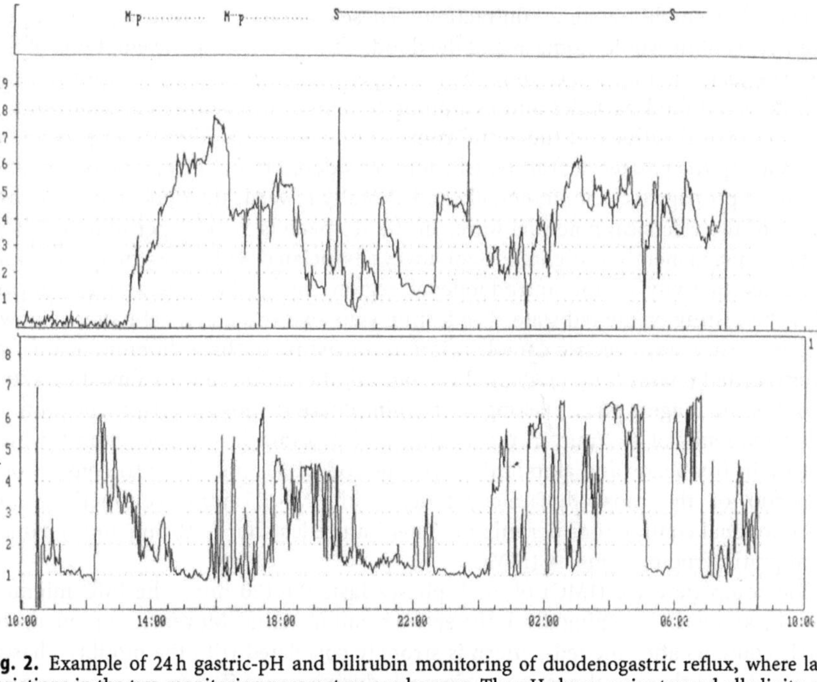

Fig. 2. Example of 24 h gastric-pH and bilirubin monitoring of duodenogastric reflux, where large variations in the two monitoring parameters can be seen. The pH shows a rise toward alkalinity, and the bilirubin monitoring exhibits an increase in absorption

(from 0.14 to 0.45 absorption values, AV) is calculated. The subjects follow a standardized protocol as mentioned above. The probes are placed in the esophageal lumen 5 cm above the lower esophageal sphincter, and in the gastric lumen 5 cm below the lower border of the lower esophageal sphincter. Fig. 2. demonstrates a 24 h circadian cycle of intragastric pH measurement as well as intragastric bilirubin monitoring as measured by the Bilitec device.

An additional system for measuring foregut motility is scintigraphy. The patient has to swallow a certain amount of food or fluid traced with technetium or iridium. Often scrambled eggs with slices of white bread are given together with water, after technetium 99 sulfocolloid (1 mCi) is injected into a freshly beaten egg prior to scrambling. A gamma camera will count the radiolabeled isotopes when they are transported through the esophagus into the stomach and further in the duodenum. Particular regions of interest in subsequent segments of the foregut can be differentiated, which allows for calculation of speed of transportation as well as reflux.

Physiological Motility

In physiological circumstances esophageal motility has the ability to empty refluxing material from the esophageal lumen into the gastric lumen with strong contractions. The proximal stomach including fundus and approximately the upper third of the corpus, serving as a reservoir, acts motorially differently from the distal stomach. The main feature of this area is a receptive relaxation with the ingestion of food and subsequently low amplitude tonic contractions. These contractions create a pressure gradient between the whole stomach and the duodenum, promoting the emptying of liquids. The distal stomach, including the lower part of the corpus and antrum, acts as a mill to grind food particles and as a pump to deliver chyme into the duodenum.

The electrical activity of the antral contractions is generated from an area in the corpus along the greater curvature, which is considered to be the gastric pacemaker. The waves propagate circumferentially and aborally towards the duodenum. The frequency of the electrical potential waves in the stomach is 3 cycles per minute. These waves are permanently present, but not always associated with a gastric contraction. Mechanical activity of the antroduodenal region shows different patterns during either the fasting or the fed state. The fasting state exhibits a cyclical pattern known as interdigestive myoelectric complex (IMC), consisting of three different degrees of activity, called phases (Fig. 1). Phase I is a period of quiescence with almost no activity and is the longest phase, lasting 45–60 min. Phase II shows intermittent contractions (frequency of 1–2/min in the antrum and 2–5/min in the duodenum), which increase in frequency and amplitude over a period of 30 min. Phase III consists of a crescendo of the most dynamic activity, with 2.5–3.5 antral contractions and 8–12 duodenal contractions per minute. This feature lasts for 5–10 min and is named the migrating motor complex (MMC).

One complete cycle (IMC) of all 3 phases lasts 90–120 min. The IMC migrates from the stomach, sweeping down the entire small intestine. Movement of remaining gastric contents after the fed-pattern is strongly correlated with the motility phases. During phase I there is almost no movement, during phase II there is more a mixing of contents than of propulsion, and phase III provides the aboral propulsion of large

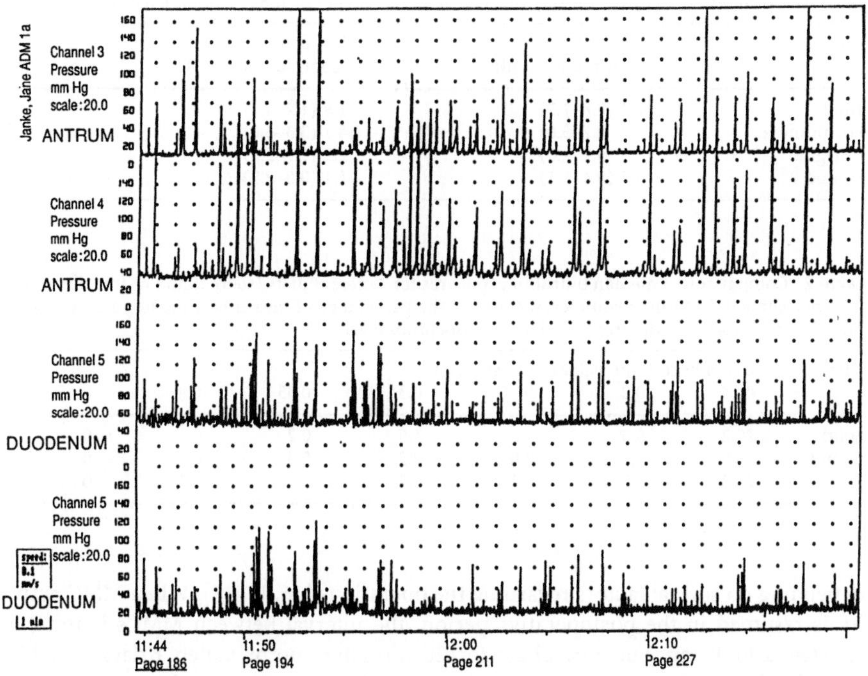

Fig. 3. Example of a normal fed pattern, showing the amplitude and frequency of contractions irregular but higher than those in interdigestive Phase 2

indigestible contents. This cyclical activity repeats itself until it is disrupted by the ingestion of food.

Typical fed-pattern motility consists of intermittent contractions similar to phase II (Fig. 3). The duration of the postprandial activity depends on the food characteristics.

Table 1 shows an overview of physiological values for antroduodenal and jejunal motility, as measured in 10 healthy volunteers. Monitoring gastric pH for 24 h shows a physiological circadian rhythm.

Bilirubin monitoring for 24 h verifies, in most volunteers, physiological bile reflux in the supine position. Table 2 shows gastric bilirubin monitoring in healthy volunteers, reflecting the value of different borderline absorption values from 0.14 to 0.45.

Early Postoperative Motility Changes

The interdigestive MMC as well as the fed-pattern is interrupted when a laparotomy is performed. When measured by electromyography, a basic electrical rhythm can be recorded, and also immediately after the operation. Several authors have used the reoccurrence of phase 3-like activity of the MMC as an indicator for resumed motor activity in the small bowel, during the postoperative phase. Controversial reports have been published about the extent of the interruption of intestinal motility,

Table 1. Normal frequency of contractions (median and range) of the antroduodenal segment

Diet	Antrum (contractions/min)	Duodenum (contractions/min)
Total	1.2 (0.8–1.7)	1.8 (1.2–4.1)
Postprandial	1.7 (0.7–3.0)	4.7 (3.3–6.0)
Upright	1.4 (0.9–2.0)	2.1 (1.1–2.8)
Supine	0.7 (0.4–1.1)	1.1 (0.5–2.3)

Table 2. Comparison of median bilirubin exposures for different diets (solid, liquid or free diet of the patients' choice), in healthy volunteers, showing the percentage of measured time of positive gastric bilirubin monitoring at different borderline absorption levels

Diet	Given borderline values of absorption						
	0.14	0.2	0.25	0.3	0.35	0.4	0.45
Solid	20.2	8.3	4.3	1.5	0.2	0	0
Liquid	20.9	6.9	2.0	0.7	0.3	0	0
Free	21.2	6.5	1.7	0.2	0.1	0.1	0

depending on several factors regarding the operations [16, 17, 18]. When MMC activity is resumed in the postoperative period, the interval between MMCs is initially shortened to 40 min but normalizes to 120 min after approximately 6 days. In addition, the first postoperative phase 3-like activity has been measured in experimental studies. The results show that after 60 min of intestinal manipulation, there is a 48 h interval (range 24–53 h) until the first phase 3-like activity reoccurs. After a small-bowel resection it takes a median of 18 h (range 3–28 h) and after a colonic resection 67 h (range 49–73 h), for detection of the first postoperative phase 3-like activity. From experimental investigations with electromyography (EMG) and from intraluminal motility studies, as well as from clinical studies using intraluminal manometry, we can observe an early postoperative reduction of motility in the stomach and small bowel [5, 10, 15, 17, 18]. The variation in resumed normal physiological activity depends on the individual, on the extent of surgery, on the extent of manipulation during the operation and, probably, on many other factors such as neurohumoral dysregulation and hemostasis.

As a consequence, when assessing postoperative motility it is very important to record all surrounding circumstances of each individual patient, to interpret the recorded data in a reasonable way. When performing studies in the early postoperative period to assess motility of the foregut, it is very difficult to establish a comparable situation for generating homogenous data, since the interindividual and even intraindividual differences may be large. This has to be kept in mind when interpreting patient-data or comparing them with data generated in the physiological situation under more standardized conditions.

Late Postoperative Problems of Foregut Motility

Following surgery to the esophagus, stomach or small bowel, such as gastric resections and vagotomies, major changes occur in the physiology of the foregut. Not only is the reservoir function of the stomach limited, but the physiological connections and feedback mechanisms of the foregut to modify motility, release bile and pancreatic juices are interrupted. As a consequence, major changes can occur in all compartments, altering pH environment and enzyme activity as well as changing motility, and neurohormonal feedback mechanisms. In the past, postgastrectomy syndrome has been the most relevant in patients with severe reduction of their quality of life [9, 11, 12, 13, 20]. Two major problems occur in this situation. The first is gastric stasis, and the second is enterogastric or duodenogastric reflux. The clinical relevance of this phenomenon has been discussed controversially in the past decades. Optimal assessment of duodenogastric reflux comprises a combination of diagnostic procedures, such as long term gastric pH and bilirubin monitoring, as well as aspiration of gastric fluid to detect pancreatic enzymes. Excessive reflux of bile and pancreatic enzymes together with acid can have a damaging effect on the gastric mucosa, especially the esophageal mucosa. Due to the variability of mucosal resistance and the extent of bile and pancreatic enzyme exposure in the stomach and esophagus, it is very difficult to establish a sharp margin between the physiological amount of reflux and its pathological borderline.

Postoperative motility of the foregut can be accurately assessed with new monitoring technology. Problems arise, on the one hand with the severely ill patient on the ICU, since monitoring-catheters could cause additional problems, and on the other hand from the lack of specific drugs to influence motility in the critically ill patient.

References

1. Baker LW, Webster DR: Postoperative intestinal motility. Br J Surg 1968, 55: 374–378
2. Bechi P: Fiberoptic measurement of 'alkaline' gastro-esophageal reflux: technical aspects and clinical indications. Dis Esophagus 1994, 7: 131–138
3. Bueno L, Ferre JP, Ruckebush Y: Effects of anaesthesia and surgical procedures on intestinal myeoelectric activity in the dog. Am J Surg 1978, 23: 690–695
4. Coelho JC, Gouma DJ, Moody FG, Li YF: Gastrointestinal myoelectric activity following abdominal operations in the opossum. World J. Surg 1985, 9: 612–618
5. Dahlgren S, Selking O: postoperative motility of the small intestine. Ups J Med Sci 1972, 217: 202–204
6. Fein M, Fuchs KH, Bohrer T, Freys SM, Thiede A: Fiberoptic technique for 24 hour bile reflux monitoring – standards and normal values for gastric monitoring. Dig Dis Sci 1996, 41(1): 216–225
7. Fuchs KH, DeMeeester TR, Hinder RA, Stein HJ, Barlow AP, Gupta NC: Computerized identification of pathological duodenogastric reflux using 24-hour gastric pH monitoring. Ann Surg 1991, 213: 13–20
8. Fuchs KH, Selch A, Freys SM, DeMeester TR: Gastric Acid Secretion and Gastric pH Measurement in Peptic Ulcer Disease. Problems in General Surgery 1992, 9: 138–151
9. Fuchs KH, Thiede A, Engemann R, Deltz E, Stremme O, Hamelmann H: Reconstruction of the food passage after total gastrectomy: randomized trial. World J Surg 1995, 19: 678–705
10. Galligan JJ, Furness JB, Costa M: Migration of the myoelectric complex after interruption of the myenteric plexus: intestinal transection and regeneration of enteric nerves in the guinea pig. Gastroenterology 1989, 97: 1135–1146
11. Heimbucher J, Fuchs KH, Freys SM et al.: Motility in the Hunt-Lawrence pouch after total gastrectomy. Am J Surg 1994, 168: 622–626

12. Hinder RA, Esser J, DeMeester TR: Management of gastric emptying disorders following the Roux-en-Y procedure. Surgery 1988, 104: 765–772
13. Mathias JR, Fernandez A, Sninsky CA, Clench MA, Davis RH: Nausea, motiting and abdominal pain after Roux-en-Y anastomosis: motility of the jejunal limb. Gastroenterology 1985, 88: 101–107
14. Müller-Lissner SA, Fraass C: Dissociation of duodenogastric marker reflux and bile salt reflux. Dig Dis Sci 1985, 30: 733–738
15. Richter HM III, Kelly KA: Effect of transection and pacing on human jejunal pacesetter potential. Gastroenterology 1986, 91: 1380–1385
16. Schippers E, Braun J, Erhard W, Schumpelick V: Frühe postoperative Motilität nach abdominalchirurgischen Eingriffen im Tierexperiment. Langenbecks Arch Chir 1990, 375: 175–180
17. Schippers E, Hölscher AH, Bollschweiler E, Siewert JR: Return of the interdigestive motor complex after abdominal surgery: end of postoperative ileus? Dig Dis Sci 1991, 36: 621–626
18. Schippers E: Pathophysiologie und Therapie chirurgisch induzierter Dünndarmmotilitätsstörungen. In: Gastrointestinale Funktionsstörungen. Hrsg.: KH Fuchs, HJ Stein, A Thiede, Springer Verlag Heidelberg 1996, 787–808
19. Soper NJ, Sarr MG, Kelly KA: Human duodenal myoelectric activity after operation and with pacing. Surgery 1990, 108: 63–68
20. Toye DKM, Alexander-William J: Postgastrectomy bile vomiting. Lancet 1965, 2: 524–526

Electrogastrography During the Early Postoperative Period

J. Maroske · J. Heimbucher · K. H. Fuchs · S. M. Freys · A. Thiede
Department of Surgery, University of Würzburg, 97080 Würzburg, Germany

Introduction

Electrogastrography (EGG) is a diagnostic procedure by which gastric myoelectrical activity is recorded noninvasively, using skin electrodes. Although documented first by Alvarez [2] in 1922, and then by other scientists [10, 11, 12, 14], it is still looked upon as an experimental procedure. In contrast to other electrophysiological diagnostic procedures, development of the EGG has made slow progress. The relatively poor quality of the original EGG signal makes it imperative that the technique of data acquisition generates a trace with an optimal signal to noise ratio. The interpretation of recorded abnormalities, as well as a doubtful correlation between electrical phenomena and real gastric motility caused further confusion. With the development of computerized analyses of the recorded data and the possibility of a 24 h monitoring period, EGG gained new clinical interest. Compared to other diagnostic motility procedures its main attraction is its noninvasive nature. The correlation of documented EGG phenomena and gastric motility is part of ongoing studies [3].

Physiological Background

The stomach is a neuromuscular organ with intrinsic electrical activity called slow waves. They originate in a pacemaker at the fundus/corpus borderline [5]. The slow waves have a frequency of 3 cycles per minute (cpm) (range: 2.5–3.5 cpm) and migrate towards the pylorus. The mechanical activity of the gastric muscle layer is not generated by the slow waves but is associated with spikes between the slow waves [4]. Both mechanical as well as electrical activity are influenced by multiple intrinsic and extrinsic factors. Modulation of the activity is due to the autonomic nervous system, influenced by hormones, and being changed by variations in nutrition; even stress and emotions may have substantial influence on gastric motility [11].

Recording of the Electrogastrogram

This chapter describes the way of adjusting the EGG to patients and volunteers. In our study we focused on three groups. Group A consisted of 11 patients, following abdominal surgery, group B comprised 8 patients after trauma surgery, and group C was made up of 10 healthy volunteers serving as controls. Measurements were taken on the first two postoperative days, between 6 a.m. and 8 a.m. and 6 p.m. to 8 p.m.

M. K. Herbert et al. (Eds.), Problems of the Gastrointestinal Tract in Anesthesia...

Data were recorded, using the portable microdigitrapper-EGG (Synectics Medical, Irvine, Texas, USA). Since motion of the individual causes imprecise recordings, the manufacturer recommended that the patient be in the resting position, starved, and isolated from electrical fields during recording [3]. Commercially available software will cut out noise and register well-defined episodes only. One neutral and two active electrodes were applied to the abdominal skin of the patients or volunteers. Prior to the attachment of the Ag-AgCl electrodes, the skin needs to be cleaned to reduce the skin resistance. The skin to electrode impedance should be lowered to approximately 10 kΩ to avoid skin potential responses that will otherwise confuse the EGG. Lowering the impedance is achieved, for example by cleaning the skin with alcohol and scrubbing or lightly abrading with fine sandpaper. For correct placement of the electrodes, ultrasound is of great benefit. Ideally, the two active Ag-AgCl electrodes should be placed along the longitudinal axis of the antrum. If ultrasound is not available, the first active electrode should be placed 3 cm to the paramedian left of the axis between xyphoid and umbilicus. The second electrode should be placed 2 cm to the paramedian right and 2 cm further caudally; the neutral electrode should be positioned at the right lower thorax aperture.

Analysis

After data transfer to a PC, the recorded curve will be screened for artifacts, which then are excluded from further analysis. The actual EGG analysis is performed in a so-called running spectral analysis mode [10]. Evaluation includes the following parameters:

1. The dominant frequency and its corresponding intensity. Slow waves have the dominant frequency, and are present with 2.5–3.5 contractions per minute. The so called tachygastria is defined as having a frequency of more than 4 cpm and bradygastria as having fewer than 2 cpm.
2. Variation in intensity of the dominant frequency. The intensity of the dominant frequency is related to the amplitude and the difference in voltage [3, 11]
3. Percentage of different frequencies.

Furthermore, a few additional parameters have been defined and used in some studies but their clinical relevance has not yet been proven.

The display of the recorded data as a running spectral analysis means that the dominant frequency as well as tachy- and bradygastria are easily visible. Available software automatically counts the different frequencies and lists them as percentages of slow waves, tachy-, and bradygastria or arrhythmia. Arrhythmia is defined as irregular slow waves, including tachyarrhythmia and bradyarrhythmia. The spectral analysis can also be analyzed for different periods such as pre– and postprandial, and for episodes where symptoms occur. The intensity of the dominant frequency can be analyzed too.

The following two statements are well known and verified:

1. With an increasing percentage of brady- and/or tachygastria, the likelihood of a gastric motility disorder is increased as well.
2. The prandial period is linked with an increase in slow waves and amplitude.

Koch et al. [7] reported mainly normal electrical gastric frequency in patients with gastroparesis due to a mechanical gastric outlet obstruction. Tachygastria and a conversion to normal slow wave rhythm have been observed in patients suffering from diabetic gastroparesis after the application of prokinetics [8]. Even in patients with documented mesenteric ischemia, the total disappearance of dysrhythmias was recorded after revascularization [9]. The clinical value of the often-noted arrhythmias in nausea and vomiting is of minor importance [1, 13, 15]. The relevance of the EGG analysis in starved patients is doubtful [3, 4]. As for the broad spectrum of the motility phenomena, an identification of pathological disorders by EGG is too inaccurate. The typical postprandial changes in the EGG have been reported in several studies [6, 8] and investigated in detail, but they are dependent on a variety of influences. Therefore, the clinical relevance of the EGG is not yet fully elucidated.

Indications

On considering the experience and reported data on EGG a few clinical aspects of this study can be found:

Due to its noninvasive nature the EGG can be applied in every individual to detect gastric motility disorders. Furthermore during the simultaneous measuring of EGG with a more invasive diagnostic procedure such as scintigraphy for gastric emptying, a correlation with EGG phenomena could be found. The success of a medical treatment, e.g. with prokinetics is an interesting indication for EGG application. A recent investigation to find the right time for enteral feeding in ICU patients with abdominal or neurological diseases or trauma did not come up with any predictive value.

References

1. Abell TL, Malagelada JR (1985) Glucagon evoked gastric dysrhythmias in humans shown by an improved electrogastrographic technique. Gastroenterology 88:1932–1940
2. Alvarez WC (1922) The electrogram and what it shows. JAMA 78:1116–1118
3. Chen JDZ, Richards RD, McCallum RW (1994) Identification of gastric contractions from the cutaneous electrogastrogram. Am J Gastroenterol 89:79–85
4. Geldof H, van der Schee EJ, Grashuis JL (1986) Electrogastrographic characteristics of the interdigestive migrating complex in humans. Am J Physiol 250:G165–171
5. Hinder RA, Kelly KA (1977) Human gastric pacesetter potential: site of origin, spread and response to gastric transsection and vagotomy. Am J Surg 133:29–33
6. Koch KL, Stern RM, Bingaman S, Eggli D (1991) Satiety, stomach and gastric myoelectrical activity during solid phase gastric emptying: a study of healthy individuals. J Gastrointest Motility 5:41–47
7. Koch KL, Bingaman S, Sperry N, Stern RM (1991) Electrogastrography differentiates mechanical vs. idiopathic gastroparesis in patients with nausea and vomiting. Gastroenterology 100:A99
8. Koch KL, Stern RM, Steward WR, Vasey MW, Sullivan ML (1989) Gastric emptying and gastric myoelectrical activity in patients with symptomatic diabetic gastroparesis: effect of long-term domperidone treatment. Am J Gastroenterology 84:1069–1075
9. Liberski SM, Koch KL, Atnip RG (1990) Ischemic gastroparesis: resolution of nausea, vomiting and gastroparesis after mesenteric artery revascularization. Gastroenterology 99:252–257
10. Schee EJ van der, Grashuis LJ (1987) Running spectrum analysis as an aid in the representation and interpretation of electrogastrographic signals. Med Biol Eng Comput 25:57–62
11. Smout AJPM, van der Schee EJ, Grashuis JL (1980) What is measured in electrogastrography? Dig Dis Sci 25:179–187
12. Stern RM (1985) A brief history of electrogastrogram. In: Stern RM, Koch KL (eds) Electrogastrography: methodology, validation and applications. Praeger, New York, pp 3–9

13. Stern RM, Koch KL, Stewart WR, Lindblad IM (1987) Spectral analysis of tachygastria recorded during motion sickness. Gastroenterology 93:92–97
14. Stern RM, Uijtdehaage SHJ, Koch KL, Hanisch H (1991) Ambulatory recording of the electrogastrogram. J Gastrointestinal Motility 3:202
15. You CH, Lee KY, Chey WY (1980) Electrogastrographic study of patients with unexplained nausea, bloating and vomiting. Gastroenterology 79:311–314

INVITED ARTICLE

Therapeutic Interventions for Improvement of Impaired Intestinal Blood Flow

G. F. E. Nöldge-Schomburg · D. A. Vagts

Anaesthesiologische Universitätsklinik, Hugstetter Str. 55, 79106 Freiburg, Germany

Introduction

There is increasing evidence that intestinal hypoperfusion with the consequence of mucosal hypoxia might play an important role in the development of systemic inflammatory response syndrome (SIRS), sepsis, and multiple organ dysfunction (MODS) or failure (MOF) (Meakins and Marshall 1984; Mythen and Webb 1994). Despite improved diagnostic monitoring and new therapeutic modalities, the mortality rate of MOF is still very high (Knaus et al. 1991) and unchanged compared to earlier studies. Thus, early detection of splanchnic organ dysoxia and early therapeutic interventions to prevent persistent splanchnic ischemia are essential to avoid the gut becoming the "motor of multiple system organ failure" (Meakins and Marshall 1984, 1989).

The splanchnic region contains about 30% (ca. 1.4 l) of blood volume in human beings (Price et al. 1966). Low flow states such as those associated with acute blood loss are primarily compensated by an increase in sympathetic nervous activity, which induces pronounced vasoconstriction, especially in the splanchnic vascular bed, acting as a blood reservoir. This so-called "autotransfusion response" (Reilly and Bulkley 1993; Xu et al. 1993) provides immediate survival by redistribution of blood away from the splanchnic organs to the vital organs. However, prolonged intestinal hypoperfusion as a consequence of persistent hypovolemia increases the risk of ischemic mucosal damage.

Not only hemorrhage, hypovolemia, or reperfusion states, but especially endotoxinemia may induce splanchnic hypoxia. Recently, it could be shown (Nöldge-Schomburg et al. 1996; Vallet et al. 1994) that endotoxinemia causes splanchnic circulatory disturbances on the macro- and microcirculatory level, and on early and sustained intestinal mucosal hypoxia. Additionally, endotoxinemia is associated with an imbalance in oxygen delivery and oxygen uptake, especially in the splanchnic region. Despite increased oxygen demand (Fong et al. 1990), the ability of the gut for oxygen uptake is diminished (Schumacker et al. 1993; Vallet et al. 1994).

It needs to be emphasized that, during all these conditions, there might be hypoperfusion in the splanchnic region, even with normal systemic blood pressure, normal or even increased cardiac output, or normal or increased mixed venous oxygen saturation (Maynard et al. 1993).

Prolonged hypoperfusion and persistent mucosal hypoxia can cause increased permeability of the gut mucosal layer with consecutive loss of the physiological barrier function and translocation of micro-organisms and endotoxins into the portal venous circulation (Meakins and Marshall 1989; Deitch 1990). This may stimulate the immune

M. K. Herbert et al. (Eds.), Problems of the Gastrointestinal Tract in Anesthesia...

system, induces sequestration and activation of granulocytes (Botha et al. 1995; Moore et al. 1994), activates hepatocytes and Kupffer's cells (Gimson 1987), and hence stimulates the release of different mediators like interleukin-1, interleukin-6, interleukin-8, and TNF. Together with bacterial endo- and exotoxins, these mediators impend endothelial and other organ cells, where organ dysfunction or even multiple organ failure may develop (Michie et al. 1989).

Anatomic and Physiologic Considerations

The gut and, particularly, the gut mucosal layer is extremely susceptible to any reduction in oxygen delivery. Therefore, it has also been called the "canary" of the body (Dantzker 1993).

This high vulnerability, especially of the intestinal mucosa to lack of oxygen, is due to special anatomical and physiological conditions:

1. Microvascular Hemodilution as a Consequence of Plasma Skimming

The intestinal villus is served by a central arteriole originating from the supplying artery in a right angle. During normal blood flow conditions, the red blood cells pass the origin of the arteriole in greater volume than plasma does. This so-called "plasma skimming" results in a villus hematocrit which is half that occurring in systemic circulation (Fink 1991a). The microvascular hematocrit is maintained until the systemic hematocrit drops below 20% (Fink 1991a). Despite the rheological advantages of microvascular hemodilution regarding flow properties, hemodilution is associated with a reduction in oxygen-carrying capacity. Any additional decrease in blood flow will further decrease oxygen delivery. Because of the high metabolic rate of the layer cells, especially at the villus tip, these cells are at risk of developing hypoxic damage due to insufficient convective oxygen transport.

2. Countercurrent Flow

The second condition favoring microvillus hypoxia is due to parallel course and proximity of the ascending villus arteriole and the descending venule. This countercurrent circulation means that oxygen tension (pO_2) is always higher at the base than at the tip of the mucosal villus (Bohlen 1980). The resulting pO_2 gradient between the villus base and the villus tip will further increase, due to diffusion from the highly oxygen-saturated arteriole outward to the low-saturated venule (oxygen shunting). This mechanism accentuates the lower oxygen pressure at the tip of the villus, where metabolic demand is highest due to uptake of nutrients and other molecules (Lundgren and Haglund 1978). Especially during low flow states, oxygen shunting is increased, since there is more time for diffusion, and oxygen tension at the villus tip will further decrease. Consequently, the risk of necrosis at the tip of the villus increases (Bohlen 1980).

3. Precapillary Sphincters

The presence of capillary and precapillary sphincters which are mainly located in the mucosal layer may be a further reason for the high susceptibility of the intestinal mucosa to any decrease in oxygen delivery. Any increase in vasoconstricting mediators will preferentially induce mucosal hypoperfusion and carries the risk of ischemic damage.

Monitoring of Intestinal Oxygenation

Detecting splanchnic ischemia is an important precondition for initiating rational therapy. There are several methods available for monitoring splanchnic perfusion and oxygenation, but only few can be used in daily, routine clinical practice. Thus, the search for the dysoxic threshold, especially in the splanchnic region, is still going on (Schlichtig 1991).

Different methods, such as duplex ultrasound (Dalton et al. 1995), laser Doppler flowmetry (Duranteau et al. 1996), different clearance methods, tissue pPO_2 measurement with pO_2 electrodes and intravital microscopy are mainly used during experimental conditions. They will possibly gain more acceptance in clinical practice in coming years, as they develop further (Kvietys et al. 1985; Sair et al. 1996).

At the moment, gastric tonometry (pHi, $piCO_2$) (Brown and Gutierrez 1997; Chang et al. 1994; Knichwitz 1998, Knichwitz et al. 1996; Marik 1998), measurement of cardiac function, volume status and liver function using a double indicator dilution technique (the COLD-system: Cardiac output – Oxygenation – Liver function/Lung water-Diagnosis) and the determination of hepatic venous oxygen saturation seem to be the methods most reliable and useful for clinical practice. These methods and their limitations have been described in detail elsewhere (de Backer and Vincent 1998; Groeneveld 1998; Knichwitz et al. 1996, 1998; Mythen and Webb 1994).

Therapeutic Possibilities to Increase Splanchnic Oxygen Delivery

Therapeutical interventions are aiming to avoid, diminish, or overcome splanchnic hypoperfusion and/or dysoxia. Considering the equation for oxygen transport capacity (Fig. 1), oxygen delivery (DO_2) to the whole body or to special organs may be increased by:

- 1. an increase in oxygen content of the blood (CaO_2), where CaO_2 is the sum of the amount of oxygen bound to hemoglobin (Hb, SaO_2) and the amount of oxygen physically dissolved (PaO_2) in plasma. The amount of O_2 bound by hemoglobin is about 50–100 times higher than the amount physically dissolved
- 2. and/or by increasing cardiac output (CO).

$$DO_2 = (Hb\ [g/dl] \times SaO_2\ [\%] \times 1.36\ [ml\ O_2/g\ Hb] + 0.003\ [ml\ O_2/dl\ blood/mmHg\ PO_2] \times PaO_2\ [mmHg])\ X\ CO\ [ml/min]$$

Fig. 1. Oxygen transport capacity. QO_2: oxygen transport capacity [ml/min]; CO: cardiac output = stroke volume × heart rate = $\Delta P/R$; Hb: hemoglobin concentration; SaO_2: arterial oxygen saturation of hemoglobin; 1.36: Hüfner's number; 0.003: solubility constant for O_2 in blood (= 0.0225 ml O_2/dl blood/kPa PaO_2); PaO_2: arterial oxygen partial pressure

Increasing Oxygen Content of the Blood

An increase in hemoglobin concentration and hematocrit (Hct), and thus in oxygen content of the blood, is possible by transfusing red blood cells. However, due to concomitant changes in viscosity, this therapeutic modality does not necessarily increase oxygen delivery. Rheological alterations may induce a decrease in blood flow, especially in microcirculation. Thus, the question of the "optimal hematocrit" has not yet been answered and is still a subject of controversy. For a long time, a Hct of 30 %–35 % respective to a hemoglobin concentration of 10 g/dl was recommended (Czer and Shoemaker 1978), based on theoretical calculations regarding viscosity, flow, and optimal DO_2. However, in a recent study (Dietrich et al. 1990), when Hb had been increased above 8.3 g/dl, no better outcome was found. Furthermore, Marik and Sibbald (1993) observed a decrease in pHi, indicating mucosal dysoxia, despite a theoretical increase in oxygen content, by transfusing stored blood older than 10 days. Van der Linden (1994) recommended an optimal hematocrit for most patients between 20 % and 30 %. Our own results have shown that, for the gut, the "critical hematocrit", indicating dependency of oxygen intake on oxygen supply, is in a range lower than 15 % (Nöldge et al. 1992; Ott et al. 1997).

In a further study, it could be demonstrated that no decrease in pO_2 in mucosal tissue could be observed until hemoglobin concentration rose above 3 g/dl (Haisjackl et al. 1997). The latter results were obtained from experiments in healthy pigs, where hematocrit was gradually lowered by normovolemic hemodilution; and it must be emphasized that care was taken to provide strict normovolemia.

There are no data showing that an increase in oxygen transport by increasing arterial oxygen saturation above 90 % (corresponding to a PaO_2 of 60 mmHg) improves results. Preliminary data obtained from our pig model show that the gut did not become oxygen-supply-dependent until arterial PaO_2 was kept above 30 mmHg. Nevertheless, in critically ill patients, oxygen saturation should not be less than 90 %, corresponding to a PaO_2 of 60 mmHg.

Increasing Cardiac Output

Volume Therapy

At the moment, there is agreement that therapy should be goal-oriented, aiming for a cardiac index (CI) not less than 4.5 l/min/m^2 body surface. The first step toward augmenting cardiac output is to increase blood volume, which has a major impact on splanchnic blood flow. It could be shown that intestinal perfusion is decreased with hypovolemia (Edouard et al. 1994), and it is important to emphasize that intestinal hypoperfusion persists, even if systemic blood volume is restored. Thus, early volume resuscitation is of primary importance to avoid sustained mucosal ischemia. In critically ill patients, intestinal hypoperfusion is mostly induced by either absolute hypovolemia following hemorrhagic shock or by relative hypovolemia following increased capillary permeability caused by endothelial lesions in septic or burned patients. There is no doubt that absolute or relative hypovolemia warrants immediate volume therapy.

The question of whether crystalloids or colloids are preferable for volume replacement has not been answered yet. Boldt (1996a, 1996b) found advantages in low molecular hydroxyethyl starch (HAES) solution over albumin, since HAES was able to increase the parameters of systemic hemodynamic and mucosal oxygenation, characterized by maintained pHi.

A beneficial effect of colloids in comparison to crystalloids could be observed in a septic sheep model, where colloids were able to slow progression of extrapulmonary tissue injury (Morisaki et al. 1994). In a porcine septic model, Fink showed that the most successful resuscitation technique was a combination of crystalloids and colloids together with dobutamine (Fink et al. 1991b).

New approaches to increase oxygen delivery by using new synthetic oxygen carriers promise benefits for splanchnic perfusion. However, it is too early to draw a final conclusion (Frankel et al. 1996; Mourelatos et al. 1996; Reah et al. 1997; Siegel et al. 1997; Xu et al. 1997). If volume therapy is not sufficient, cardiac output and thus oxygen transport capacity can be increased additionally by catecholamine therapy.

Catecholamines

The choice of a special catecholamine depends on the specific clinical situation of the patient, especially with regard to cardiac contractility, and systemic and pulmonary vascular resistance. In general, we need to differentiate between β-adrenergic stimulation, which increases cardiac output by improving myocardial contractility and reducing systemic vascular resistance, and α-adrenergic stimulation, which elicits vasoconstriction with potential reduction of blood flow. The relative adrenergic receptor activity is summarized in Table 1. Under physiological conditions, β-adrenergic and dopaminergic stimulation increases splanchnic blood flow, and α-

Table 1. Action of catecholamines on different receptors

Catecholamine	Receptor α	β_1	β_2	D
Epinephrine	+++	+++	++	-
Norepinephrine	+++	++	+	-
Dobutamine	+	+++	++	-
Dopamine				
< 3 μg/kg/min	–	-	–	+++
2–10 μg/kg/min	+	++	+	++
> 10 μg/kg/min	++	++	+	+
Dopexamine	–	+	+++	++

adrenergic stimulation decreases it (Braatvedt et al. 1993; Kvietys et al. 1982). However, in critically ill patients, the suspected physiological response to catecholamines can be modified by altered volume status, receptor downregulation, underlying altered pathophysiological conditions such as distributive shock, and circulating vasodilating mediators. Additionally, the therapeutic effects of the different catecholamines on splanchnic perfusion may be influenced by the dose used and by the possible administration of other vasoactive drugs which may counteract the physiological effects.

Dobutamine

According to several authors (Dhainaut et al. 1990; Reinhart et al. 1990; Shoemaker et al. 1989, 1993), dobutamine seems to be the catecholamine of choice because of its β1-adrenergic stimulation. According to several authors, dobutamine increased splanchnic blood flow in nonseptic animals (Drexler et al. 1987; Liang et al. 1981; Robie and Goldberg 1975; Wanless et al. 1987). However, it did not have any effect on reversing PEEP-induced depression of mesenteric blood flow (Azar et al. 1996). Additionally, in our own experiments using acutely instrumented healthy pigs, dobutamine did not have any positive effect on superior mesenteric arterial blood flow, despite a pronounced increase in CO and DO_2 (Priebe et al. 1995).

In combination with adequate volume resuscitation, dobutamine increased CO and DO_2 in experimental septic shock (Vincent et al. 1987). In animal and clinical studies, Vincent (1987, 1990) and Gilbert (1986) showed that the increase in DO_2 by dobutamine was associated to an increase in oxygen uptake. Whereas red blood cell transfusion and 5 μg/kg/min dobutamine increased DO_2 by the same amount in septic patients (Silverman and Tuma 1992), only dobutamine increased a low pHi as well.

This was consistent with findings of other groups, where dobutamine increased splanchnic blood flow and increased pHi in endotoxic animal models (Fink et al. 1991b; De Backer and Vincent 1998; Nevière 1997). In other studies, dobutamine did not increase VO_2, but did increase pHi (Gutierrez et al. 1994).

In contrast to the latter studies, dobutamine did not increase splanchnic blood flow, mucosal blood flow (Karzai et al. 1996), or pHi (Parviainen et al. 1995; Uusaro et al. 1996) in patients with acute pancreatitis (Ruokonen et al. 1997) and patients with congestive heart failure (Leier 1988), and after cardiac surgery.

Because of lack of methods for continuous, simultaneous monitoring of splanchnic flow in human patients, it is difficult to decide whether an increase in pHi, reflecting improvement of mucosal perfusion, is the result of increased systemic hemodynamic parameters or whether it is caused by selective action on splanchnic vessels. There are at least hints that, in septic patients, there is no specific action on splanchnic vessels (Reinelt et al. 1997), and a dobutamine-induced increase in splanchnic blood flow results from increased cardiac output.

There have been only a few clinical studies concerning the effects of dobutamine on mucosal blood flow. Despite still controversial results, a greater number of studies and the latest one showed improvement of mucosal blood flow in endotoxic rats and pigs during application of dobutamine (Neviére et al. 1997; Secchi et al. 1997).

In summary, dobutamine might be able to increase splanchnic perfusion and mucosal blood flow as a result of increasing systemic DO_2 without having a specific effect on splanchnic circulation. However, it has to be emphasized that most results have been taken from animal models (healthy pig, dog, sheep, or as models for sepsis), where regional flows could be measured using invasive methods. Whether the conclusions from one or the other study can be transferred to critically ill humans has to be proven in future clinical studies. Additionally, most of the older studies did choose pHi as an indicator of mucosal perfusion and oxygenation. However, there is increasing evidence that determination of intestinal mucosal pCO_2 is a better parameter for detecting mucosal ischemia. Thus, future clinical human studies will be necessary to characterize and quantify the effects of vasoactive drugs by determining intestinal mucosa pCO_2.

Dopamine

Dopamine is a precursor of norepinephrine and epinephrine. It binds to all subtypes of adrenergic receptors. At low doses (1–3 μg/kg/min), there is mainly an effect on dopaminergic receptors, which can be found not only at renal, but also mesenteric vessels (Goldberg 1972). At higher doses (3–8 μg/kg/min), the β-adrenergic effect causes an increase in cardiac output. In high doses (> 10 μg/kg/min), α-adrenergic stimulation becomes overwhelming.

Dopamine (at 15 μg/kg/min) increased superior mesenteric arterial and portal venous blood flow in healthy pigs by 30 % but decreased hepatic arterial blood flow by the same amount (Priebe et al. 1995). Compared to dobutamine and norepinephrine, dopamine was the only drug which was able to increase both systemic and splanchnic oxygen delivery. Additionally, it was able to decrease the mesenteric oxygen extraction rate (Priebe et al. 1995).

In general, the data regarding the effects of dopamine on splanchnic blood flow and especially on mucosal oxygenation are still controversial. Some studies did confirm the observation that dopamine increases total splanchnic blood flow (Germann et al. 1997a; 1997b; Giraud and Mac Cannel 1984; Johnson et al. 1991; Pearson et al. 1996; Robie and Goldberg 1975; Schmidt et al. 1996; Winsö et al. 1995), while others could not prove it (Azar et al. 1996; Bersten et al. 1992; Breslow et al. 1987; Cheung et al. 1997). The results regarding the oxygen supply/demand relationship during administration of dopamine are equivocal. Royblat (1989) found increased liver but unchanged gut O_2 consumption. Segal (1992) observed detrimental effects of dopamine on critical O_2 delivery in case of hemorrhage. Hannemann (1995) showed that patients in septic shock treated with dopamine did not show improvement of splanchnic microcirculation; however, they had higher heart rates, filling pressures, and higher intrapulmonary shunts compared to patients treated with a combination of dobutamine and norepinephrine. Therefore, the combination of dobutamine and norepinephrine was favored, since, there were more disadvantages with dopamine, such as increased myocardial oxygen demand and impaired pulmonary gas exchange.

Results regarding the effects of dopamine on mucosal perfusion and oxygenation are even more controversial. It is possible to find "positive" results, like delayed onset of villus ischemia (Schmidt et al. 1996) and increased gut mucosal pO_2 with up to 16 μg/kg/min dopamine in pigs (Germann et al. 1997a, b) as well as decreased mucosal blood flow and decreased intestinal O_2 extraction in dogs (Giraud and Mac Cannel 1984). Additionally, dopamine neither increased pHi in cardiac surgical patients (Gärdebäack et al. 1995) nor in septic patients (Marik and Mohedin 1994; Maynard et al. 1995; Meier-Hellmann et al. 1997; Nevière et al. 1996; Olson et al. 1996).

Vincent et al. (1987) and Shoemaker et al. (1989) speculated that higher doses of dopamine might be potentially detrimental for microcirculation, due to α-mimetic effects. Recent studies not only failed to show a beneficial effect of dopamine on pHi, but even reported a decrease in pHi (Marik and Mohedin 1994) or reduction in gut mucosal blood flow (Nevière et al. 1996). On the other hand, some studies indicate that dopamine might have a protective effect on the mucosa regarding translocation of endotoxins (MacNaughton and Wallace 1989).

In conclusion, dopamine seems to be able to increase total splanchnic blood flow, but its effects on mucosal blood flow remain unclear. When thinking of indications for the use of dopamine in critically ill patients, we need to keep in mind the other adverse effects of dopamine, like impaired activity of macrophages and lymphocytes, suppression of pituitary function (Lucas et al. 1990; Van den Berghe et al. 1994 a, b), and its influence on thyroid function (Van den Berghe et al. 1994b).

Thus, there is no indication for routine use of low-dose dopamine with the intention to raise intramucosal gastric pHi (Olson et al. 1996).

Dopexamine

Dopexamine is a synthetic catecholamine with strong action on β_1-, β_2- and DA_1-receptors, and no stimulation of α-receptors (Stephan et al. 1990). Thus it elicits systemic vasodilatation (Mousdale et al. 1985) and reduces afterload, resulting in increased CO. The resistance of hepatosplanchnic vessels is markedly reduced (Moss et al. 1990). Theoretically, the properties of dopexamine offer many advantages as an ideal catecholamine for improving splanchnic perfusion.

Dopexamine increased splanchnic blood flow in critically ill patients (Leier 1988; Maynard et al. 1995; Reinelt et al. 1997; Uusaro et al. 1996) and in animals (Germann et al. 1997; Steinberg et al. 1996; Schmidt et al. 1996; Tighe et al. 1993), elevated mucosal pO_2 in rabbits (Lund et al. 1995), and decreased lactate production of the gut (Cain and Curtis 1991). Additionally, it increased pHi in septic patients (Maynard et al. 1995; Smithies et al. 1994).

A new study (Temmesfeld-Wollbrück et al. 1998) indicates that dopexamine might be able to improve regional oxygen delivery to the upper gastrointestinal tract in septic patients, as measured with reflectance spectrophotometry.

In conclusion, dopexamine improves splanchnic perfusion and oxygenation in animal models and perfusion in men; but further studies examining the influence of dopexamine on $piCO_2$, must be done before a final conclusion can be drawn on its usefulness regarding mucosal perfusion.

Epinephrine

Epinephrine is a potent ß-adrenergic drug at low doses, and a predominantly potent α- adrenergic stimulants in higher doses. There are only a few studies available which focus on the effects of epinephrine on splanchnic perfusion, and, again, the results are not clear, either (Bersten et al. 1992; Cheung et al. 1997). Meier-Hellmann et al. (1997) found that, in patients with septic shock, splanchnic perfusion was impaired, lactate increased transiently, and the ratio of splanchnic blood flow to CO was reduced. This is in agreement with the results of a recently published study (Day et al.

1996), in which treatment with epinephrine resulted in increased plasma lactate levels. The work of Levy et al. (1997 a, b) showed that, in patients treated with epinephrine, pHi decreased. Some patients who required very high doses of epinephrine due to cardiac failure in sepsis did show beneficial effects from the additional infusion of low doses of dobutamine (5 μg/kg/min) regarding lactate levels and pCO_2 gap. Lactate levels and pCO_2 gaps decreased in epinephrine-treated patients during dobutamine infusion, indicating improved splanchnic perfusion (Levy et al. 1997 a, b).

In summary, the increasing number of new studies showing no beneficial or even detrimental effects of epinephrine on splanchnic oxygenation, especially in patients with septic shock, do not make epinephrine the drug of choice, especially when maintenance or improvement of hepatosplanchnic oxygenation is desired.

Norepinephrine

Norepinephrine has mainly α-adrenergic properties and acts as a vasoconstrictor at the splanchnic vessels (Hirsch et al. 1976). From a theoretical point of view, norepinephrine might have detrimental effects on splanchnic circulation. Thus, it is not surprising that such effects could be observed in some studies (Breslow et al. 1987; Richardson et al. 1980; Ryan and Gisolfi 1995). But again, the results are not univocal (Bersten et al. 1992; Galindo 1965; Hussain et al. 1988; Kvietys et al. 1983). In other studies, norepinephrine increased liver blood flow in endotoxic dogs, increasing hepatic arterial blood flow (Zhang et al. 1997), and increased hepatic venous oxygen saturation and decreased pHi, indicating improvement of hepatosplanchnic blood flow in septic shock patients (Ruokonen et al. 1993; Meier-Hellmann et al. 1996).

Recently, Tighe et al. (1998) showed that the α_1-adrenergic agonist methoxamine and the β_2-receptor antagonist ICI 118551 both augmented hepatic injury in their porcine model of fecal peritonitis. The effects on liver ultrastructure were comparable to those seen in septic patients after treatment with norepinephrine and/or dobutamine.

In summary, despite inconsistent results in experimental studies and the theoretical, potential disadvantages of predominantly vasoconstricting drugs, the beneficial effect of norepinephrine seem to outweigh the potential negative effects, especially in critically ill, septic patients.

Other Therapeutic Modalities to Improve Splanchnic Oxygen Delivery

Vasodilation

Results with prostacyclin or its analogues are promising (Kiluchi et al. 1994; Radermacher et al. 1996; Raper et al. 1991; Rasmussen et al. 1992; Seelig et al. 1981) but need further evaluation. Vlatten et al. (1998) and Träger et al. (1998a) recently reported that iloprost, a prostacyclin analogue, did not improve intestinal blood flow in a porcine endotoxic shock model when given as treatment, but it prevented endotoxin-induced decease in lactate clearance. A similar effect could be observed after treatment with the combined thromboxane receptor antagonist and synthase inhibitor DTTX30 (Träger et al. 1998b).

Nitric oxide is a potent vasodilator and has a key role in regulation of splanchnic perfusion (Ayuse et al. 1995), but its mechanisms of action are not fully understood yet. Infusion of NO donors (GTN, sodium nitroprusside) induces vasodilation and can diminish mucosal damage caused by endotoxin (Allman et al. 1996; Boughton-Smith et al. 1990; Fan et al. 1996; Zhang et al. 1996). Consequently, inhibition of NO decreased splanchnic perfusion (Allmann et al. 1996; Booke et al. 1996; Fan et al. 1996; Mendez et al. 1997; Pilette et al. 1996; Spain et al. 1994; Walker et al. 1995).

It is unclear whether the mucosal protection is due to improved mucosal perfusion and oxygenation or inhibition of the inflammatory cascade (Gauthier et al. 1994). The protective effects of NO on the gut mucosa (Bougthon-Smith et al. 1990; Sorells et al. 1996; Vollmar et al. 1994), such as maintained impermeability (Schleiffer and Raul 1996) and reduced bacterial translocation (Adawi et al. 1997), seem to overwhelm the detrimental effects (Salzman et al. 1995; Vollmar et al. 1994).

Other vasodilators like adenosine and isoprenaline might increase macrocirculation but can lead to splanchnic steal and redistribution of blood flow (Leier 1988; Parviainen et al. 1996; Sheperd et al. 1984).

ACE inhibitors (enalaprilat) showed modest improvements on splanchnic perfusion (Leier 1988; Parviainen et al. 1995). The idea behind this approach is to antagonize angiotensin, one of the strongest vasoconstricting drugs. Although the etiology of gut hypoperfusion after shock and resuscitation is still unclear, experimental and clinical data support the idea of an important role for angiotensin (Bailey et al. 1982; Gasic et al. 1989; McNeill et al. 1970). Hesse et al. (1986) showed that ACE inhibitors can attenuate splanchnic vasoconstriction during systemic hypotension.

However, until now there is a lack of sufficient studies focusing on the effects of ACE inhibitors on splanchnic circulation in septic or critically injured patients, except for one study proving the positive effect of enalaprilat on mucosal pHi in human shock patients after resuscitation (Kincaid et al. 1998). According to this study, enalaprilat could increase pHi when a low pHi was due to decreased perfusion (low flow state), as detected by an increase in the arterial mucosal pCO_2 gradient. There was no effect when low pHi was due to low arterial bicarbonate concentration representing an open system with anaerobic metabolism.

Epidural Anesthesia

Regional hypoperfusion is mainly caused by local vasoconstriction generated through enhanced nervous sympathetic activity and increased plasma levels of catecholamines. Therefore, it might be reasonable to induce regional vasodilation by locally blocking the sympathetic nervous system with epidural anesthesia. Recently, the results of a small prospective study were published, indicating benefits of epidural anesthesia on the outcome after emergency abdominal surgery (Jomura et al. 1997).

Already in 1964, Fine described a decrease from 80 % to 20 % in mortality of dogs and rabbits in which the splanchnic viscera had been surgically denervated before induction of endotoxic shock. This beneficial outcome might have been due to immune modulation of the spleen and liver, elicited by sympathicolysis and/or reduced sympathetic activity by blocking the sympathetic outflow from the spinal cord and the adrenal glands. In our own recent study we found that, in healthy pigs, epidural anesthesia (EA) of the splanchnic region (T5–T10) induced hypotension associated with pronounced mesenteric vasodilation. Thus, despite a decrease in perfusion pressure, mesenteric blood flow did not change significantly and mucosal tissue pO_2 and pCO_2 were maintained (Vagts et al. 1998a, b). Lactate metabolism of the gut remained unchanged. Volume loading prior to EA in order to overcome EA-induced hypotension did not improve splanchnic blood flow, but also disturbed mucosal oxygenation by hypervolemic hemodilution. But maintaining mean arterial pressure with dopamine to overcome EA-induced hypotension was able to decrease mucosal $piCO_2$ (Vagts et al. 1998c). In conclusion, these experiments showed that EA did not improve splanchnic perfusion or oxygenation in healthy pigs. However, the pronounced decrease in blood pressure did not show any detrimental effect, either, as long as mean arterial pressure was maintained above 60 mm Hg.

Future studies will be done to investigate whether a positive effect of EA can be shown during endotoxemia to overcome initially observed, marked vasoconstriction (Nöldge-Schomburg et al. 1996).

Arachidonic Acid Metabolites and Antioxidants

Mediators of arachidonic acid metabolism, such as prostaglandins, thromboxane A2, and leukotrienes are potent vasoconstrictors. Inhibition of the arachidonic acid metabolism by blockers like ibuprofen or meclofenamat could increase systemic and mesenteric DO_2 and reduce VO_2 (Fink et al. 1989). Antioxidants like N-acetylcysteine improved oxygen extraction after endotoxemia, but had no influence on splanchnic perfusion during reperfusion (Zhang et al. 1995).

Although the complement system has been shown to play an important role in disturbances of regional perfusion, Schmidt et al. (1998) failed to demonstrate a positive effect of C1-esterase inhibitor on mucosal tissue oxygenation in endotoxic rats.

Nutrition

Perioperative feeding with an arginine-enriched diet improved mucosal perfusion in critically ill patients (Braga et al. 1996). This effect could be due to increased formation of NO but to other, unknown factors, as well. Cancer patients perioperatively fed with immunonutrition showed increased intestinal oxygen tension, measured continuously by an implanted polarographic oxygen microprobe catheter, and improved outcome (Braga et al. 1998).

Early feeding seems to provide many benefits. Nevertheless, until now, there are no studies focussing on the effects of feeding on splanchnic perfusion in critically ill patients. Early feeding probably increases splanchnic perfusion; however, it also increases regional oxygen demand. Thus, feeding may be detrimental if it is started when mucosal DO_2 and VO_2 are mismatched. In dogs, no harmful effect could be observed when feeding was started within 1 h after ischemia and reperfusion (Dubin et al. 1998). Further studies are required to get more knowledge about the effects of early enteral nutrition on splanchnic oxygenation.

Conclusion

There is agreement (De Backer and Vincent 1998; Rudis et al. 1996; Meier-Hellmann et al. 1998) that improvement of splanchnic oxygen delivery by different means of treatment, especially the choice of a catecholamine after volume resuscitation, is a very complex affair. Additionally, we have to keep in mind that improvement of splanchnic perfusion does not necessarily mean improvement of oxygenation or function. Structural integrity is not guaranteed by maintenance of organ flood flow (Webb et al. 1991; Tighe et al. 1998). It is important to recognize that the goal of our treatment is not just improved perfusion and "adequate" oxygenation, but even more: functional integrity. We still do not have devices sophisticated enough to monitor splanchnic function online and noninvasively, and we do not have a specific drug to influence perfusion and oxygenation of each organ concerned in an optimal way.

Therefore, until now, it is only possible to recommend several potential ways, but not the only therapeutic modality to improve splanchnic oxygenation and function.

References

1. Adawi D, Kasravi FB, Molin G, Jeppson B (1997) Effect of Lactobacillus supplementation with and without arginine on liver damage and bacterial translocation in acute liver injury model in rat. Hepatology 25:642–647
2. Allman KG, Stoddart AP, Kennedy MM, Young JD (1996) L-arginine augments nitric oxide production and mesenteric blood flow in ovine endotoxemia. Am J Physiol 271:H1296-H1301
3. Ayuse T, Revelly JPP, Boitnott JK, Robotham JL (1995) Role of nitric oxide in porcine liver circulation under normal and endotoxemic conditions. J Apppl Phyiol 78: 1319–1329
4. Azar G, Love R, Choe E, Flint L, Steinberg S (1996) Neither dopamine nor dobutamine reverses the depression in mesenteric blood flow caused by positive end-expiator pressure. J Trauma 40:679–687
5. Bailey RW, Bulkley GB, Levy KI, Anderson JH, Zuidema GD (1982) Pathogenesis of nonocclusive mesenteric ischemia: studies in a porcine model induced by pericordial tamponade. Surg Forum 33:194–196
6. Bersten AD, Hersch M, Cheung H, Rutledge FS, Sibbald WJ (1992) The effects of various sympathomimetics on the regional circulations in hyperdynamic sepsis. Surgery 112:549–561
7. Bohlen HG (1980) Intestinal tissue pO_2 and microvascular response during glucose exposure. Am J Physiol 238:H164–H171
8. Boldt J, Heesen M, Müller M, Pabsdorf M, Hempelmann G (1996) The effect of albumin versus hydroxyethyl starch solution on cardiorespiratory and circulatory variables in critically ill patients. Anesth Analg 83:254–261
9. Boldt J, Müller M, Menges T, Papsdorf M, Hempelmann G (1996) Influence of different volume therapy regimes on regulators of the circulation in the critically ill. Br J Anaesth77:480–487
10. Botha AJ, Moore FA, Moore EE, Sauaia A, Banerjee A, Peterson VM (1995) Early neutrophil sequestration after injury: A pathogenic mechanism for multiple organ failure. J Trauma 39:411–417
11. Booke M, Hinder F, McGuire R, Traber LD, Traber DL (1996) Nitric oxide synthase inhibition versus norepinephrine in ovine sepsis: effects on regional blood flow. Shock 5:362–370
12. Boughton-Smith NK, Hucheson IR, Deaking AM, Whittle BJR, Moncada S (1990) Protective effect of S-nitroso-N-acetyl-penicillamine in endotoxin-induced acute intestinal damage in the rat. Eur J Pharmacol 191:485–488
13. Braatvedt GD, Flynn MD, Stanners A, Halliwell M, Corall RJM (1993) Splanchnic blood flow in man: evidence for mediation via a (-adrenergic) mechanism. Clin Sci 84:201–207
14. Braga M, Gianotti L, Cestari A, Vignali A, Pellegatta F, Dolci A, Di Carlo V (1996) Gut function and immune and inflammatory response in patients perioperatively fed with supplemented enteral formulas. Arch Surg 131:1257–1265
15. Braga M, Gianotti L, Vignali (1998) Artificial nutrition after major abdominal surgery: impact of route of administration of the diet. Crit Care Med 26:24–30

16. Breslow MJ, Miller CF, Parker SD, Walman AT, Traystman RJ (1987) Effect of vasopressors on organ blood flow during endotoxin shock in pigs. Am J Physiol 252:H291–H300
17. Brown SD, Gutierrez G (1997) Tonometry revisited. Curr Opin in Anaesthesiol 10:77–85
18. Cain SM, Curtis SE (1991) Systemic and regional oxygen uptake and delivery and lactate flux in endotoxic dogs infused with dopexamine. Crit Care Med 19:1552–1560
19. Chang MC, Cheatham ML, Nelson LD, Rutherford EJ, Morris JA (1994) Gastric tonometry supplements information provided by systemic indicators of oxygen transport. J Trauma 37:488–494
20. Cheung PY, Barrington KJ, Pearson RJ, Bigam DL, Finer NN, Van Aerde JE (1997) Systemic, pulmonary, and mesenteric perfusion and oxygenation effcts of dopamine and epinephrine. Am J Respir Crit Care Med 155:32–37
21. Czer LS, Shoemaker WC (1978) Optimal hematocrit value in critically ill postoperative patients. Surg Gynecol Obstet 147:363–368
22. Dalton JM, Gore DC, Makhoul RG, Fisher MR, DeMaria EJ (1995) Decreased splanchnic perfusion measured by duplex ultrapound in humans undergoing small volume hemorrhage. Crit Care Med 23:491–497
23. Day NP, Phu NH, Bethell DP, Mai NT, Chau TT, Hien TT, White NJ (1996) The effects of dopamine and adrenaline infusions on acid/base balance and systemic haemodynamics in severe infection. Lancet 348:219–223
24. Dantzker DR (1993) The gastrointestinal tract. The canary of the body? JAMA 270:1247–8
25. De Backer D, Vincent JL (1998) Pharmacologic modulation of splanchnic blood flow. Current Opinion in Intensive Care 104–110
26. Deitch EA (1990) The role of intestinal barrier failure and bacterial translocation in the development of systemic infection and multiple organ failure. Arch Surg 125:403–404
27. Dhainaut JF, Edwards JD, Grootendorst AF (1990) Practical aspects of oxygen transport: conclusions and recommendations of the Round Table Conference. Int Care Med 16:179–180
28. Dietrich KA, Conrad SA, Hebert CA, Levy GL, Romero MD (1990) Cardiovascular and metabolic response to red blood cell transfusion in critically ill volume-resuscitated nonsurgical patients. Crit Care Med 18:940–944
29. Drexler H, Höing S, Faude F, Wollschläger H, Just H (1987) Central and regional vascular hemodynamics following intravenous milrinone in the conscious rat: comparison with dobutamine. J Cardiovasc Pharmacol 9:563–569
30. Dubin A, De Paula J, Estenssoro E, Barán M, Laporte M, Murias G, Badie J, Sottile P, Canales H, Diaz Rivas M, Pálizas F, Barrio MG (1998) Absence of harmful effects of enteral nutrition on tissue oxygenation of ischemic gut. (abstract) Intensive Care Med 24:S13
31. Duranteau J, Sitbon P, Vicaut E, Descorps-Declere A, Vigue B, Samii K (1996) Assessment of gastric mucosal perfusion during simulated hypovolaemia in healthy volunteers. Am J Respir Crit Care Med 154:1653–1657
32. Edouard AR, Degremont A-C, Duranteau J, Pussard E, Berdeaux A, Samii K (1994) Heterogenous regional vascular responses to simulated transient hypovolaemia in man. Intensive Care Med 20:414–420
33. Fan WQ, Smolich JJ, Wild J, Yu VYH, Walker AM (1996) Nitric oxide modulates regional blood flow differences in the fetal gastrointestinal tract. Am J Physiol 271:G598–G604
34. Fine J (1964) Denervation of the splanchnic viscera for the treatment of shock. Am J Surg 107:723–724
35. Fink MP (1991a) Gastrointestinal mucosal injury in experimental models of shock, trauma, and sepsis. Crit Care Med 19:627–641
36. Fink MP, Kaups KL, Wang H, Rothschild HR (1991b) Maintenance of superior mesenteric arterial perfusion prevents increased intestinal mucosal permeability in endotoxic pigs. Surgery 110:154–161
37. Fink MP, Rothschild R, Deniz YF, Wang H, Lee PC, Cohn SM (1989) Systemic and mesenteric O_2 metabolism in endotoxic pigs: effect of ibuprofen and meclofenamate. J Appl Physiol 67:1950–1957
38. Fong Y, Marano MA, Moldawer LL, Calvano SE, Kenney JS, Allison AC, Ceramin A, Shires GT, Lowri SF (1990) The acute splanchnic and peripheral metabolic response to endotoxin in humans. J Clin Invest 85:1896–1904
39. Frankel HL, Nguyen HB, Shea-Donohue T, Aiton LA, Ratigan J, Malcolm DS (1996) Diaspirin cross-linked hemoglobin is efficacious in gut resuscitation as measured by GI tract optode. J Trauma 40:231–241
40. Gärdebäack M, Sittergren G, Öhquist G, Tiren C (1995) Effect of dopexamine on calculated low gastric intramucosal pH following valve replacement. Acta Anaesthesiol Scand 39: 599–684
41. Galindo A (1965) Hepatic circulation and hepatic function during anesthesia and surgery. Can Anaesth Soc J 12:262–274

42. Gasic S, Heinz G, Kleinbloesem C, Korn A (1989) Effects of ace inhibition with cilazapril on splanchnic and systemic haemodynamics in man. Br J Clin Pharmacol 27:225S–234S
43. Gauthier TW, Davenpeck KL, Lefer AM (1994) Nitric oxide attenuates leukocyte-endothelium interaction via P-selectin in splanchnic ischemia reperfusion. Am J Physiol 267:G562–G568
44. Germann R, Haisjackl M, Schwarz B, Deusch E, Meusburger S, Gruber E, Pajk W, Hausdorfer H, Bonatti J, Furtner B, Ulmer H, Hasibeder W (1997) Inotropic treatment and intestinal mucosal tissue oxygenation in a model of porcine endotoxemia. Crit Care Med 25:1191–1197
45. Germann R, Haisjackl M, Schwarz B, Salak N, Deusch E, Pajk W, Wolf HJ, Riedmann B, Hasibeder W (1997) Dopamine and intestinal mucosal tissue oxygenation in a porcine model of haemorrhage. Br J Anaesth 79:357–362
46. Gilbert EM, Haupt MT, Mandanas RY, Huaringa AJ, Carlson RW (1986) The effect of fluid loading, blood transfusion, and catecholamine infusion on oxygen delivery and consumption in patients with sepsis. Am Rev Respir Dis 134:873–878
47. Gimson AES (1987) Hepatic dysfunction during bacterial sepsis. Intensive Care Med 13:162–166
48. Giraud GD, Mac Cannell KL (1984) Decreased nutrient blood flow during dopamine- and epinephrine-induced intestinal vasodilation. J Pharmacol Exp Ther 230:214–220
49. Goldberg LI (1972) Cardiovascular and renal actions of dopamine: potential clinical applications. Pharmacol Rev 24:1–29
50. Groeneveld ABJ (1998) Measuring splanchnic perfusion. Curr Opin Crit Care 4:111–115
51. Gutierrez G, Clark C, Brown SD, Price K, Ortiz L, Nelson C (1994) Effect of dobutamine on oxygen consumption and gastric mucosal pH in septic patients. Am J Respir Crit Care 150:324–329
52. Haisjackl M, Luz G, Sparr H, Germann R, Salak N, Friesenecker B, Deusch E, Meusburger S, Hasibeder W (1997) The effects of progressive anemia on jejunal mucosal and serosal tissue oxygenation in pigs. Anesth Analg 84:538–544
53. Hannemann L, Reinhart K, Grenzer O, Meier-Hellmann A, Bredle DL (1995) Comparison of dopamine to dobutamine and norepinephrine for oxygen delivery and uptake in septic shock. Crit Care Med 23:1962–1970
54. Hesse B, Stadaeger C, Rasmussen S, Henriksen O, Bonde-Petersen F (1986) The influence of the renin-angiotensin system on adrenergic vasoconstrictor responses in the forearm and splanchnic region in sodium-depleted man. J Hypertension 4:S402-S405
55. Hirsch LJ, Ayabe T, Glick D (1976) Direct effects of various catecholamines on liver circulation in dogs. Am J Physiol 77:432–438
56. Hussain SNA, Rutledge F, Roussos C, Magder S (1988) Effects of norepinephrine and fluid administration on the selective blood flow distribution in endotoxic shock. J Crit Care 1:32–42
57. Johnson DJ, Johannigman JA, Branson RD, Davis K, Hurst JM (1991) The effect of low dose dopamine on gut hemodynamics during PEEP ventilation for acute lung injury. J Surg Res 50:344–349
58. Jomura K, Hamada T, Sugiki K, Ito Y (1997) [Epidural anesthesia reduces mortality rate in the patients after emergency abdominal surgery. Abstract] [Japanese]. Japanese Journal of Anesthesiology 46:1602–8
59. Karzei W, Lötte A, Günnicker M, Vorgrimler-Karzei UM, Priebe HJ (1996) Dobutamine inreases oxygen consumption during constant flow cardiopulmonary bypass. Br J Anaesth 76:5–8
60. Kiluchi E, Fukui H, Matsumoto M, Tsujita S, Matsumura M, Uemura M, Tsujii T (1994) Effects of prostaglandin E_1 on experimantal acute hepatic failure in rabbits: prostaglandin E_1 prevents the development of multiple organ failure. J Hepatol 20:478–482
61. Kincaid EH, Miller PR, Meredith JW, Chang MC (1998) Enalaprilat improves gut perfusion in critically injured patients. Shock 9:79–83
62. Knaus WA, Wagner DP, Draper EA, et al (1991) The APACHE III prognosis systrem: risk prediction of hospital mortality for critically ill hospitalized adults. Chest 100:1619–1631
63. Knichwitz G, (1998) Kontinuierliche intramukosale pCO_2 -Messung: Entwicklung und Stellenwert eines neuen Verfahrens. AINS 33:S78–S84
64. Knichwitz G, Rötker J, Brüssel T, Kuhmann M, Mertes N, Möllhoff T (1996) A new method for continuous intramucosal pCO_2 measurement in the gastrointestinal tract. Anesth Analg 83:6–11
65. Kvietys PR, Granger DN (1982) Vasoactive agents and splanchnic oxygen uptake. Am J Physiol 243:G1-G9
66. Kvietys PR, Perry MA, Granger DN (1983) Intestinal capillary exchange capacity and oxygen delivery-to-demand ratio. Am J Physiol 245:G635–640
67. Kvietys PR, Shepherd AP, Granger DN (1985) Laser-Doppler, H2 clearance and microsphere estimate of mucosal blood flow. Am J Physiol 249:G221-G227
68. Leier CV (1988) Regional blood flow responses to vasodilators and inotropes in congestive heart failure. Am J Cardiol 62:86E-93E

69. Levy B, Bollaert PE, Charpentier C, Nace L, Audibert G, Bauer P, Nabet P, Larcan A (1997a) Comparison of norepinephrine and dobutamine to epinephrine for hemodynamics, lactate metabolism, and gastric tonometric variables in septic shock: a prospective, randomized study. Intensive Care Med 23:282–287
70. Levy B, Bollaert PE, Lucchelli J-P, Sadoune L-O, Nace L, Larcan A (1997b) Dobutamine improves the adequacy of gastric mucosal perfusion in epinephrine-treated septic shock. Crit Care Med 25:1649–1654
71. Liang CS, Yi JM, Sherman LG, Black J, Gavras H, Hood WB (1981) Dobutamine infusion in conscious dogs with and without acute myocardial infarction: effects on systemic hemodynamics, myocardial blood flow, and infarct size. Circ Res 49:170–180
72. Lucas A, Baker BA, Cole TJ (1990) Plasma prolactin and clinical outcome in preterm infants. Arch Dis Child 65:977–983
73. Lund N, De Asla RJ, Cladis F, Papadakos PJ, Thorborg PAJ (1995) Dopexamine hydrochloride in septic shock: effects on oxygen delivery and lactate flux in endotoxic dogs infused with dopexamine. J Trauma 38:767–775
74. Lundgren O, Haglund U (1978) The pathophysiology of the intestinal countercurrent exchanger. Life Sciences 23:1411–1422
75. MacNaughton WK, Wallace JL (1989) A role for dopamine as an endogenous protective factor in the rat stomach. Gastroenterology 96:1165–1169
76. Marik P (1998) Gastric tonometry: the canary sings once again. Crit Care Med 26:809–810
77. Marik PE, Mohedin M (1994) The contrasting effects of dopamine and norepinephrine on systemic and splanchnic oxygen utilization in hyperdynamic sepsis. JAMA 272:1354–1357
78. Marik PE, Sibbald WJ (1993) Effect of stored-blood transfusion on oxygen delivery in patients with sepsis. JAMA 269:3024–3029
79. Maynard N, Bihari D, Beale R, et al (1993) Assessment of splanchnic oxygenation by gastric tonometry in patients with acute circulatory failure. JAMA 270:1203–1210
80. Maynard ND, Bihari DJ, Dalton RN, Smithies MN, Mason RC (1995) Increasing splanchnic blood flow in the critically ill. Chest 108:1684–1654
81. McNeill JR, Stark RD, Greenway CV (1970) Intestinal vasoconstriction after hemorrhage: roles of vasopressin and angiotensin. Am J Physiol 219:1342–1347
82. Meakins JL, Marshall JC (1984) The gastrointestinal tract: The "motor" of multiple organ failure. Arch Surg 121:197–201
83. Meakins JL, Marshall JC (1989) The gut as the motor of multiple system organ failure. In: Marston A, Bulkley GB, Fiddian-Green RG et al (eds) Splanchnic ischemia and multiple organ failure. Edwart Arnold, London, S 339–348
84. Meier-Hellmann (1998) Aspekte zu Überwachungs- und Therapiemöglichkeiten einer gastrointestinalen Minderperfusion bei Sepsis. AINS 33:S60–S69
85. Meier-Hellmann A, Specht M, Hannemann L, Hassel H, Bredle DL, Reinhart K (1996) Splanchnic blood flow is greater in septic shock treated with norepinephrine than in severe sepsis
86. Meier-Hellmann A, Reinhart K, Bredle DL, Specht M, Spies CD, Hannemann L (1997) Epinephrine impairs splanchnic perfusion in septic shock. Crit Care Med 25:399–404
87. Mendez A, Casadevall M, Wachter CH, Elizalde JI, Del Rivero M, Heinemann A, Holzer P, Quintero E, Pique JM (1997) Gastric mucosal blood flow regulation in response to different stimuli. Digest Dis Sci 42:1873–1879
88. Michie HR, Guilluon PJ, Wilmore DW (1989) Tumor necrosis factor and bacterial sepsis. Br J Surg 76:670–671
89. Moore EE, Moore FA, Franciose RJ, Kim FJ, Biffl WL, Banerjee A (1994) The postischemic gut serves as a priming bed for circulating neutrophils that provoke multiple organ failure. J Trauma 37:881–887
90. Morisaki H, Bloos F, Keys J, Martin C, Neal A, Sibbald MJ (1994) Compared with cristalloids, colloid therapy slows progression of extrapulmonary tissue injury in septic sheep. J Appl Physiol 77:1507–1518
91. Moss R, Tighe D, Haywood GA, et al (1990) The differing effects of dopexamine, dobutamine, and placebo on the histology of the liver in pig peritonitis. Intensive Care Med 16 (Suppl 1):66
92. Mourelatos MG, Enzer N, Ferguson JL, Rypins EB, Burhop KE, Law WR (1996) The effects of diaspirin cross-linked hemoglobin in sepsis. Shock 5:141–148
93. Mousdale S, Clyburn PA, Mackie A, et al (1985) Comparison of the effects of dopamine, dobutamine, and dopexamine upon renal blood flow: a study in normal healthy volunteers. Br J Clin Pharmacol 85:609–619
94. Mythen MG, Webb AR (1994) The role of gut mucosal hypoperfusion in the pathogenesis of postoperative organ dysfunction. Intensive Care Med 20:203–209

95. Neviére R, Chagnon JL, Lebleu N, Wattel F (1996) The contrasting effects of dobutamine and dopamine on gastric mucosal perfusion in septic patients. Am J Respir Crit Care Med 154:1684–1688.
96. Neviére R, Chagnon JL, Vallet B, Lebleu N, Marechal X, Mathieu D, Wattel F, Dupuis B (1997) Dobutamine improves gastrointestinal mucosal blood flow in a porcine model of endotoxic shock. Crit Care Med 25:1371–1377
97. Nöldge GFE, Priebe HJ, Geiger K (1992) Splanchnic hemodynamics and oxygen supply during acute normovolemic hemodilution alone and with isoflurane-induced hypotension in the anesthetized pig. Anesth Analg 75: 666–674
98. Nöldge-Schomburg GFE, Priebe H-J, Armbruster K, Pannen B, Haberstroh J, Geiger K (1996) Different effects of early endotoxaemia on hepatic and small intestinal oxygenation in pigs. Intensive Care Med 22:795–804
99. Olson D, Pohlmann A, Hall JB (1996) Administration of low dose dopamine to nonoliguric patients with sepsis syndrome does not raise intramucosal gastric pH nor improve creatinine clearance. Am J Respir Crit Care Med 154:1664–1670
100. Ott A, Nöldge-Schomburg GFE, Armbruster K, Haberstroh J, Göpfert A, Geiger K (1997) Unterschiede in der kritischen Sauerstoffversorgung von Leber und Dünndarm unter normovolämischer Hämodilution. AINS 32: S20
101. Parviainen I, Ruokonen E, Takala J (1995) Dobutamine-induced dissociation between changes in splanchnic blood flow and gastric mucosal pH after cardiac surgery. Br J Anaesth 74:277–282
102. Parviainen I, Ruokonen E, Takala J (1996) Sodium nitroprossude after cardiac surgery: systemic and splanchnic blood flow and oxygen transport. Acta Anaesth Scand 40:606–611
103. Pearson RJ, Barrington KJ, Jirsch DW, Cheung PY (1996) Dopaminergic receptor-mediated effects in the mesenteric vasculature and renal vasculature of the chronically instrumented newborn piglet. Crit Care Med 24:1706–1712
104. Pilette C, Kirstetter P, Sogni P, Cailmail S, Moreau R, Lebrec D (1996) Dose-dependent effects of a nitric oxide biosynthesis inhibitor on hyperdynamic circulation in two models of portal hypertension in conscious rats. J Gastroenterol Hematol 11:1–6
105. Price HL, Deutsch S, Marshall BE, Stephen GW, Behar MG, Neufeld GR (1966) Hemodynamic and metabolic effects of hemorrhage in man, with particular reference to the splanchnic circulation. Circ Res 18:469–474
106. Priebe H-J, Nöldge GFE, Armbruster K, Geiger K (1995) Differential effects of dobutamine, dopamine, and noradrenaline on splanchnic haemodynamics and oxygenation in the pig. Acta Anaesthesiologica Scandinavica 39:1088–96
107. Radermacher P, Buhl R, Santak B, Klein M, Kniemeyer HW, Becker H, Tarnow J (1996) The effects of prostacyclin on gastric intramucosal pH in patients with septic shock. Intensive Care Med 21:414–421
108. Raper RF, Sibbald WJ, Hzobson J, Rutledge FS (1991) Effect of PGE_1 on altered distribution of regional blood flows in hyperdynamic sepsis. Chest 100:1703–1711
109. Rasmussen I, Arvidsson D, Zak A, Haglund UH (1992) Splanchnic and total body oxygen consumption in experimental fecal peritonitis in pigs: effects of dextran and iloprost. Circ Shock 36:299–306
110. Reah G, Bodenham AR, Mallick A, Daily EK, Przybelski RJ (1997) Initial evaluation of diaspirin cross-linked hemoglobin (DCLHbTM) as a vasopressor in critically ill patients. Crit Care Med 25:1480–1488
111. Reinelt H, Rademacher P, Fischer G, Geisser W, Wachter U, Wiedeck H, Georgieff M, Vogt J (1997) Effects of a dobutamine-induced increase in splanchnic blood flow on hepatic metabolic activity in patients with septic shock. Anesthesiology 86:818–824
112. Reinhart K, Hannemann L, Kuss B (1990) Optimal oxygen delivery in critically ill patients. Intensive Care Med 16 (Suppl 2):149–155
113. Reilly PM, Bulkley GB (1993) Vasoactive mediators and splanchnic perfusion. Crit Care Med 21:S55-S68
114. Richardson PDI, Granger DN, Kvietys PR (1980) Effects of norepinephrine, vasopressin, isoproterenol, and histamine on blood flow, oxygen uptake, and capillary filtration coefficient in the colon of the anesthetized dog. Gastroenterology 78:1537–1544
115. Robie NW, Goldberg LI (1975) Comparative systemic and regional hemodynamic effects of dopamine and dobutamine. Am Heart J 90:340–345
116. Royblat L, Gelman S, Bradley EL, Henderson T, Parks D (1989) Dopamine and hepatic oxygen supply/demand relationship. Can J Physiol Pharmacol 68:1165–1169
117. Rudis MI, Basha MA, Zarowitz BJ (1996) Is it time to reposition vasopressors and inotropes in sepsis? Crit Care Med 24:525–537

118. Ruokonen E, Takala J, Kari A, Saxen H, Mertsola J, Hansen EJ (1993) Regional blood flow and oxygen transport in septic shock. Crit Care Med 21: 1296–1303
119. Ruokonen E, Uusaro A, Alhava E, Takala J (1997) The effect of dubutamine infusion on splanchnic blood flow and oxygen transpport in patients with acute pancreatitis. Crit Care Med 23:732–737
120. Ryan AJ, Gisolfi CV (1995) Responses of rat mesenteric arteries to norepinephrine during heat stress and acidosis. J Appl Physiol 78:38–45
121. Sair M, Winlove CP, Evans TW (1996) Microcirculation in sepsis: experimental methods and pathophysiological observations. Clin Sci 91:131–139
122. Salzman AL, Menconi MJ, Unno N, Ezzel RM, Casey DM, Gonzalez PK, Fink MP (1995) Nitric oxide dilates tight junctions and depletes ATP in cultured Caco-2BB intestinal epithelial monolayers. Am J Physiol 268:G361-G373
123. Schleiffer R, Raul F (1996) Prophylactic administration of L-arginine improves the intestinal barrier function after mesenteric ischemia. Gut 39:194–198
124. Schlichtig R (1991) In search of a dysoxic threshold. Intensive Care Med 17: 313–314
125. Schmidt H, Secchi A, Wellmann R, Böhrer H, Bach A, Martin E (1996) Effect of low dose dopamine on intestinal villus microcirculation during normotensive endotoxemia in rats. Br J Anaesth 76:707–712
126. Schmidt W, Stenzel K, Walther A, Gebhard MM, Martin E, Schmidt H (1998) Influence of C_1-esterase inhibitor on tissue oxygenation of jejunal mucosa during endotoxemia. Intensive Care Med 24:S127
127. Schumacker PT, Kazaglis J, Conolly HV, Samsel RW, O'Connor MF, Umans JG (1995) Systemic and gut O_2 extraction during endotoxemia. Role of nitric oxide synthase. Am J Respirat Crit Care Med 151:107–115
128. Secchi A, Wellmann R, Martin E, Schmidt H (1997) Dobutamine maintains intestinal villus blood flow during normotensive endotoxemia: an intravital microscopic study in the rat. J Crit Care 12:137–141
129. Seelig RF, Kerr JC, Hobson RW, Machiedo GW (1981) Prostacyclin (epoprostenol): its effects on canine splanchnic blood flow during hemorrhagic shock. Arch Surg 116:428–430
130. Segal JM, Phang PT, Walley KR (1992) Low dose dopamine hastens onset of gut ischemia in a porcine model of hemorrhagic shock. J Appl Physiol 73:1159–1164
131. Shepherd AP, Riedel GL, Maxwll LC, Kiel JW (1984) Selective vasodilators redistribute intestinal blood flow and depress oxygen uptake. Am J Physiol 247:G377-G348
132. Shoemaker WC, Appel PL, Kram HB, Bishop M, Abraham E (1993) Hemodynamic and oxygen transport monitoring to titrate therapy in septic shock. New Horiz 1:145–159
133. Shoemaker WC, Appel PL, Kram HB, Duarte D, Harrier HD, Ocampo HA (1989) Comparison of hemodynamic and oxygen transport effects of dopamine and dobutamine in critically ill surgical patients. Chest 96:120–126
134. Siegel JH, Fabian M, Smith JA, Costantino D (1997) Use of recombinant hemoglobin solution in reversing lethal hemorrhagic hypovolemic oxygen debt shock. J Trauma 42:199–212
135. Silverman HJ, Tuma P (1992) Gastric tonometry in patients with sepsis. Effects of dobutamine infusions and packed red blood cell transfusions. Chest 102:184–188
136. Smithies M, Yee TH, Jackson L, Beale R, Bihari D (1994) Protecting the gut and the liver in the critically ill: effects of dopexamine. Crit Care Med 22:789–795
137. Sorells DL, Friend C, Koltuksuz U, Courcoulas A, Boyle P, Garett M, Watkins S, Rowe MI, Ford HR (1996) Inhibition of nitric oxide with aminoguadine reduces bacterial translocation after endotoxin challenge in vivo. Arch Surg 131:1155–1163
138. Spain DA, Wilson MA, Bar-Natan MD, Garrison RN (1994) Nitric oxide synthase inhibition aggravates intestinal microvascular vasoconstriction and hypoperfusion of bacteremia. J Trauma 36:720–725
139. Steinberg S, Azar G, Love R, Lee R, Choe E, Flint L (1996) Dopexamine prevents depression of mesenteric blood flow caused by positive end-expiratory pressure in rats. Surgery 120:597–602
140. Stephan H, Sonntag H, Henning H, et al (1990) Cardiovascular and renal haemodynamic effects of dopexamine: Comparison with dopamine. Br J Anaesth 65:380–387
141. Temmesfeld-Wollbrück, Mayer K, Seeger W, Grimminger F (1998) Abnormalities of gastric mucosal oxygenation in septic shock. Am J Resp Crit Care Med 157:1586–1592
142. Tighe D, Moss R, Bennett D (1998) Adrenergic receptor (1) agonist and (2) antagonist increase hepatic injury during sepsis (abstract). Intensive Care Med 24:S128
143. Tighe D, Moss R, Haywood G, Webb A, Al-Saadi N, Heath F, Bennett D (1993) Dopexamine hydrochloride maintains portal blood flow and attenuates hepatic ultrastructural changes in a porcine peritonitis model of multiple system organ failure. Circ Shock 39:199–206

144. Träger K, Vlatten A, Matejovic M, Zülke C, Altherr J, Georgieff M, Radermacher P (1998) Hepatic O_2 exchange and liver energy balance in hyperdynamic porcine endotoxin shock: effects of iloprost (abstract). Intensive Care Med 24:S21
145. Träger K, Vlatten A, Matejovic M, Zülke C, Altherr J, Georgieff M, Radermacher P (1998) Hepatic O_2 exchange and liver energy balance in hyperdynamic porcine endotoxin shock: effects of the TXA_2-inhibitor DTTX30 (abstract). Intensive Care Med 24:S128
146. Uusaro A, Ruokonen E, Takala J (1996) Splanchnic oxygen transport after cardiac surgery: evidence for inadequate tissue perfusion after stabilization of hemodynamics. Intensive Care Med 22:26–33
147. Vagts DA, Iber T, Haberstroh J, Nöldge-Schomburg GFE: Dopamine in combination with thoracic epidural anaesthesia improves liver perfusion and oxygenation in healthy pigs A.P.I.C.E. Book of Selected Papers 1998; Vol. 13:35–36
148. Vagts DA, Iber T, Puccini M, Haberstroh J, Villinger F, Nöldge-Schomburg GFE: Effects of thoracic epidural anaesthesia on hepatic oxygenation and function in healthy pigs. AINS 1998, 33:619
149. Vagts DA, Puccini M, Haberstroh J, Iber T, Villinger F, Nöldge-Schomburg GFE: Gut oxygenation during thoracic epidural anaesthesia. AINS 1998, 33:619
150. Iber T, Vagts DA, Haberstroh J, Amann S, Nöldge-Schomburg GFE: thoracic epidural anaesthesia combined with dopamine does improve intestinal perfusion and oxygenation in healthy pigs. A.P.I.C.E. Book of Selected Papers. 1998; Vol. 13:31–35.
151. Vallet B, Lund N, Curtis SE, Kelly D, Cain SM (1994) Gut and muscosal tissue pO_2 in endotoxemic dogs during shock and resuscitation. J Appl Physiol 76:793–800
152. Van den Berghe G, de Zegher F, Lauwers P (1994) Dopamine and the sick euthyreot syndrome in critical illness. Clin Endocrinol Oxf 41:731–737
153. Van den Berghe G, de Zegher F, Lauwers P, Veldhuis JD (1994) Growth hormone secretion in critical illness: effect of dopamine. J Clin Endocrinol Metab 79:1141–1146
154. Van der Linden P (1994) The optimal hematocrit. In: Vincent JL (Hrsg) Yearbook of Intensive Care and Emergency Medicine. Springer, Berlin, S227–235
155. Vincent JL, Roman A, Kahn RJ (1990) Dobutamine administration in septic shock: addition to a standard protocol. Crit Care Med 18:689–693
156. Vincent JL, Van der Linden P, Domb M, Blecic S, Azimi G, Bernard A (1987) Dopamine compared with dobutamine in experimental septic shock: relevance to fluid administration. Anest Analg 66:565–571
157. Vlatten A, Träger K, Matejovic M, Zülke C, Altherr J, Georgieff M, Radermacher P (1998) Intestinal O_2 exchange and energy balance in hyperdynamic porcine endotoxin shock: effects of iloprost (abstract). Intensive Care Med 24:S21
158. Vollmar B, Lang G, Menger MD, Mesmer K (1994) Hypertonic hydroxyethyl starch restores hepatic microvascular perfusion in hemorrhagic shock. Am J Physiol 266:H1927–H1934
159. Walker TA, Curtis SE, King-Vanvlack CE, Chapler CK, Vallet B, Cain SM (1995) Effects of nitric oxide synthase inhibition on regional hemodynamics and oxygen transport in endotoxic dogs. Shock 4:415–420
160. Wanless RB, Anand IS, Gurden J, Harris P, Poole-Wilson PA (1987) Regional blood flow and hemodynamics in the rabbit with adriamycin cardiomyopathy: effects of isosorbide dinitrate, dobutamine, and captopril. J Pharmacol Exp Ther 243:1101–1106
161. Webb AR, Moss RF, Tighe D, Al-Saady N, Bennett ED (1991) The effects of dobutamine, dopexamine, and fluid on hepatic histological responses to porcine faecal peritonitis. Intensive Care Med 17:487–493
162. Winsö O, Biber B, Martner J (1995) Does dopamine suppress stress-induced intestinal and renal vasoconstriction? Acta Anaesth Scand 29:508–514
163. Xu D, Qi L, Guillory D, Cruz N, Berg R, Deitch EA (1993) Mechanisms of endotoxin-induced intestinal injury in a hyperdynamic model of sepsis. J Trauma 34:676–682
164. Xu L, Rollwagen FM, Li Y, Pacheco ND, Pikoulis E, Leppäniemi A, Sloltero R, Burris D, Malcolm D, Nielsen TB (1997) Cellular responses to surgical trauma, hemorrhage, and resuscitation with diaspirin cross-linked hemoglobin in rats. J Trauma 42:32–41
165. Zhang H, Rogiers P, Friedman G, Preiser JC, Spapen H, Buurman WA, Vincent JL (1996) Effects of nitric oxide donor SIN-1 on oxygen availability and regional blood flow during endotoxic shock. Arch Surg 131:767–774
166. Zhang H, Smail N, Cabral A, Rogiers P, Vincent JL (1997) Effects of norepinephrine on regional blood flow and oxygen extraction capabilities during endotoxic shock. Am J Respir Crit Care Med 155:1965–1971
167. Zhang H, Spapen H, Nguyen DN, Rogiers P, Bakker J, Vincent JL (1995) Effects of N-acetyl-L-cysteine in regional blood flow during endotoxic shock. Eur J Surg 9:236–243

Influence of Dopexamine on Splanchnic Perfusion During Cardiac Surgery

F. Bach · M. Silomon · T. Graeter · R. Larsen · U. Grundmann

Clinic for Anesthesiology and Critical Care Medicine, University of the Saarland, 66421 Homburg/Saar, Germany

Gastrointestinal complications following major surgery, including cardiac surgery requiring cardiopulmonary bypass (CPB), have been associated with splanchnic ischemia. Because of the annual increase in the number of CPB procedures including elderly patients with a higher incidence of existing diseases, the importance of CPB-related gastrointestinal complications has become more pronounced. Severe intestinal complications after CPB such as nonocclusive mesenteric ischemia are, fortunately, rare but seem to be a trigger mechanism for mucosal barrier breakdown, translocation of endotoxin, and systemic inflammatory response. Therefore, a severe course of intestinal ischemia is associated with high mortality [1, 2].

Regional tissue hypoxia following CPB may develop despite apparently stable systemic hemodynamic conditions as shown by gastric acidosis [3] and direct measurement of splanchnic blood flow [4]. It is concluded that a mismatch between splanchnic oxygen delivery and demand following cardiac surgery may be responsible for tissue hypoxia [4]. Furthermore, gut permeability is increased after CPB, as shown by the ratio of absorbed lactulose to L-rhamnose [5]. There is absolute consensus concerning the need for improvement in regional blood flow to prevent tissue hypoxia [6]. The recommendations to prevent and correct tissue hypoxia are optimization of oxygen delivery to the tissue and reduction of oxygen demand.

Supply of oxygen and removal of metabolic products are basic factors to ensure function of the mammal cell. Particularly after trauma or major surgery, tissue oxygen demand is increased and oxygen delivery possibly limited by hemorrhage or decreased cardiac output, and a deterioration of tissue oxygen balance may occur. The gastrointestinal tract (GIT) is one of the most vulnerable organ systems for hypoxia in the organism. The microvasculature of the villus is characterized by a countercurrent exchange mechanism of oxygen from the inflow to the outflow vessels of the villus, resulting in a descending gradient of tissue pO_2 from the base to the tip of the villus [7–10]. The oxygen supply of the gut mucosa is further limited by a phenomenon called “plasma skimming”, which decreases the effective hematocrit of the blood reaching the villus [8]. Moreover, the mesenteric vessels are disproportionately sensitive to effects of angiotensin II and other vasoconstrictors, compared to other vascular beds [9].

Hypoperfusion and heterogeneity of microvascular perfusion of the gut mucosa are associated with the development of tissue hypoxia and implicated in the pathogenesis of multiple organ failure. Efforts have been made to improve splanchnic perfusion, i.e., by fluid resuscitation and the use of vasoactive drugs. One pharmacological approach is intestinal vasodilation to improve splanchnic tissue oxygenation by

M. K. Herbert et al. (Eds.), Problems of the Gastrointestinal Tract in Anesthesia...

increasing splanchnic blood flow as well as mucosal blood flow without increasing tissue oxygen demand. Therefore a promising approach seems to be the use of so-called "inodilators". These drugs increase cardiac output by positive inotropy and reduce the afterload by means of arterial vasodilation.

Dopexamine hydrochloride (Dopacard) is a catecholamine for short-term intravenous administration with inodilator properties, whereby an improved cardiac output is mediated by a positive inotropic effect and afterload reduction [11]. It was first designed for use in low cardiac output states. The vasodilator effects of dopexamine are a consequence of a β_2 adrenoceptor and post-synaptic DA_1 receptor stimulation causing relaxation of the vascular smooth muscle [12, 13]. Due to its β_2- and dopamine-agonistic activity, dopexamine has been found to improve intestinal blood flow in patients without sepsis [14]. It also seems to be suitable for improving splanchnic blood flow and increasing splanchnic oxygen delivery in patients undergoing cardiac surgery. The positive inotropic effect by cardiac stimulation is mediated by indirect stimulation of cardiac β_1-adrenoceptors as a consequence of uptake-1-inhibition of endogenous catecholamines and direct stimulation of β_2-adrenoceptors as well as by a reflex mechanism (baroreceptor activation). Direct α-adrenoceptor agonistic activities with vasoconstriction are not known for dopexamine.

There is growing evidence that the occurrence of gut mucosal hypoperfusion is common during cardiac surgery and may result in translocation of endotoxins with an activation of inflammatory pathways. By the use of gastric laser Doppler flowmetry, Ohri et al. showed that during hypothermic nonpulsatile CPB, a significant intestinal hypoperfusion occurred despite acceptable hemodynamic performance [15]. In an animal study, the same study group demonstrated that at the beginning of the hypothermic phase of CPB, mucosal blood was reduced [16]. Furthermore, gut mucosal hypoxia was present in the rewarming phase of CPB, during which a disparity between mesenteric oxygen consumption and oxygen delivery with villus tip ischemia occurred. Moreover, the values of jejunal tonometry were unaffected during the hypothermic phase of CPB and decreased with the onset of rewarming from hypothermia.

After the approval by the local ethics committee, we studied the influence of perioperative dopexamine application in patients undergoing elective coronary bypass surgery. Twenty eight patients were randomly assigned to receive perioperatively either dopexamine (Dopacard) at a dose of 1 μg/kg/min or an equal volume of 0.9 % NaCl as placebo. The cardiopulmonary bypass was performed with a nonpulsatile flow rate of 2.4 $l/min/m^2$ in moderate hypothermia (33 °C rectal).

In addition to arterial cannulation, all patients received a central venous line and a pulmonary artery catheter. Furthermore, a hepatic venous catheter and a nasogastric tonometer tube were inserted. Gastric $prCO_2$ was measured by gas tonometry (Tonocap, Datex, Finland) and the difference between the mucosal $prCO_2$ and arterial pCO_2 was calculated as the CO_2 gap. Hepatic blood flow was estimated with the indocyanine green dye (ICG) clearance technique [17]. Cardiac output was measured by means of thermodilution with the pulmonary artery catheter. Blood gases and hematocrit were measured using a blood gas analyser. Hepatosplanchnic blood flow was assumed to be equal to the measured hepatic blood flow. Splanchnic oxygen delivery and consumption were calculated using standard formulas.

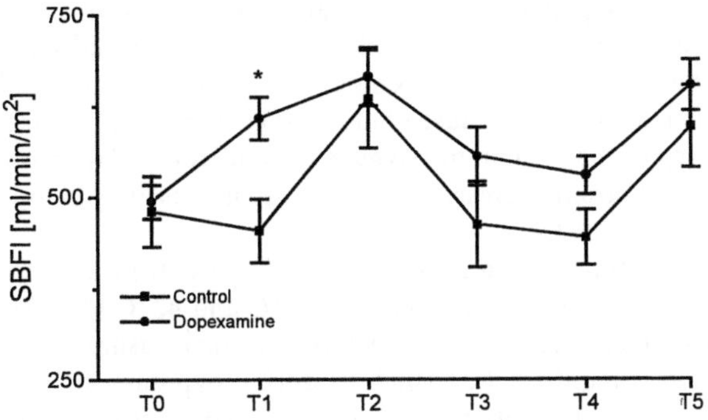

Fig. 1. Splanchnic blood flow index (SBFI) as determined by ICG clearance technique performed at the different time points (T0-T5) in the control group and in dopexamine-treated patients. Data are mean ± SEM; *: $p < 0.05$

The measurements were performed at the following times:

- T0: after induction of anesthesia when all catheters had been inserted
- T1: after 1 h of steady state conditions
- T2: 30 min after induction of CPB
- T3: 30 min after the end of CPB
- T4: 4 h after surgery
- T5: 18 h after surgery

The main observation in our study was an improvement of splanchnic blood flow and splanchnic oxygen supply following CPB by the perioperative application of dopexamine (Fig. 1). Furthermore, a beneficial effect of dopexamine on splanchnic mucosal blood flow assessed with gastric tonometry was seen (Fig. 2). Cardiac index was significantly increased up to 1 h during steady state conditions in dopexamine-treated patients. This was mediated by an increase of the heart rate as well as stroke volume. During CPB, splanchnic blood flow was well-maintained in both groups; nevertheless, splanchnic oxygen delivery decreased as a result of hemodilution during CPB. Moreover, the CO_2 gap, which seems to be the most reliable parameter of gastric tonometry [18, 19] and which was used for the evaluation of gastric mucosal blood flow, was decreased during CPB in both groups. Therefore, no impairment of splanchnic blood flow and gastric mucosal blood flow during CPB was seen in this study.

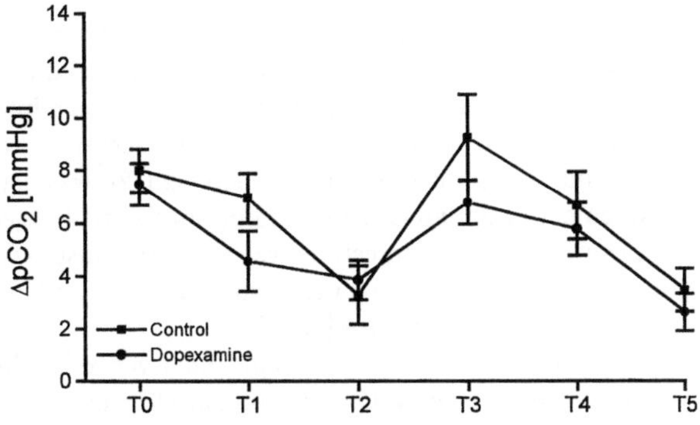

Fig. 2. The influence of dopexamine treatment on the CO_2 gap (ΔCO_2) as the difference between $prCO_2$ and $paCO_2$ determined by gastric tonometry and arterial blood gas monitoring at the different time points (T0-T5). Data are mean ± SEM

Cardiopulmonary bypass can be described as an open system for CO_2. During steady state conditions, gastric mucosal $prCO_2$ reflects the balance of production by the regional tissue and removal by the gastric mucosal blood flow. CO_2, which may increase locally because of mucosal acidosis, can be washed out and eliminated by the lung or the membrane oxygenator if microcirculation is not impaired [12, 13]. Therefore, a strong increase in the CO_2 gap is caused by blood flow stasis or anaerobic generation of CO_2.

As evaluated in an in vitro study, $prCO_2$ measurements are independent of the temperatures ranging between 33 °C and 42 °C [20]. The lower temperature during CPB therefore does not affect tonometric measurements, and no temperature correction is required. Nevertheless, during hypothermic CPB, pCO_2 in the blood is corrected for the patient temperature, in contrast to mucosal $prCO_2$. Therefore, the calculated CO_2 gap during CPB has to be interpreted with caution.

Following CPB, splanchnic oxygen consumption was significantly increased relative to baseline in both groups. Although there was no marked difference in cardiac output between the groups after CPB, splanchnic blood flow and splanchnic oxygen delivery were substantially increased in the dopexamine group. However, splanchnic oxygen consumption was not further increased by dopexamine treatment. Gastric mucosal blood flow as assessed by gastric tonometry seems to be improved by infusion of dopexamine following CPB. However, the decrease in the CO_2 gap, mediated by perioperative dopexamine treatment, was not significant.

The result of this study strengthens the hypothesis that a regional mismatch of oxygen delivery and consumption persists or develops following open-heart surgery, despite stabilization of systemic hemodynamics [4]. The efficacy of dopexamine treatment regarding improvement of the splanchnic oxygen balance and mucosal blood flow was shown in a prospective study on patients with sepsis syndrome [21], as well as in a randomized study on patients undergoing elective cardiac surgery [22]. Gardebäck et al. found a decrease in pHi but no significant change in the pH gap in dopexamine-treated patients following open-heart surgery [23]. They explained their results with the vasodilator effect of dopexamine leading to a more rapid washout of acid metabolites from tissues that had been relatively hypoperfused during hypothermic CPB.

In the present study, an increased splanchnic metabolic demand was observed in both groups following CPB. Nevertheless, splanchnic blood flow as well as splanchnic oxygen delivery were decreased up to 4 h after CPB. Therefore, a mismatch between splanchnic oxygen delivery and demand occurred, resulting in increased oxygen extraction with a corresponding decrease in liver venous oxygen saturation. Furthermore, gastric mucosal blood flow seems to be diminished, as reflected by an increased CO_2 gap. Possibly, the mucosal injury was reinforced by deterioration of the splanchnic oxygen balance and regional CO_2 accumulated because of impaired washout. The intestinal mucosal injury following CPB was determined in other studies by measurement of gut absorption and permeability. Immediately after CPB, there was significant reduction in intestinal transcellular transport of monosaccharides and significant increase in intestinal permeability, as assessed by the differential urine excretion of lactulose/L-rhamnose [5, 15].

In the dopexamine-treated patients, however, splanchnic blood flow was substantially increased following CPB as compared to the control group. Furthermore, the oxygen balance of the splanchnic bed was also improved in the dopexamine group, since oxygen delivery was increased without an increase in oxygen consumption. This was reflected by a higher liver venous oxygen saturation following CPB in the dopexamine group. Possibly, the higher liver venous oxygen saturation could be achieved by blood shunting in the mesenteric and liver microcirculation due to the dopexamine treatment. Nevertheless, there was no difference in the lactate concentration in liver venous blood samples between the groups (data not shown) and therefore no indication for anaerobic metabolism. Furthermore, gastric mucosal blood flow as assessed by gastric tonometry seems to be improved by dopexamine treatment. Therefore, splanchnic blood flow and splanchnic oxygen delivery as well as mucosal blood flow seem to be improved perioperatively by the application of dopexamine.

During the third European Consensus Conference in Intensive Care Medicine in 1996, it was defined that there is a relationship between oxygen delivery and mortality and that critically ill patients with normal or supranormal oxygen delivery are more likely to survive than patients with less than normal O_2 delivery [6]. An optimization of oxygen delivery should be achieved using fluid resuscitation and vasoactive drugs. Mythen and Webb showed that perioperative plasma volume expansion reduces the incidence of gut mucosal hypoperfusion and improves outcome of cardiac surgery patients [27].

Against the background of data from other studies, the results of the present investigation suggest that the phase of rewarming during CPB and early reperfusion after CPB is the most critical for splanchnic perfusion during cardiac surgery. Impairment of intestinal blood flow results in a mismatch of the splanchnic oxygen balance. Furthermore, the perioperative use of inodilator dopexamine in patients undergoing elective cardiac surgery improves splanchnic blood flow and splanchnic oxygen balance as well mucosal blood flow as assessed by gastric tonometry. Therefore, it seems an interesting approach to improving splanchnic perfusion in critically ill patients, beside volume expansion. Nevertheless, more clinical studies are required to elucidate whether the application of dopexamine reduces the incidence of nonocclusive mesenteric ischemia and improves the outcome of patients undergoing cardiac surgery, particularly in critically ill patients with a preexisting decrease of intestinal microperfusion or a congestive heart failure.

References

1. Mythen MG, Webb AR (1994) The role of gut mucosal hypoperfusion in the pathogenesis of postoperative organ dysfunction. Intensive Care Med 20:203–209
2. Ohri SK, Bjarnason I, Pathi V, Somasundaram S, Bowles CT, Keogh BE, Khaghani A, Menzies I, Yacoub MH, Taylor KM (1993) Cardiopulmonary bypass impairs small intestinal transport and increases gut permeability. Ann Thorac Surg 55:1080–1086
3. Fiddian-Green RG, Baker S (1987) Predictive value of the stomach wall pH for complications after cardiac operations: comparison with other monitoring. Crit Care Med 15:153–156
4. Uusaro A, Ruokonen E, Takala J (1996) Splanchnic oxygen transport after cardiac surgery: evidence for inadequate tissue perfusion after stabilisation of hemodynamics. Intensive Care Med 22:26–33
5. Sinclair DG, Houldsworth PE, Keogh B, Pepper J, Evans TW (1997) Gastrointestinal permeability following cardiopulmonary bypass: a randomised study comparing the effects of dopamine and dopexamine. Intensive Care Med 23:510–516
6. Third European Consensus Conference in Intensive Care Medicine (1996) Tissue Hypoxia. How to detect, how to correct, how to prevent. Am J Respir Crit Care Med 154:1573–1578

7. Kampp M, Lungren O, Nilsson NJ (1968) Extravascular shunting of oxygen in the small intestine of the cat. Acta Physiol Scand 72:396–403
8. Fink MP (1991) Why the GI tract is pivotal in trauma sepsis, and MOF. J Crit Illness 6:253–276
9. Landow L, Andersen LW (1994) Splanchnic ischaemia and its role in multiple organ failure. Acta Anaesthesiol Scand 38:626–639
10. Takala J (1996) Determinants of splanchnic blood flow. Br J Anaesth 77:50–58
11. Hurley J, McDonagh P, Cahill M, White M, Luke D, McGovern E, Pehelan D (1995) The haemodynamic effect of prophylactic peri-operative dopexamine in coronary artery bypass patients. European Heart Journal 16:1705–1709
12. Leier CV (1988) Regional blood flow responses to vasodilators and inotrops in congestive heart failure. Am J Cardiol 62:86E-93E
13. Smith GW, O'Connor SE (1988) An introduction to the pharmacologic properties of dopacard (dopexamine hydrochloride). Am J Cardiol 62:9C–17C
14. Leier CV, Binkley PF, Carpenter J, Randolph PH, Underferth DV (1988) Cardiovascular pharmacology of dopexamine in low output congestive heart failure. Am J Cardiol 62:94–99
15. Ohri SK, Somasundraram S, Koak Y, Macpherson A, Keogh BE, Taylor KM, Menzies IS, Bjarnason I (1994) The effect of intestinal hypoperfusion on intestinal absorption and permeability during cardiopulmonary bypass. Gastroenterology 106:318–323
16. Ohri SK, Becket J, Brannan J, Keogh BE, Taylor KM (1994) Effects of cardiopulmonary bypass on gut blood flow, oxygen utilization, and intramucosal pH. Ann Thorac Surg 57:1193–1199
17. Soons PA, De Boer A, Cohen AF Breimer DD (1991) Assessment of hepatic blood flow in healthy subjects by continuous infusion of indocyanine green. Br J Pharmac 32:697–704
18. Knichwitz G, van Aken H, Brüssel T (1998) Gastrointestinal monitoring using measurement of intramucosal pCO_2. Anesth Analg 87:134–142
19. Russell JA (1997) Gastric tonometry: does it work? Intensive Care Med 23:3–6
20. Barry B, Mallick A, Hartley G, Bodenham A, Vucevic M (1998) Comparison of air tonometry with gastric tonometry using saline and other equilibrating fluids: an in vivo and in vitro study. Intensive Care Med 24:777–784
21. Smithies M, Yee TH, Jackson L, Beale R, Bihari D (1994) Protecting the gut and the liver in the critically ill: effects of dopexamine. Crit Care Med 22:789–795
22. Sinclair DG, Haslam PL, Quinlan GJ, Pepper JR, Evans TW (1995) The effect of cardiopulmonary bypass on intestinal and pulmonary endothelial permeability. Chest 108:718–724
23. Gardebäck M, Settergren G, Öhquist G, Tirén C (1995) Effect of dopexamine on calculated low gastric intramucosal pH following valve replacement. Acta Anaesth Scand 39:599–604
24. Mythen MG, Webb AR (1995) Perioperative volume expansion reduces the incidence of gut mucosal hypoperfusion during cardiac surgery. Arch Surg 130:423–429

Postoperative Intestinal Ischemia in Cardiac Surgical Patients

J. Neumann · H.-D. Unrein
Herz-und-Gefäß-Klinik, Salzburger Leite 1, 97616 Bad Neustadt/Saale, Germany

Introduction

An acute abdomen after heart surgery is a rare but often highly dramatic disease. In a retrospective study at our hospital, all patients were included who had a laparotomy after heart surgery due to an acute abdomen.

Out of 37,787 patients undergoing cardiac surgery with extracorporeal circulation between July 1984 and May 1998 in our department, 133 patients had abdominal operations (0.35%) within the early postoperative period. Intraoperative findings were: (1) ileus in 39 patients; (2) inflammation of intraabdominal organs in 22 cases; (3) bleeding in 27; and (4) peptic ulcers in 21. In 24 patients, ischemia of the ileum and/or the colon was found.

An intestinal ischemia was found in 18% of the patients with the help of laparotomy. The blood circulation disturbance of the intestine, related to the total number of the heart surgery patients is, with 0.06%, not substantially higher than in the patient group of general surgical hospitals, which – depending upon literature specification – varies between 0.01% and 0.05% [15].

Clinical Process

Patients

The patients presenting with intestinal ischemia included 8 women and 16 men, with an average age of 69.1 years. The youngest patient was 60 years old, the eldest 78. Fourteen patients were preoperatively in NYHA stage IV and were operated on the heart urgently or in emergency with different attending diseases (Table 1). Our patients were compared with a representative sample of 1,000 patients who were consecutively operated on the heart in 1994, when most of them developed intestinal ischemia.

Heart Surgical Procedure

The heart operations (Table 2) were executed under extracorporeal circulation and general and local hypothermia. The bypass time averaged 101 min and was thereby 31 min or almost 50% longer than in the control group. Clamping time took 36 min

M. K. Herbert et al. (Eds.), Problems of the Gastrointestinal Tract in Anesthesia...

Table 1. Preoperative data of patients with intestinal ischemia as compared with a control group of 1,000 patients with heart surgery

Male:female ratio	1.67:1	(2.82:1)
Mean age (years)	68.6; 59–78	(63.3; 16–84)
Diabetes	10 patients	(41.7% vs. 21.7%)
Hypertension	18 patients	(75.0% vs. 61.0%)
Peripheral occlusive disease	12 patients	(50.0% vs. 12.0%)
Stroke syndrome, cerebrovascular accident	6 patients	(25.0% vs. 4.9%)
Reduced ejection fraction	11 patients	(45.8% vs. 34.8%)
Myocardial infarction	9 patients	–
Arrhythmia	14 patients	(58.3% vs. 8.2%)
Anamnestic laparotomy	11 patients	–

Table 2. Cardiac surgical procedures

Coronary artery bypass grafting	10 patients
Coronary artery bypass grafting and aortic valve replacement	5 patients
Coronary artery bypass grafting and mitral valve reconstruction	2 patients
Coronary artery bypass grafting and carotid thromboendarterectomy	2 patients
Coronary artery bypass grafting and ascending aortic aneurysm resection	1 patient
Aortic and mitral valve replacement	1 patient
Mitral valve reconstruction	1 patient
Aortic valve replacement	2 patients

Table 3. Intraoperative data of patients with intestinal ischemia (control group)

	Average	Minimum	Maximum
Operating time (min)	195 (160)	110 (65)	470 (600)
Cardiopulmonary bypass time (min)	101 (70)	39 (17)	391 (321)
Aortic cross-clamp time (min)	36 (28)	14 (0)	79 (100)

and the lowest rectal temperature averaged 29.2 °C (Table 3). In one patient whose ascending aorta was replaced, the intervention was executed during the deadlock in 18 min at a temperature of 22 °C.

Postoperative Process

Low cardiac output syndrome, rethoracotomy, respiratory insufficiency, acute renal failure, and neurological deficits were the complications registered after cardiac surgical intervention. Only two patients had an uneventful recovery until the onset of abdominal symptoms. Three patients had one complication, five patients had two, three or four complications: and four patients had all five of the complications mentioned above.

Sixteen patients developed a low cardiac output requiring catecholamine support, often over several days. These make up 66.7%, as compared to 5.2% in the control group. Thirteen of these patients needed continuous adrenaline infusion for at least 12 h. Two other patients received adrenaline as bolus. In one patient, an intraaortic balloon pump was implanted for 24 h and removed during laparotomy. Six patients

(25.0 % vs. 4.4 % in the control group) had to be rethoracotomized because of bleeding, tamponade, or myocardial ischemia. Six patients (25.0 % vs. 4.4 %) suffered an apoplectic stroke postoperatively.

Nineteen patients (79.2 % vs. 9.9 %) developed respiratory insufficiency, defined by postoperative artificial respiration for more than 24 h or by reintubation in the further postoperative process. Eleven patients were not extubated until the laparotomy. Two patients had to be artificially respirated for more than 24 h before they could be extubated. Only eleven patients could be taken away from the artificial respiration machine at the normal time. Eight of the 13 extubated patients had to be reintubated before the formation of abdominal symptomatology. In twelve patients, tracheotomy was necessary because of long-term artificial respiration. The duration for artificial respiration averaged 13.5 days.

A postoperative renal insufficiency with oliguria or anuria as well as an increase in creatinine of at least 1.8 mg/dl was noted in 18 patients. Without exception, all patients with intestinal ischemia had an increase in creatinine after the heart surgery. So preoperatively the creatinine was on average 1.2 mg/dl (0.8–1.8 mg/dl) and postoperatively 2.5 mg/dl (1.0–4.9 mg/dl). Ten out of 18 patients needed hemofiltration. Seventy five per cent of our patients developed intestinal ischemia in the first postoperative week.

Abdominal pain, pain after pressure, and/or distension of the abdomen were documented with almost all patients (Table 4). In six patients, not including those with a postoperative apoplectic stroke, psychologically conspicuous findings in the sense of a passage syndrome or an organic brain syndrome were described. Chemically, leukocytosis with an average value of 18,600 white blood cells/nl was noticed in 18 patients, metabolic acidosis in twelve patients, and amylasemia in eleven.

Eleven patients had a hemoglobin value of less than 10 mg/dl at the time of the laparotomy. Only in eight patients was the serum lactate determined, whereby six pathological values showed up. In the sonographic investigation which was carried out with 20 patients before the laparotomy, there were signs of an ileus in the form of expanded, standing, or liquid-filled loops of intestine, with or without pendulum movements in 14 patients. Furthermore, in the case of two patients pericholecystitis, ascites, or hepatomegaly was found. Sonography did not produce a concrete suspicion diagnosis with any of the patients.

Table 4. Symptoms and laboratory findings

Abdominal pain	23 patients	96 %
Distension	22 patients	92 %
Aperistalsis	18 patients	75 %
Oliguria or anuria	18 patients	75 %
Nausea or vomiting	15 patients	62 %
Obstipation	10 patients	42 %
Diarrhea	8 patients	33 %
Gastrointestinal bleeding	6 patients	25 %
Rectal bleeding	2 patients	8 %
Leukocytosis	18 patients	75 %
Metabolic acidosis	12 patients	50 %
Amylasemia	11 patients	46 %
Anemia (with hemoglobin < 10 mg/dl)	11 patients	46 %
Pyrexia (temperature > 38.5 °C)	7 patients	29 %

Gastroscopy executed preoperatively in five patients showed esophagitis or erosive and ulcerous modifications in the fundus and corpus area of the stomach. Abdominal x-rays with proof of nonspecific modifications, such as small intestinal mirrors, were taken in seven patients. Angiography of the mesenteric vessels was not possible in any of our multimorbid patients requiring intensive care.

The time interval from the beginning of documented clinical symptomatology to laparotomy amounted to less than 6 h in eleven patients and up to three days in five.

Surgical Procedure and Etiology

The laparotomies were terminated in six patients prematurely due to incurable findings. In these patients, necrosis of parts of the duodenum and jejunum, the entire ileum, as well as parts of the cecum and colon was found. These patients died within the following hours. In one patient with an ischemia of the small intestine, a finding similar to that of the patients with explorative laparotomy, an embolectomy of the arteria mesenterica superior was executed. A second intervention 12 h later showed a subtotal ischemia of the loops of the small intestine with inclusion of the right hemicolon. This patient also deceased a few hours later.

An intestinal resection with anastomosis of the remaining intestinal loops was executed in seven patients. In one patient, a terminal jejunostomy was performed after the intestinal resection, in five an ileostomy, and in four patients a colostomy was done. In seven patients from the same session, a cholecystectomy due to necrosis or gangrene or empyema of the gall bladder, a hydrocholecystis, or cholelithiasis was executed.

Evaluation of the etiology was based either on intraoperative or histological findings. Arterial embolic or thrombotic causes were present in twelve patients, venous thrombosis in four, and nonocclusive disease in eight patients, which indicates an ischemic injury to the intestinal mucosa without proof of mesenteric vascular disease in eight patients.

Seven patients deceased on the operation day. Six further patients died within the first three days. Altogether, 17 patients deceased within the first two weeks. Two patients were moved into their home hospitals 19 and 26 days after the laparotomy and died a few weeks later. In ten patients, autopsy could be performed. With all of them, shock-associated lungs, liver, and kidney modifications were found, so that the main cause of death was caused by multiorgan failure due to protracted septic shock.

Furthermore, all patients presented substantial general arteriosclerosis with high grade areally ulcerated and calcified atheromatosis, particularly of the abdominal aorta, partially with ulceration and partial thrombosis. In four of ten patients, high grade proximal stenosis was found in all visceral branches of the celiac axis, the superior or inferior mesenteric artery, with vascular insufficiency in the respective supply area. In the other patients, the larger blood vessels were free; however, histologically, three patients showed expanded atheromatous and cholesterol microembolisms in the submucosal arterioles of the intestine with expanded mucosa necrosis and fibrinopurulent peritonitis.

Only three of the 24 patients survived the intervention, whereby the time interval between the beginning of the symptoms and laparotomy amounted to 3 h in one, 18 h in another, and 26 h in a third. All three of these patients underwent intestinal resection, and histology showed that one had an expanded hemorrhagic infarction with initial gangrene of the small intestine, the second had a segmental hemorrhagic infarction of the terminal ileum with secondary ischemic mucosa necrosis and initial peritonitis, and the third had segmental ischemic colitis at the cecum and ascending colon with expanded ischemic mucosa necrosis. In none of these three patients was a thrombus or embolus found in preparation.

Conclusions

The list of all preoperative specifications and findings for the examined patients shows that, apart from the heart disease, several other diseases existed, e.g., absolute arrhythmia with atrial fibrillation, arterial occlusion disease, and cerebral apoplexy.

During the time between heart-surgery and the occurrence of abdominal symptomatology requiring an operation, no clear hint of intestinal ischemia could be deduced from changed laboratory parameters, in particular during the early phase. In keeping with the literature, it is necessary to refer again to the fact that a rise in serum-lactate does not necessarily indicate intestinal ischemia, since an increase of lactate is also found after shock conditions or reanimation. On the other hand, the increase of lactate can be small, despite intestinal necrosis [6].

A substantial pathogenetic factor in the development of intestinal ischemia in our polypathic patients is hypotension and hypoperfusion of the visceral organs occurring during extracorporeal circulation [2, 3, 5, 7, 14]. Opiates have a negative influence on intestinal motility, and digitalis can lead to a decrease in mesenteric blood circulation. Catecholamine therapy, in particular with adrenaline, may cause constriction of the mesenteric vessels.

Under compromised circulatory conditions, the intestine is a very vulnerable organ and can release and maintain a shock condition [1, 11, 16]. This fact is indicated by a number of experimental investigations on animals and clinical studies using continuous, intramucosal pCO_2 measurement and pHi calculation [4, 8, 10, 12, 13]. The volume distribution and oxygen accommodation in the splanchnic area and their changes by therapeutic intervention and in morbid states, such as cardiogenic and hemorrhagic shock, hypovolemia, and hypoxemia, as well as endotoxemia, must also be considered, although they are not specific for the diagnosis of intestinal ischemia.

So far the clinical diagnosis of intestinal ischemia is not possible before the occurrence of abdominal symptomatology, because specific pathognomonic parameters are missing and, even in cases of suspicion, angiography and endoscopy may not be possible due to the frequently critical state of the patients.

In summary, the results from our patient group show that rapid laparotomy should take place after the occurrence of acute abdominal symptomatology. This leads to safe diagnosis, surgical treatment, and the start of intensive therapy without delay. Thus, progressing peritonitis, intoxication with septic shock, and finally multiorgan failure can be reduced. A reduction of mortality, consistently high for many years – between 80 % and 100 % [6, 7, 9] – will only be possible if easily feasible, meaningful and adequate methods of intensive care can be developed and transferred into practice to facilitate early recognition of intestinal ischemia.

References

1. Allen KB, Salam AA, Lumsden AB (1992) Acute mesenteric ischemia after cardiopulmonary bypass. J Vasc Surg 16:391–396
2. Bailey RW, Hamiltor SR (1986) Pathogenesis of nonocclusive ischemic colitis. Ann Surg 203:590–599
3. Christianson JT, Schmuziger M, Maurice J, Simonet F, Velebit V (1994) Gastrointestinal complications after coronary artery bypass grafting. J Thorax Cardiovasc Surg 108:899–906
4. Fiddian-Green RG, Baker S (1987) Predictive value of stomach wall pH for complications after cardiac operations: Comparison with other monitoring. Crit Care Med 15:153–156
5. Gandhi SK, Hanson MM, Vernava AM, Kaminski DL, Longo WE (1996) Ischemic colitis. Dis Colon Rectum 39:88–100
6. Gauß A, Drück A, Hemmer W, Georgieff M (1994) Abdominelle Komplikationen nach kardiochirurgischen Eingriffen. Anästhesiol Intensivmed Notfallmed Schmerzther 29:23–29
7. Gennaro M, Ascer E, Matano R, Jacobowitz IJ, Cunningham JN, Uceda P (1993) Acute mesenteric ischemia after cardiopulmonary bypass. Am J Surg 166:231–239
8. Hamulu A, Atay Y, Yagdi T, Discigil B, Bakalim T, Buket S, Bilkay Ö (1998) Effects of flow types in cardiopulmonary bypass on gastric intramucosal pH. Perfusion 13:129–135
9. Häring R, Zilch H (1986) Chirurgie. de Gruyter Verlag, Berlin, New York
10. Knichwitz G (1998) Kontinuierliche intramukosale pO_2-Messung: Entwicklung und Stellenwert eines neuen Verfahrens. Anästhesiol Intensivmed Notfallmed Schmerzther 33:606
11. Moneta GL, Misbach GA, Ivey TD (1985) Hypoperfusion as a possible factor in the development of gastrointestinal complications after cardiac surgery. Am J Surg 149:648–650
12. Mythen MG (1998) Gastric intramucosal tonometry. Anästhesiol Intensivmed Notfallmed Schmerzther 33:606
13. Nöldge-Schomburg GFE (1998) Therapeutische Strategien zur Verbesserung der gestörten Darmperfusion. Anästhesiol Intensivmed Notfallmed Schmerzther 33:606
14. Rocke DA, Gaffin SL, Wells MT, Koen MSY, Brock-Utine JG, RN, PAA (1987) Endotoxemia associated with cardiopulmonary bypass. J Thorax Cardiovasc Surg 93:832–837
15. Serfling HJ, Schober KL, Schmitt W (1990) Spezielle Chirurgie. Johann Ambrosius Barth Verlag, Leipzig 1990
16. Zeeb I, Pfenninger E, Grünert A (1990) Der Darm als Ischämieorgan. Anaesthesist 39:343–352

Gastrointestinal Complications After Cardiopulmonary Bypass

J. Rötker[1] · M. Erren[1,2] · G. Knichwitz[1,3] · R. Tandler[1] · N. Roeder[1] · M. C. Deng[1]
D. Hammel[1] · H. H. Scheld[1]

[1] Department of Cardiothoracic Surgery, Westphalian Wilhelms-University of Münster, Albert-Schweitzer-Str. 33, 48129 Münster, Germany
[2] Institute of Laboratory Medicine, Westphalian Wilhelms-University of Münster, Münster, Germany
[3] Department of Anesthesiology, Westphalian Wilhelms-University of Münster, Münster

Introduction

Abdominal complications after extracorporeal circulation occur in 0.3%–2.3% of patients [1–14]. They carry significant mortality, up to 67% in some reports [1].

Since clinical signs of gastrointestinal complications after cardiopulmonary bypass are often subtle, specifically in the setting of an intensive care unit, where the patient receives sedatives and is on respirator support, a risk score that predicts which patient will probably develop a gastrointestinal complication may be helpful.

Methods

Five thousand five hundred ninety-five consecutive patients undergoing cardiopulmonary bypass from Jan. 1 1993 to Sept. 30 1997 were investigated for gastrointestinal complications in the postoperative period. All data were acquired prospectively by an on-line computer-based data system. GICs (gastrointestinal complications) were classified as follows: (1) upper gastrointestinal bleeding, manifested by hematemesis or melena, associated with a decrease in the hemoglobin level of 2 g/dl and confirmed by endoscopy, (2) pancreatitis, manifested by elevated serum amylase and lipase levels in the presence of abdominal pain or tenderness and/or confirmed by computed tomographic findings of the upper abdomen, (3) acute cholecystitis, manifested by abdominal pain and tenderness and positive ultrasonographic or computed tomographic findings, (4) ischemic or infarcted gut confirmed by laparotomy or autopsy, and (5) paralytic ileus that lasted for more than 4 days after surgery, despite adequate medical treatment, and required operative intervention.

For statistical analysis, binary variables were evaluated by Chi^2-Test with Yates correction or Fisher's exact test. Continuous variables were analyzed by Wilcoxon-Mann-Whitney rank sum test. Univariate testing was performed for all variables. A probability value less than 0.05 was regarded as significant. The relative risk (RR) for each variable with a p value less than 0.05 was estimated as follows: (percent of GIC if variable is present)/(percent of GIC if variable is absent). On the basis of these relations, a risk factor selection scale was developed. Weights (W) for variables were assigned: $1 < RR \leq 2.5$:W = 1; $2.5 < RR \leq 5.0$: W = 2; $5 < RR \leq 10$: W = 3; RR>10: W = 4. Weights were summed up to obtain a risk score for each individual patient.

M. K. Herbert et al. (Eds.), Problems of the Gastrointestinal Tract in Anesthesia...

Results

Clinical Outcomes

From Jan. 1 1993 to Sept. 30 1997, 59 patients among 5,595 consecutive patients developed GIC, an incidence of 1.05 %. Twenty patients with a GIC died within 30 days of surgery, corresponding to a mortality rate of 33.9 %. Patients with a GIC died significantly more often than patients without one ($p < 0.001$; odds ratio: 10.0; 95 % confidence interval: 5.5 to 18.2). The overall 30day mortality for the whole group of patients studied was 3.6 %. Therefore, 10.0 % of all deaths were in some way associated with GIC. Among the 59 patients with GIC, there were 28 with intestinal paralysis (47.5 %), 14 with intestinal ischemia or infarction (23.7 %), seven with acute cholecystitis (11.9 %), 10 with gastrointestinal bleeding (16.9 %), three with an acute pancreatitis (5.1 %), and two had pseudoperitonitis (3.4 %). Four patients with acute cholecystitis and one with acute pancreatitis had intestinal paralysis as well.

Patients with gastrointestinal bleeding or acute pancreatitis were usually treated conservatively.

Patients with refractory intestinal paralysis, despite maximum conservative treatment and with additional clinical suspicion of gastrointestinal ischemia, underwent laparotomy and a cecal fistula was usually placed. At laparotomy, 14 patients showed intestinal ischemia or infarction. Nine of these had intestinal resection and four of them survived. In four patients, the whole bowel was infarcted at the time of laparotomy, and no further treatment was applied. A cholecystectomy was performed in all patients with acute cholecystitis.

Risk Factors

Analysis of thirty pre-, intra-, and postoperative variables was performed to identify risk factors for GIC after CPB (cardiopulmonary bypass). Two groups of patients, i.e., patients with and without GIC, were compared; and each variable was tested by univariate analysis. No association of GIC with age ($p = 0.24$), height ($p = 0.61$), weight ($p = 0.34$), body mass index ($p = 0.41$), sex ($p = 0.99$), nicotine use ($p = 0.72$), diabetes ($p = 0.34$), hypertension ($p = 0.98$), atrial fibrillation ($p = 0.16$), previous pacemaker implantation ($p = 0.35$), previous cardiac surgery ($p = 0.09$), concomitant central neurological disease ($p = 0.22$), valve surgery ($p = 0.81$), combined coronary vascularization and valve surgery ($p = 0.33$), surgery of thoracic aneurysms ($p = 0.59$), aortic crossclamp time ($p = 0.72$), or deep sternal wound infection ($p = 0.69$) was detected. Patients with coronary artery revascularization had significantly less GIC than patients only with other kinds of cardiac surgery ($p < 0.001$).

Seventeen pre-, intra-, and postoperative variables had a significant correlation ($p < 0.05$) to postoperative GIC. Analysis of variables revealed that (1) a history of cardiac decompensation prior to surgery ($p = 0.007$), (2) emergency surgery ($p = 0.001$), (3) renal ($p = 0.034$), and (4) concomitant pulmonary disease ($p = 0.023$), (5) ejection fraction below 50 % ($p = 0.014$), (6) final diastolic pressure above 15 mmHg ($p = 0.012$), (7) type of surgery performed (transplantation; ($p < 0.001$), (8) implantation of a left ventricular assist device ($p < 0.001$), (9) prolonged bypass time (> 100 min-

Table 1. Pre-, intra-, and postoperative risk factors associated with GIC after CPB

	Variable	Relative risk	95 % confidence interval
Preoperative	Concomitant pulmonary disease	2.5	1.2–5.0
	Concomitant renal disease	2.1	1.1–4.3
	Ejection fraction < 50 %	2.6	1.3–5.9
	LVEDP > 15 mmHg	2.4	1.2–5.0
	Cardiac decompensation	3.9	1.6–9.2
	Emergency status	2.6	1.5–4.7
Intraoperative	Transplantation	6.9	2.9–16.6
	Implantation of a LVAD	20.9	8.9–49.0
	Bypass time > 100 min	3.2	1.7–5.8
	Implantation of an IABP	5.8	3.1–11.1
Postoperative	Rethoracotomy	4.9	2.3–10.2
	CPR	11.4	5.6–23.6
	Arrhythmia	4.3	2.4–13.5
	Perioperative infarction	4.7	1.7–13.5
	Low-output-syndrome	15.1	8.3–27.0
	Respiratory failure	5.5	2.3–13.0
	Central neurologic deficit	7.5	4.0–14.1

CPR, Cardiopulmonary resuscitation; LVAD, left ventricular assist device; IABP, intraaortic balloon pump; LVEDP, left ventricular enddiastolic pressure

utes) ($p< 0.001$), (10) implantation of an intraaortic balloon pump ($p< 0.001$), (11) rethoracotomy ($p< 0.001$), (12) cardiopulmonary resuscitation ($p< 0.001$), (13) perioperative cardiac infarction ($p = 0.014$), (14) postoperative low-output-syndrome ($p< 0.001$), (15) respiratory failure ($p = 0.001$), (16) arrhythmia ($p< 0.001$), and (17) a new central neurologic deficit ($p = 0.001$) were significantly associated with gastrointestinal complications in the postoperative course. The relative risks and the 95 % confidence intervals are displayed in Table 1.

For each patient, weights were summed up to obtain a risk score for each individual patient. If all variables were included in the risk score, specificity was 91.1 % and sensitivity was 66.7 %, with a diagnostic efficiency of 90.8 %.

Patients with a postoperative GIC stayed significantly longer in the intensive care unit compared to patients without GIC (12.6 ± 12.5 vs. 1.4 ± 2.9 days respectively).

Comments

Although GICs are relatively rare, they are associated significantly with overall postoperative mortality in open heart surgery. Intestinal paralysis and intestinal ischemia were the most serious kinds of complication. Of the 20 patients with GIC who died, 19 had intestinal paralysis or intestinal ischemia.

Risk factors for GIC after operations using CPB have been reported in the literature [1–4, 10, 11]. Comparison between these reports is often difficult because of different perioperative management of patients and the different kinds of operations performed.

In the last decade, the spectrum of patients has changed in most major centers. More and more terminally ill patients are referred to procedures such as transplantation and implantation of a left ventricular assistance device (LVAD) or on an emergency status [15]. We report on a consecutive cardiac surgery commonly performed in a major, contemporary academic cardiac surgery department. Although transplantation and implantation of LVADs made up only 3.0 % of all procedures, these operations accounted for 22.9 % of all GICs in our series.

Most risk factors are attributable to a pre-, intra-, or postoperative state of hemodynamic instability. This is obvious for patients with cardiac decompensation or emergency status. Patients requiring cardiac transplantation or implantation of an LVAD are also preoperatively in an unstable circulatory state. In the postoperative period, cardiopulmonary resuscitation, rethoracotomy due to cardiac tamponade or excessive bleeding, and implantation of an assist device are also indicative of hemodynamic instability.

Clinical signs of gastrointestinal complications after cardiopulmonary bypass are often subtle and nonspecific. This is especially true in the setting of an intensive care unit while the patient receives sedatives and is on respirator support. Therefore, diagnosis and treatment of GIC is often delayed until signs of intraabdominal sepsis and multisystem organ failure are present, leading to the high mortality observed in these patients. The physician needs a high level of suspicion for timely diagnosis and treatment. Therefore, a risk score that predicts which patient will probably develop a gastrointestinal complication may be of value in these circumstances.

References

1. Wallwork J, Davidson KG (1980) The acute abdomen following cardiopulmonary bypass surgery. Br J Surg 67:410–412
2. Lawhorne TW, Davis JL, Smith GW (1978) General surgical complications after cardiac surgery. Am J Surg 136:254–256
3. Hanks JB, Curtis SE, Hanks BB, Andersen DK, Cox JL, Jones RS (1982) Gastrointestinal complications after cardiopulmonary bypass. Surgery 92:394–400
4. Reath DB, Maull KI, Wolfgang TC (1983) General surgical complications following cardiac surgery. Am Surg 49:11–14
5. Aranha GV, Pickleman J, Pifarre R, Scanlon PJ, Gunnar RM (1984) The reason for gastrointestinal consultation after cardiac surgery. Am Surg 50:301–304
6. Moneta GL, Misbach GA, Ivey TD (1985) Hypoperfusion as a possible factor in the development of gastrointestinal complications after cardiac surgery. Am J Surg 149:648–650
7. Welling RE, Rath R, Albers JE, Glaser RS (1986) Gastrointestinal complications after cardiac surgery. Arch Surg 121:1178–1180
8. Leitman IM, Paull DE, Barie PS, Isom OW, Shires GT (1987) Intra-abdominal complications of cardiopulmonary bypass operations. Surg Gynecol Obstet 165:251–254
9. Krasna MJ, Flancbaum L, Trooskin SZ, et al (1988) Gastrointestinal complications after cardiac surgery. Surgery 104:773–780
10. Huddy SP, Joyce WP, Pepper JR, et al (1991) Gastrointestinal complications in 4,473 patients who underwent cardiopulmonary bypass surgery. Gut mucosal ischemia during normothermic cardiopulmonary bypass results from blood flow redistribution and increased oxygen demand. Br J Surg 78:293–296
11. Ohri SK, Desai JB, Gaer JA, et al (1991) Intra-abdominal complications after cardiopulmonary bypass. Ann Thorac Surg 52:826–831
12. Tsiotos GG, Mullany CJ, Zietlow S, van Heerden JA (1994) Abdominal complications following cardiac surgery. Am J Surg 167:553–557
13. Lazar HL, Hudson H, McCann J, et al (1995) Gastrointestinal complications following cardiac surgery. Cardiovasc Surg 3:341–344
14. Christenson JT, Schmuziger M, Maurice J, Simonet F, Velebit V (1994) Gastrointestinal complications after coronary artery bypass grafting. J Thorac Cardiovasc Surg 108:899–906
15. Deng MC, Breidhardt G, Scheld HH (1995) Interdisciplinary heart failure and transplant program Münster: a 5 year experience. Int J Cardiol 50:7–17

FREE COMMUNICATION

The "Laparoscopic Window": A New Laparoscopic Bedside Technique for Second Look Intervention

A. van Ophoven · B. Patel · H. G. Schindler

Paracelsusklinik der Stadt Marl, Abteilung für Gefäss- und Thoraxchirurgie, Venerologie, Lipper Weg 11, 45770 Marl, Germany

Introduction

"Second look" laparotomy following surgical treatment of bowel ischemia is not always performed as a routine procedure. Although the literature reports up to 30 % recurrence of bowel necrosis after primary resection with bowel revascularization, a second laparotomy is often not performed, due to the patient's age and cardiovascular disease.

In order to avoid additional laparotomy and its implicit risks, we developed a new, minimal invasive technique in the field of second look laparoscopy which we call the "laparoscopic window".

Laparoscopy for second look interventions has become an alternative to surgical re-exploration for several years. The common "pneumoperitoneum technique" has certain hazards and disadvantages, e.g., a second general anesthesia and trauma by trocars. In contrast, the presented "laparoscopic window" technique allows us to carry out a safe and diagnostic procedure within a few minutes at bedside or in the ICU.

Laparoscopic Technique

Because of the risks associated with extensive bowel resection, at the end of our open laparatomies we placed a 30 Ch flexible, transparent drainage tube into the abdomen near the site of revascularization. The tube is formed into a U-shape by anchoring its midportion to the mesentery near the reconstructed area and bringing out both open ends through the skin and suturing them in place (Fig. 1). This provides an aseptic access to the abdominal cavity for inspection using a flexible laparoscope. The laparoscope can be placed into either open end of the drainage tube and directed easily to the reconstructed area for inspection of the bowel.

This can be done for general follow-up and especially in cases of suspected bowel necrosis. The tube can be left in for several days for repeated use and delayed diagnosis. This can be done quickly and simply, without anesthesia or additional incisions, and at the bedside.

M. K. Herbert et al. (Eds.), Problems of the Gastrointestinal Tract in Anesthesia...

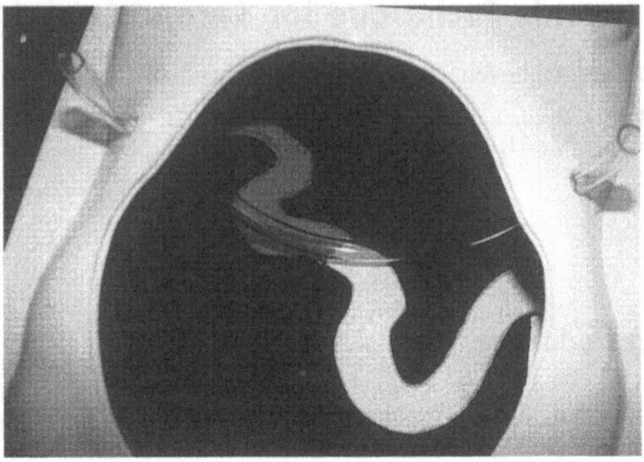

Fig. 1. Drainage tube placement at the site of bowel reanastomosis

Clinical Experience

We used our new technique on 12 patients presenting with the following vascular diseases: three patients with mesenteric arterial embolus, three patients with mesenteric arterial thrombosis, two patients with mesenteric venous thrombosis, and four patients with suspected vascular compromise in the descending colon and sigmoid during aortobifemoral graft placement. In all twelve patients, bowel viability was examined 6 to 12 hours postoperatively using the above technique.

In two patients, bowel necrosis was diagnosed after 12 hours, leading to subsequent surgical revision.

The remaining patients were noted to have a viable bowel after 24 to 48 hours, requiring no further intervention for easy removal of the drainage tube. The first four tubes were removed under direct vision using the laparoscope through the tube. Only minimal tears and hemorrhages were noted at the anchoring suture site upon removal of the tube. No abdominal cavity infections or infections at the point of the tube insertion in the skin occurred. None of the patients showed signs of sepsis or extended ileus.

Of the two patients diagnosed laparoscopically with bowel necrosis, one patient died. This was secondary to progressive and irreversible intestinal infarction which could not be medically or surgically prevented.

Conclusions

We have shown a simple, safe, and cost-effective method of monitoring and diagnosing postoperative bowel necrosis in patients at high risk. The procedure can be performed with minimal ancillary support, no anesthesia, and at bedside, even in critically ill patients. A quick decision can then be made on whether or not the patient requires further surgical intervention. This method can be used potentially in multiple clinical settings requiring minimal invasive diagnosis in major surgeries.

References for Further Reading

1. Beger HG, Schoenberg MH (1994) Second-Look-Laparoskopie nach Mesenterialinfarkt. Langenbecks Arch Chir 379(2):65
2. Bickel A, Daud G, Vaksman I, Eitan A (1996) A technique for second-look laparoscopy in the obese patient. J Laparoendosc Surg 6(2):113–115
3. Chagla L, Kiff R (1994) "Second-look" laparoscopy in the management of acute mesenteric ischemia. Br J Surg 81(7):1083
4. Glattli A, Seiler C, Metzger A, Stirnemann P, Baehr HU (1994) Die Second-Look-Laparoskopie nach Mesenterialinfarkt. Langenbecks Arch Chir 379(2):66–69
5. Greene FL, Brown PA, (1994) Laparoscopic approaches to abdominal malignancy. Sem Surg Onc 10(6):386–90
6. Iberti TJ, Salky BA, Onofrey D (1989) Use of bedside laparoscopy to identify intestinal ischemia in postoperative cases of aortic reconstruction. Surgery 105:686–689
7. MacSweeny ST, Postlethwait JC (1994) "Second-look" laparoscopy in the management of acute mesenteric ischemia. Br J Surg 81(1):90
8. Nassar A (1994) "Second-look" laparoscopy in the management of acute mesenteric ischemia. Br J Surg 81(7):1083
9. Nassar AH, Htwe T, Hefny H, Kholeif Y (1996) The abdominal drain. A convenient port for second look laparoscopy. Surg Endos 10(11):1114–1115
10. Paolucci V, Gutt CN, Schaeff B, Encke A (1995) Gasless laparoscopy in abdominal surgery. Surg Endosc 9(5):497–500
11. Sackier JM (1994) "Second-look" laparoscopy in the management of acute mesenteric ischemia. Br J Surg 81(10):1546
12. Slutzki S, Halpern Z, Negri M, Kais H, Halevy A (1996) The laparoscopic second look for ischemic bowel disease. Surg Endosc 10(7):729–731
13. Tola M, Portoghese A, Maniga AM (1997) Il "second-look" laparoscopico nell'ischemia intestinale acuta. Minerva Chir 52(2):527–530

PART V

Postoperative Nausea and Vomiting

INVITED ARTICLE

Postoperative Nausea and Vomiting

P. L. R. Andrews

Department of Physiology, St. George's Hospital Medical School, Cranmer Terrace, Tooting, London SW17, ORE, United Kingdom

Introduction

There is not an *a priori* reason why anesthesia and surgery should induce nausea and vomiting both of which have evolved as components of the body's defensive system against accidentally ingested toxins. It is indeed interesting that nausea and vomiting are such common symptoms of diverse diseases and treatments. For nausea and vomiting to be induced, the only requirement is for some component of the operative environment (e.g., a pharmacological effect of the anesthetic or a mechanical effect of the surgery) to cause activation of one of the afferent pathways which can trigger the response. In the case of a food-ingested toxin, both nausea and vomiting are viewed as being "appropriate". Nausea generates a memory which leads to an aversion to that stimulus (i.e., the food) when encountered again and vomiting which expels the toxin. Provided that the toxin has not been absorbed or triggered, a secondary systemic process is self-limiting. Considering clinical stimuli, such as anticancer chemotherapy or anesthesia and surgery, both nausea and vomiting are "inappropriate". Nausea may generate an aversion which in the case of anticancer chemotherapy can lead to the genesis of anticipatory nausea and vomiting, whereas vomiting does not lead to ejection of the stimulus which is systemic (i.e., not in the gut lumen); hence, vomiting may be protracted.

Nausea and vomiting have long been associated with anesthesia and surgery, as have attempts to alleviate them. Snow in 1848 proposed wine and Battley's solution was opium as postoperative treatment. It can be argued that progress in reducing postoperative nausea and vomiting (PONV) has been more from the improvement in anesthetic techniques (masks vs endotracheal tubes), anesthetics (volatile vs injectable) and surgical techniques (reduction of trauma and time required for surgery) rather than an understanding of the mechanisms responsible, in turn leading to the identification of rational antiemetic treatment. Patient predictive factors (e.g., age, gender, stage of menstrual cycle) are still a matter of debate (see chapter by Apfel) and the precise efficacy (if any) of well-established antiemetic treatments in PONV is still being quantified [1]. Mechanistically, PONV is in a confused state. In addition, in contrast to numerous other clinical emetic triggers (e.g., anticancer chemotherapy) there is no animal model of PONV in which the mechanism(s) can be investigated (see below). This review attempts to provide insights into PONV by reviewing knowledge of the emetic mechanisms, identifying features of the operative environment which could activate these pathways and finally reviewing approaches to "universal" antiemetics.

M. K. Herbert et al. (Eds.), Problems of the Gastrointestinal Tract in Anesthesia...

The Events Comprising PONV

The events comprising PONV are discussed in the approximate temporal order in which they occur; however, according to the present author's knowledge, there are no quantitative descriptions of the natural time course and intensity of nausea, retching, and vomiting comprising PONV under controlled conditions (i.e., same surgery, anesthesia, patient population, etc.). Such studies could give insights into mechanisms and help identify whether there may be separate phases (with different predominant mechanisms) as is the case for chemotherapy-induced emesis where anticipatory, acute, and delayed phases with different mechanisms, but a common initiator (i.e., the chemotherapeutic agent), are identified [2].

Nausea

Nausea is derived from the Greek word for seasickness (*nautia*) which is itself derived from the word for ship (*naus*). It can be defined as a self-reported subjective sensation [3], often diffusely related to the epigastrium and abdomen, that emesis is imminent or that there is an urge to vomit. Other descriptions include "queasiness" or "sick-to-the-stomach" sensation. Its subjective nature has made research into this area very difficult and this is compounded by the lack of generally accepted instruments for assessment. Determining the precise mechanism by which the sensation of nausea is generated is also compounded by the problem of studying it in animals. Whereas nausea is difficult to study in man, in animals it is arguably impossible to do so because of its subjective, self-reported nature. In animals, particularly the ferret, a number of behaviors (e.g., walking backwards, rubbing chin on the ground, intense licking) have been observed [4] both preceding and concomitant with retching and vomiting and arguably can be considered as "equivalents", "correlates", or "surrogates" of nausea. Even if a unique set of behaviors were identified which were induced only by emetic agents and had the correct temporal association to retching and vomiting, it would still be impossible to know the sensations perceived by the animal. A similar argument applies to the study of pain in which, although the behavioral responses to noxious stimuli are similar to those observed in man (e.g., writhing, vocalization and limb withdrawal or tensing), it is impossible to know what the animal is experiencing. Studying the sensations of nausea and pain in neonates has many of the same problems as the same studies in animals. It would be of interest to investigate whether adult humans exhibit specific behaviors prior to the onset of retching and vomiting.

Nausea has a clear relevant biological function when induced by "toxins" accidentally ingested with food [i.e., if it is not detected prior to ingestion by vision (e.g., bright color), smell (unpleasant), or taste (bitter). The unpleasant sensation will reduce or stop ingestion of the contaminated food if the "toxin" is detected promptly, although the onset of nausea may be temporarily dissociated from ingestion if, for example, the toxin is generated by a bacterial contaminant once it is in the body. In general, nausea is induced by less intense activation of emetic pathways than are required to induce vomiting and this is consistent with its "warning" function.

A more important function of nausea is to generate a conditioned aversion linking the nausea to the taste or sight of the food. Thus, when encountered on a future occasion the animal will promptly reject the food. Such food-specific aversions can be induced in species which lack a vomiting reflex (e.g., rats, rabbits) and have been demonstrated in a range of species with a vomiting reflex ranging from fish to humans. The aversion may be lifelong as confirmed by the experience of humans who as a child became ill after eating shellfish and have an aversion to shellfish lasting into adulthood [5]. The advantage of such responses in uncontrolled settings is clear, but such aversions can also be induced in the clinic because, unfortunately, some therapies activate the emetic mechanism. Most notable among them are anticancer chemotherapeutic agents and particularly the highly emetic agents, such as cisplatin, which if adequate antiemetic cover is not given during the acute and delayed phases of emesis can lead to the development of anticipatory nausea and vomiting. In this type of aversive response a linkage is made between nausea, the treatment (i.e., the anticancer drug), and features associated with treatment (e.g., needles, the smell or sight of a hospital, the oncology staff, food given in close temporal association to therapy) [6]. Such aversions have led to the refusal of potentially curative therapy or reduced compliance with treatment schedules. As mentioned previously, PONV is a predictor of subsequent PONV; hence, anticipatory responses analogous to those with chemotherapy may be induced by untreated PONV. This requires formal investigation.

Whereas the function of nausea is clear and beneficial, the mechanism by which the sensation is generated is unclear. The importance of understanding this is of considerable clinical significance because, as far as can be ascertained presently, antiemetic agents are usually more efficacious against retching and vomiting than against nausea (e.g., 5-hydroxytryptamine 3 receptor antagonists). What then is known about the physiology and pharmacology of nausea?

Pathways for Induction

Although nausea and vomiting can occur in isolation (e.g., raised intracranial pressure and pyloric obstruction can induce sudden projectile vomiting with little if any nausea), nausea can be induced by activation of the same pathways as retching and vomiting (see below). Studies of motion sickness indicate that nausea requires less intense activation for induction than does vomiting, and this would be consistent with its proposed warning function. In addition, there must be a temporal dimension to the stimulus because even with intense emetic stimuli the onset of nausea precedes that of retching and vomiting. Whereas nausea continues between bouts of vomiting, a frequently encountered anecdotal comment is that vomiting reduces or even abolishes the sensation of nausea and a sense of well-being may be experienced suggesting the release of an endogenous opioid. This phenomenon has not been systematically documented, nor has the mechanism been investigated, but from a teleological perspective it can be argued that the act of vomiting is being "rewarded" or "reinforced" by the proposed opioid release because the act of vomiting is removing the toxin from the system. Some indirect evidence which supports the involvement of an endorphin is that naloxone reduces the time for subjects exposed to provocative motion to reach Malaise level III and the discomfort lasts up to 3 days, something not observed in placebo-treated subjects [7].

The precise mechanism by which the sensation of nausea is generated is not known, but studies predominantly in the past 10 years have characterized numerous endocrine, gastric, and more general autonomic nervous-system-mediated changes which occur in association with nausea [8]. These are described before giving a concluding overview of nausea.

Endocrine Changes

The endocrine changes which accompany nausea are complex [3, 8–11] and it is difficult to distinguish the changes which are specific to nausea and which may contribute to its genesis, and those which are a component of a response to the "stress" of nausea (e.g., cortisol, ACTH) or general autonomic arousal (e.g., adrenaline, pancreatic polypeptide). The most consistent endocrine change is a massive increase (up to 50 times maximal antidiuretic levels) in plasma antidiuretic hormone (ADH) and vasopressin, but not in oxytocin. Increases in ADH have been reported in subjects made nauseous by apomorphine, illusory selfmotion, ipecac, cholecystokinin, and anticancer chemotherapy drugs. In the ferret an increase in ADH was induced by apomorphine and electrical stimulation of the abdominal vagal afferents [8]. The function of such a massive release of vasopressin is unclear, although the levels would be sufficient to promote fluid retention in advance of the expected loss by vomiting and the diarrhea which often accompanies it, and also to contribute to the peripheral vasoconstriction. If the ADH is involved in the genesis of the sensation of nausea apart from an effect on the gut itself leading to the epigastric discomfort, the most likely mechanism is via the area postrema. Antidiuretic hormone has been shown to act on the area postrema to modulate the arterial baroreceptor reflex via its connections with the nucleus tractus solitarius which receives baroreceptor inputs [12]; thus, circulating ADH could act on the area postrema to influence the nucleus tractus solitarius. If the effect was on nucleus tractus solitarius neurons receiving a vagal or splanchnic afferent input from the gut, then activation would mimic the effect of their activation, including evoking a sensation (which would appear to have originated in the gut) via activation of the projections from the nucleus tractus solitarius to the cerebral cortex.

Antidiuretic hormone secretion is not an absolute requirement for the genesis of nausea, because patients with diabetes insipidus can experience nausea [13].

Gastric Motor Changes

An increase in the frequency of the gastric electrical slow wave from $\sim$ 3 to 4–9 cpm has been reported in association with nausea induced by illusory selfmotion, pregnancy (first trimester), gastroparesis (diabetic, idiopathic), functional dyspepsia, peptic ulcer disease, and gastric surgery [3, 8]. This phenomenon has been studied most extensively during illusory self-motion where the gastric frequency increase begins a few minutes after the start of drum rotation and precedes the onset of reported nausea (6.1 ± 1.1 min) by a few minutes [8]. Plasma ADH was elevated by the time nausea was reported and increased further as drum rotation continued. The motor correlate of the electrical events could contribute to the sensation of nausea by activation of mechanoreceptors, but alternatively the dysrhythmias could be secondary to the endocrine changes (e.g., adrenaline, β endorphin) or an abnormal autonomic outflow to the stomach [8].

Sympathetic activation heightens the perception of experimental intestinal distension in humans [14], and as sympathetic activation is associated with nausea, such a heightened perception of events in the gut could contribute to the sensation of epigastric awareness during nausea.

Autonomic Changes

Associated with nausea are numerous responses mediated by the autonomic nervous system and which are suggestive of autonomic arousal [9]. These responses are, as far as can be ascertained, not responsible for the genesis of the sensation of nausea, although they temporally coexist with nausea. The main responses are salivation frequently accompanied by repetitive swallowing, tachycardia, cutaneous vasoconstriction (giving rise to pallor), sweating (together with cutaneous vasoconstriction producing the cold and clammy feel of the skin), and pupil dilatation.

Outstanding Problems

Understanding the mechanism(s) underlying the genesis of the sensation of nausea is probably the most significant challenge in emesis research. Although plasma ADH and gastric dysrhythmias provide useful markers, their utility as objective measures is limited unless they can either be causally linked or shown to be predictably correlated to the subjective reports of nausea.

Improved quantification of the temporal characteristics of nausea is needed to understand the anecdotal reports that it occurs in "waves". What is their periodicity and do they increase in intensity until vomiting occurs, and what factors are involved in the transition from nausea to retching and vomiting?

Progress is being made towards identifying the cerebral regions where the conscious sensation may be generated. Using magnetic source imaging (MSI) activation (assessed by the presence and number of dipoles) of the inferior frontal gyrus occurred in subjects who reported nausea induced by either vestibular stimulation or oral syrup of ipecac [15]. The number of dipoles was related to the intensity of the nausea. Understanding the cortical site at which the sensation is generated may provide a novel target for drugs which selectively target nausea. The importance of this should not be underestimated because patients generally find nausea more distressing than retching and vomiting, it is more protracted in contrast to the brief episodes of retching and vomiting and antiemetics are usually more effective against retching and vomiting than against nausea.

Mechanics of Retching and Vomiting

The mechanical events comprising retching and vomiting are well characterized, particularly in experimental animals such as the dog and the cat where activity of the various muscles can be measured. The more limited studies in humans suggest that the major features seen in animals occur in humans. The mechanics of retching and vomiting have been reviewed extensively [16–18] and therefore are only described briefly herein.

Prior to the Onset of Retching

Before the dramatic motor events of retching and vomiting are apparent, preparatory changes have already taken place in the gastrointestinal tract. The first event is relaxation of the proximal stomach [14]. This occurs under the influence of vagal efferents activating intramural neurons using non-adrenergic non-cholinergic inhibitory neurotransmitters, probably nitric oxide and vasoactive intestinal peptide. The second major event is a retrograde giant contraction originating in the mid- to lower small intestine. It is under vagal control and can be blocked by atropine indicating its mediation by acetylcholine acting on a muscarinic receptor [20]. This large amplitude contraction sweeps towards the stomach and it probably contributes to the frequent presence of bile in vomit. From a biological perspective these motor events are proposed to contribute to the protective function of vomiting. The gastric relaxation will delay the emptying of any toxin-contaminated food and provide a reservoir for any contaminated gastric contents already emptied which will be returned to the stomach by the retrograde giant contraction. Relaxation of the proximal stomach may also place the stomach in a mechanically advantageous position for compression by the somatic muscles (see below) and together with esophageal motor activity contribute to the formation of a "funnel" in the region of the gastroesophageal junction. Neither the gastric relaxation nor the retrograde giant contraction are essential for retching and vomiting to occur, but retching does not begin until the retrograde contraction has reached the stomach.

Retching and Vomiting

Ejection of gastric contents is brought about by retching and vomiting and, in contrast to the events described previously, they are under the control of the somatic division of the nervous system. Retching and vomiting both involve contraction of the abdominal muscles and the diaphragm [16, 17]. The function of retching is unclear, but it has been proposed to be involved in overcoming the antireflux mechanism present at the gastroesophageal junction [20]. Very little is known of the factors regulating retching and the transition from retching to vomiting. Preclinical studies [21] have shown that more retches occur prior to a vomit at low gastric volumes, and vice versa, and that the transition from retching to vomiting may be dependent on arterial blood-gas tensions (see below) [22]. During retching the entire diaphragm and the anterior abdominal muscles contract synchronously, but during vomiting the periesophageal region of the diaphragm does not contract because the phrenic nerve fibers supplying that region are selectively inhibited [16, 17]. Ejection is also accompanied by shortening of the esophagus and activation of the internal intercostal muscles, laryngeal and pharyngeal muscles and the external anal and urethral sphincters [23, 24].

The autonomic and somatic nervous activity driving the motor events described previously is generated and coordinated in the brainstem. Although the term "vomiting center" is a useful shorthand to describe the neurons responsible for the motor program, such a region with this as its sole function has not been identified, although a region of the reticular formation dorsomedial to the retrofacial nucleus [25] and part of the nucleus tractus solitarius have both been proposed as sites for the "central pattern generator" for emesis.

The Inputs Triggering Nausea and Vomiting

The inputs triggering nausea and vomiting have been the subject of numerous reviews [2, 18] and are only outlined briefly here to provide a background against which some of the possible mechanisms involved in the genesis of PONV can be discussed. Whatever the key elements of the operative environment responsible for the induction of PONV, they are likely to be triggering the response via one of the pathways described herein. However, in contrast to many other forms of emesis (e.g., anticancer chemotherapy), it is not possible to say which pathway is predominantly or exclusively involved in PONV due to the lack of an animal model (see below) of PONV itself.

Abdominal Vagal Afferents

Retching and vomiting can readily be induced by intense stimulation of the abdominal vagal afferents even under anesthesia [26]. The abdominal vagal afferents convey information from both mechanoreceptors and chemoreceptors principally to the nucleus tractus solitarius in the brainstem [27]. The mechanoreceptors have receptive fields in the muscle and discharge in response to contraction and distension of the muscle from the stomach to the first part of the colon. The chemoreceptors have receptive fields in the mucosa and respond to numerous features of the luminal environment including hypertonic and irritant solutions (e.g., copper sulfate). They also respond to mucosal stroking.

Both types of afferents are involved in the physiological control of gut function and both are also capable of inducing nausea, retching, and vomiting. The muscle mechanoreceptors are the most likely candidates for the emetic response to distension, particularly of regions such as the gastric antrum and duodenum which have relatively little capacity for accommodation. The mucosal afferents are the most likely candidates for triggering the emetic response to hypertonic solutions and irritant chemicals. The mucosal chemoreceptors differ from the mechanoreceptors in that the afferent axon itself is not the detector. It is proposed that the detector is an enteroendocrine cell which when appropriately stimulated at the luminal surface releases a neuroactive agent which then activates receptors on the afferent axon terminating in close proximity. 5-Hydroxytryptamine (5-HT) from the enterochromaffin cells and acting on 5-HT_3 receptors has been implicated in the responses to mucosal stimulation, but cholecystokinin and substance P are other likely candidates [2, 27].

The mucosal afferents have also been implicated in the emetic response to anticancer chemotherapy drugs (e.g., cisplatin) and radiation as the enterochromaffin cells appear to be particularly sensitive to both stimuli, which are proposed to generate free radicals leading to influx of calcium ions and exocytosis of 5-HT and other neuroactive substances to act on receptors located on the vagal afferent terminals [28].

The Area Postrema

The area postrema is located at the caudal extremity of the floor of the fourth ventricle and is one of a group of circumventricular organs which share a common feature of being outside the blood-brain barrier. This feature makes them accessible to substances in the blood (e.g., gut peptides). Numerous lesion studies have implicated the area postrema in the emetic response to substances in the circulation leading to it being called the "chemoreceptor trigger zone (CTZ) for emesis" [2]. Unfortunately, this nomenclature led to the assumption (not intended by the original authors of the studies) that all systemic chemicals inducing emesis acted via this route. This is not necessarily the case as some chemical stimuli (e.g., cisplatin) act via the gut afferents [2]. In addition, the precise role of the area postrema itself is under reassessment with some considering it as the transducer and others as providing a window in the blood-brain barrier by which systemic agents can gain access to receptors located on dendrites of the subjacent nucleus tractus solitarius [29]. The two possibilities are not mutually exclusive. What is clear is that nausea, retching, and vomiting can be induced by systemic agents (e.g., apomorphine) acting on the area postrema and/or the superficial nucleus tractus solitarius. The retching and vomiting induced by opioids can be blocked by lesions directed at this region, whereas they are not blocked by abdominal vagotomy [29, 30].

The Vestibular System

The pathway by which motion can induce vomiting by activation of the vestibular system and a sensory conflict or mismatch between the vestibular and visual systems is well described [31], and considerable progress has been made in describing the pharmacology of the vestibular system which may help in the design of new drugs for motion sickness [32]. The vestibular system is a potent site from which nausea and vomiting can be induced as confirmed by the severe symptoms which can be caused by motion exposure or labyrinthitis; however, the function (if any) of motion sickness is unclear. It has been argued from an evolutionary perspective that it is also a component of the body's defensive system as toxins affecting the nervous system could modify locomotion sufficiently to activate the vestibular system, and the concomitant sensation of nausea would encourage the animal to seek refuge.

Although the vestibular system would not appear to be a likely site from which systemic agents could induce emesis, agents accessing the vestibular labyrinths could modify the chemical transmission (glutamate) between the vestibular receptor hair cells and the vestibular nerve giving rise to an inappropriate signal [32].

Higher Regions of the CNS

Electrical stimulation studies have shown that vomiting preceded by quiescence, pallor, sweating, and salivation can be evoked in the monkey by stimulation in the amygdala, ventralis anterior, anterior perforated area, and the hippocampus [33]. Similar findings have been reported in humans [34].

Others

Nausea and vomiting can be induced from ventricular cardiac afferents, auricular vagal afferents, pharyngeal afferents and the taste buds, although in the case of the latter it is unclear whether this is a primary response or secondary to an association between the taste and illness experienced from a previous exposure [35].

Intrinsic Antiemetic Mechanisms

One relatively neglected aspect of emetic research is the study of intrinsic mechanisms which may inhibit emesis rather than cause activation. Such mechanisms are of interest because if they could be accessed or mimicked pharmacologically, they could provide a basis for novel antiemetic agents.

The Function of Intrinsic Antiemetic Mechanisms

Intrinsic mechanisms for the modulation of the emetic reflex can be argued to have several possible functions:

1. They permit the sensitivity of the reflex to be set by either suppressing or facilitating transmission at a critical point(s) in the emetic pathway. For example, the nucleus tractus solitarius in the brainstem is a key integrative and relay nucleus for the emetic reflex; modulation of transmission here would be expected to have a marked effect on the reflex. It has been proposed that the nucleus tractus solitarius has a "switching" function which as one of its functions selects between different respiratory pattern generators [36]. Suppression of the emetic reflex may be important if parts of the neural circuitry required for emesis was required for a more pressing function (e.g., cough as airway obstruction could kill within minutes, whereas retaining an orally ingested toxin for a few additional minutes is unlikely to have such a serious effect).
2. By reducing intrinsic inhibitory tone the sensitivity of the emetic reflex could be enhanced. For example, once an animal has been exposed to an emetic challenge

it would be logical for the system to become sensitized either by increasing the sensitivity of the detectors (e.g., vagal afferents) so they are activated by lower levels of the stimulus or there is a reduction in the central "set point" for induction of emesis. Little is known about mechanisms of vagal afferent sensitization at their peripheral terminals, although this phenomenon is well characterized for cutaneous nociceptors. Changes in "set points" are a well-characterized feature of physiological systems and are not described further.

3. Triggering the emetic reflex should be seen in the context of the "cost" of ejecting the last meal which may be eaten by another animal (as occurs in cryptoparasitism, for example, in some species of birds and during which the animal may have exposed itself to considerable danger and expended considerable energy to obtain especially when the prey may be encountered infrequently). It is therefore likely that as with many other reflex systems the trigger has both intensity and temporal elements to prevent accidental activation. This can be illustrated using activation of the emetic reflex in anesthetized animals by electrical stimulation of the abdominal vagal afferents. Using stimulus voltages sufficient to activate all the afferents and frequencies equivalent to or greater than those recorded in single abdominal vagal afferents, retching requires approximately 15 s of stimulation for induction.

The Nature of Intrinsic Antiemetic Mechanisms

A role for endogenous opioids in the modulation of emesis comes from several studies (reviewed in [37]; see below) but principally from studies of the effects of the opioid receptor antagonist naloxone. This agent is itself capable of inducing emesis in some species, increasing the magnitude of the emetic response to apomorphine, copper sulfate, cisplatin, and radiation in the ferret, and increases nausea and vomiting induced by cisplatin in patients [37]. These observations indicate that there is an endogenous opioid-mediated antiemetic tone, and from such studies it has been proposed that there is an "antiemetic" center (c.f. "vomiting" center). Although the anatomical location of the "antiemetic" center has not been identified, the parabrachial nucleus has a marked modulatory effect on the nucleus tractus solitarius and would be a likely candidate.

In anesthetized and decerebrate animals retching and vomiting can be relatively easily evoked by electrical stimulation of the abdominal vagal afferents. In contrast, similar stimulation of the cervical vagi (which contain the abdominal vagal afferents projecting to the brainstem as well as vagal afferents from thoracic structures) usually fails to induce an emetic response. Emesis induced by abdominal vagal afferent stimulation (dog), xylazine (cat, an alpha adrenoceptor agonist acting via the area postrema) and motion (monkey) can be prevented by cervical vagal afferent stimulation [38]. The effect on nausea (if any) is not known. It has been proposed that it is the pulmonary vagal afferents which are responsible for this effect, and although this has not been investigated directly, it is consistent with the anecdotal observation that deep inspiration may temporarily alleviate the urge to vomit.

Studies in the dog have implicated blood gas levels in the transition from retching to vomiting [22]. It was reported that during retching $PaCO_2$ increased and PaO_2 decreased, probably leading to activation of central and peripheral arterial chemoreceptors which in turn facilitated the transition from retching to vomiting. Electrical stimulation of the carotid sinus nerve afferents in paralyzed, artificially ventilated decerebrate dogs during induced retching was able to trigger the transition from induced retching to induced vomiting. Whereas these observations require further investigation, particularly in humans, they highlight the importance of regulation of blood gases in the postoperative period.

In the same way that higher regions of the brain (e.g., amygdala) are able to access brainstem sites to induce emesis, it appears likely that there are equivalent mechanisms by which emesis can be suppressed. This has not been the subject of formal investigation, although there are anecdotal reports from the Second World War of air and naval gunners who quickly overcame motion sickness to challenge a sudden attack. In chemotherapy there is evidence for a relationship between patients' expectation of having nausea and its actual development [39], although it is not known whether vomiting itself can also be influenced. It has been proposed by Morrow et al. [6] that psychological interventions (described by some as a "verbal placebo" [40]) could be used to enhance positive expectations. Studies of the pathway involved could provide a novel pharmacological mechanism by which nausea could be reduced.

Potentially Emetic Stimuli in the Operative Environment

Many features of the operative environment have been identified which are either emetic themselves or may predispose to emesis. During the course of induction, anesthesia, and surgery different factors are implicated and these are summarized in Table 1. Epidemiological studies have identified that some factors make a greater contribution than others [see chapter by Apfel], however, in most studies only the incidence of PONV is investigated not its duration or intensity. A detailed review of the mechanisms by which the numerous components of the operative environment may induce PONV via the pathways described above has already been published [18], so this review focuses on relatively neglected or newer aspects.

The Patient

Whereas it is clear that the trigger for the induction of PONV is some feature of the anesthetic and/or surgical environment, the observation that only a proportion of patients treated in a similar way have PONV clearly implicates patient-specific factors in determining whether PONV will occur. Numerous patient-predictive or predisposing factors have been identified (e.g., female gender, age, emetic history; see chapter by Apfel) but little attention has been given to the underlying mechanisms. The patient-predictive factors broad encompass two types, intrinsic (e.g., genetically determined anatomical or neurochemical differences) and acquired (e.g., alcohol intake), although in some cases the former could lead to the latter as can be illustrated with motion sickness. For example, in a particular individual subtle differences in the anatomy of the vestibular system could make it particularly sensitive to motion stimuli, possibly resulting in an increased sensitivity to motion sickness. The frequent occurrence of motion sickness (particularly as a child) could result in a sensiti-

Table 1. Summary of factors which may contribute to post-operative nausea and vomiting (PONV; see text and [18] for details)

Pre-operative factors

Psychological stress (e.g., release of ACTH, adrenaline, increased sympathetic activity
Gender (e.g., females *appear* more sensitive to a range of emetic stimuli than males)
Emetic history (e.g., motion sensitivity, previous PONV, pregnancy sickness)
Food [e.g., if food present, emesis more likely during induction; activates gut afferents, releases gut hormones (gastrin, CCK, PYY) and 5-HT]
Hydration
"Dehydration" (rise in ADH)
Glycemic state (mild hypoglycemia may induce nausea; in females more than males?)
Reason for surgery (patients with gastrointestinal or central nervous system problems may have a sensitized emetic reflex)

Peri-operative factors

Intubation (e.g., gag reflex; pharyngeal irritation)
Drugs (e.g., atropine-like agents: may contribute to post-surgical reduction in gastric emptying)
Opioid analgesics: dose-related emetic and anti-emetic effects
- Sensitize vestibular system
- Release ADH
- Release EC cell 5-HT
- Decrease gastric emptying

Intra-operative factors

Anesthesia (e.g., immobility reduces vestibular input; anesthesia itself tends to be anti-emetic but emesis is still possible with intense stimulation)
Anesthetic
Physical effect: gut distension by volatile anesthetics
- Pharmacological effects: catecholamine release; allosteric modulation of 5-HT_3 and other receptors; inhibition of "anti-emetic" center?; modulation of transmitter release in emetic pathway; ADH release; reduced gut motility and LOS tone; hypotension from spinal anesthesia

Surgery
General effects
Reduced gastrointestinal motility via autonomic reflexes
Release of numerous hormones, e.g., ADH
Specific types of surgery
Activation of afferents during surgery, probably leading to post-surgical sensitization centrally and peripherally: ophthalmic; ear, nose, and throat; gastrointestinal; gynecological

Post-operative factors

Accumulation of pre-, peri-, and intra-operative factors
Pain (e.g., activation of splanchnic afferents; adrenaline secretion)
Prolonged disruption of gastric emptying (e.g., distension induced activation of vagal afferents)
Movement (e.g., activation of "rested" and sensitized vestibular system by movement)
Conscious perception of abnormal state (e.g., disorientation)

zation of the central emetic pathways leading to a reduced threshold to other emetic stimuli such as PONV. Any emetic stimulus to which the patient has been frequently exposed (e.g., migraine, food allergens) is likely to influence the sensitivity of the response to clinically relevant stimuli and hence consideration should be given to taking a more extensive emetic history. Recent studies have shown racial differences in the nausea response induced by illusory self-motion with Chinese subjects being more sensitive than Caucasian and African-American subjects [41]. Studies of specific subgroups of patients undergoing surgery would be of considerable interest because pilots, astronauts, and sailors whose jobs all necessitate a low sensitivity to motion would be expected to have a lower incidence of PONV than the general population.

Identification of factors which may protect the patient against emesis have been relatively neglected in PONV. High alcohol consumption is a protective factor in anticancer chemotherapy-induced emesis [42], and although damage to the central emetic pathways has been suggested as a mechanism, the effect may be more subtle because ethanol has significant allosteric interactions with the 5-HT_3 receptor [43].

The effect of smoking on the incidence of PONV would be interesting for two reasons: firstly, the nicotinic acetylcholine receptor like the 5-HT_3 receptor is a member of the ligand-gated ion channel superfamily and hence can be modulated by anesthetics; secondly, nicotine can induce nausea and vomiting and hence it can be argued that tobacco smokers may have a downregulated emetic system and this may be reflected in a reduction in the sensitivity to PONV in comparison with non-smokers.

The Anesthetic

Anesthetics can have multiple pharmacological effects which could contribute to the genesis of PONV, but no common feature has emerged (Table 1) [18]. Recent studies of the electrophysiological properties of the 5-HT_3 receptor in cell lines and the nodose ganglion have studied the effects of anesthetic halogenated alcohols (e.g., trichloroethanol [44]) and volatile (e.g., halothane, isoflurane) and injectable (thiopental, propofol, ketamine) anesthetics [43]. These complex and continuing studies can be summarized by stating that they have shown varying degrees of positive allosteric modulation of the 5-HT_3 receptor. Such interactions with this (and probably other ion channels) receptor in the brainstem, on the vagal afferents or the enterochromaffin cell, could play an important role in the genesis of PONV. However, it is likely that this is not the only mechanism in view of the relatively low efficacy of 5-HT_3 receptor antagonists in PONV. The anesthetic may serve to prime the system to some of the stimuli outlined in Table 1.

An Overview of Mechanisms

Studies in *Suncus murinus* (house musk shrew) have demonstrated that emesis can be induced in this species by 10 min exposure to 1 % halothane in 80 % nitrous oxide and 20 % oxygen and the response was antagonized by a 5-HT_3 receptor antagonist or an NK_1 receptor antagonist [45]. This model may provide important insights into the mechanism of PONV, but some caution should be exerted because shrews have an acute olfactory system and it is not known whether the animals were responding to a noxious odor rather than specifically the anesthetic. *Suncus* is particularly sensitive to motion requiring only a few minutes of exposure for emesis to be induced [46]. As motion sickness is one of the more reliable predictive factors for PONV in man, perhaps the sensitivity of *Suncus* to the anesthetic is to be expected. In ferrets premedicated with ketamine and anesthetized with halothane (1–2 %) nitrous oxide and oxygen and undergoing abdominal surgery (e.g., abdominal vagotomy or splanchnic nerve section, fundoplication), postoperative emesis is rare (Andrews and Richardson, unpublished observations) suggesting that in this species factors in addition to the anesthetic and surgery are necessary to induce emesis.

It is highly unlikely that a single feature of the operative environment is responsible for the induction of PONV, but the anesthetic probably plays a key role, probably involving allosteric modulation of one or more ligand-gated ion channel receptors. The way in which this influences the emetic pathways is unclear, but it appears reasonable to suggest that if it sensitized the system then this would provide a background against which the other factors could act. The probability of inducing emesis would be determined by the sensitivity of the system prior to exposure to the anesthetic (e.g., determined by the emetic history of the patient or genetic factors) and the emetic burden to which the patient is exposed during surgery with some factors (e.g., type of surgery) probably making a greater contribution than others (e.g., concomitant medication). Postoperative nausea and vomiting most likely involves activation of several emetic inputs (e.g., area postrema, vagal afferents, vestibular system) with each making a different contribution depending on the stimulus (e.g., anesthetic distension of the stomach activating vagal afferents, morphine acting on the brainstem). Whereas preventing allosteric interactions could perhaps provide an approach to treating PONV, such interactions may be a fundamental property of anesthetics linked to their ability to induce anesthesia. A more rational approach considering the complex nature of the emetic stimuli in the operative environment would be to identify agents able to block all forms of emesis irrespective of the cause. Such "broad spectrum" or "universal" antiemetics are the subject of the next section.

Current and Novel Pharmacological Approaches to Antiemesis

This section reviews one current (5-HT_3 receptor antagonist) and three relatively novel (opioid and 5-HT_{1A} receptor agonists and NK_1 receptor antagonists) approaches to antiemetics, primarily from a preclinical perspective, to illustrate that considerable progress has been made towards the identification of "universal" or "broad spectrum" antiemetics.

5-Hydroxytryptamine$_3$ Receptor Antagonists

The identification of the antiemetic potential of selective, potent 5-HT_3 receptor antagonists (e.g., granisetron, ondansetron, tropisetron) and their subsequent clinical development (e.g., Kytril, Navoban, Zofran) represents a major advance in understanding the neuropharmacology of emetic mechanisms. This class of agent has revolutionized the treatment of the acute emesis induced by anticancer drugs, such as cisplatin. However, their spectrum of antiemetic effect is limited as was expected based on the originally proposed site and mechanism of action [47]. In chemotherapy and radiotherapy-induced emesis there is a considerable body of evidence implicating 5-HT in the emetic response in addition to amelioration or blockade of emesis by 5-HT_3 receptor antagonists. This evidence includes: (a) the presence of 5-HT in the emetic pathway; (b) the presence of 5-HT_3 receptors in the emetic pathway; (c) the induction of emesis by 5-HT_3 receptor agonists when injected to the site of interest; and (d) the release of 5-HT in the appropriate location by chemotherapeutic drugs and radiation [2]. To be as confident as possible of the involvement of a particular neurotransmitter and receptor in any form of emesis (e.g., PONV), all these criteria should be fulfilled. For the acute phase of emesis induced by the anticancer drug cisplatin all the criteria have been fulfilled [47]. Whereas the 5-HT_3 receptor antagonists ondansetron (Zofran) and granisetron (Kytril) have some efficacy in PONV and this in itself suggests an involvement of 5-HT in PONV, other supportive evidence is lacking. The apparently lower efficacy of 5-HT_3 receptor antagonists investigated in PONV suggests that 5-HT_3 receptors play a far less crucial role in PONV in comparison with emesis induced by anticancer therapies. It is important to appreciate that this does not preclude an involvement of 5-HT in PONV by acting on one or more of the other subtypes of 5-HT (5-HT_1, 5-HT_2, 5-HT_4, 5-HT_6, 5-HT_7) receptors. The lower efficacy may also reflect a mechanism other than blockade of 5-HT_3 receptors is responsible for their antiemetic action in PONV. For example, ondansetron (but not granisetron) can stimulate gastric emptying in the guinea pig [48], and recent studies indicate that this effect could be due to an agonist action at the 5-HT_{2B} receptor [49]. If such an effect occurs in patients, it could contribute to reducing postoperative gastric stasis, thus reducing the probability of nausea and vomiting. Further studies are required to define precisely the efficacy of various 5-HT_3 receptor antagonists in well-characterized patient groups with PONV and to investigate 5-HT metabolism (e.g., 5-HIAA levels) in different surgical/anesthetic combinations. If 5-HT acting on 5-HT_3 receptors is involved in PONV, it is most likely that this occurs in conjunction with abdominal and perhaps pelvic surgery as manipulation and transient ischemia of the gut can induce 5-HT release into the hepatic portal vein [50]. Other studies have shown that 5-HT can activate 5-HT_3 receptors on vagal [51] and splanchnic [52] afferent terminals providing a mechanism for the induction of emesis or sensitization of central pathways.

Activation of gastric mechanoreceptors by distension caused by volatile anesthetics has been implicated in PONV [18]. In volunteers nausea and gastric dysrhythmias induced by gastric antral distension were not affected by granisetron [53]. Such a mechanism could contribute to the reduced efficacy of 5-HT_3 receptor antagonists in PONV. In addition, as steroids (e.g., dexamethasone) enhance the antiemetic efficacy of 5-HT_3 receptor antagonists in patients (particularly females) undergoing anticancer chemotherapy, studies of combination therapy in PONV should be considered. Such studies are of particular relevance to PONV as steroids including dexamethasone have been shown to allosterically modulate the activity of the 5-HT_3 receptor which, as discussed previously, is also modulated by some alcohols and anesthetics.

Opioid Receptor Agonists

The role of opioids in emesis is complex and can be illustrated by studies of the relationship between the dose of morphine and the magnitude of the emetic response in the ferret. At "low" doses, morphine induces an emetic response which is dose related but as the dose is increased the magnitude of the response decreases as does the number of animals responding. The "bell-shaped" dose-response curve also occurs with loperamide, and to a lesser extent with morphine-6-glucuronide. In simple terms the dose-response curve has been explained by morphine acting at different doses on different populations of opioid receptors with different effects. At "low" doses the predominant effect is induction of emesis with μ, κ, and δ receptors all implicated [37], whereas at "higher" doses activation of opioid receptors (μ or κ) probably in a different location leads to a blockade of emesis. The antiemetic effect of morphine or more selective opioid receptor agonists is not confined to morphine with antiemetic effects being demonstrated against apomorphine, copper sulfate, nicotine, and cisplatin [37]. This antiemetic effect of opioids is consistent with the emetic effects of naloxone discussed previously and has led to the proposal that opioids with a more selective receptor profile could provide a novel basis for a broad spectrum anti-emetic agent. Based on the current animal studies this is a realistic possibility, but clinical testing awaits further understanding of the receptor subtype(s) involved and the design of potent selective brain penetrant compounds.

5-Hydroxytryptamine$_{1A}$ Receptor Agonists

Agonists acting at the 5-HT$_{1A}$ receptor (e.g., buspirone, 8-OH-DPAT, LY301317) have been shown to have antiemetic effects in the cat, dog, ferret, pigeon and *Suncus murinus* (house musk shrew) [36, 54] when tested against stimuli including motion (cat), cisplatin (dog, pigeon), 5-HT$_3$ receptor agonist (pigeon), conditioned emesis (pigeon), oral ipecac (dog), oral copper sulfate (ferret, *Suncus*), morphine (ferret) and vagal afferent stimulation (cat). The site of action has not been identified, although post-synaptic 5-HT$_{1A}$ receptors in the nucleus tractus solitarius have been proposed [36]. These preclinical studies demonstrate that 5-HT$_{1A}$ agonists have broad-spectrum antiemetic effects. The time course of the antiemetic effects suggests that they are not secondary to the anxiolytic and antidepressant effects of this class of agent. Clinical studies with 5-HT$_{1A}$ agonists as antiemetics are very limited and, as far as the present author is aware, have only been undertaken with buspirone which had no effect against acute cisplatin-induced emesis [55]. However, the potential of this class of agent should not be dismissed until studies have been undertaken with more potent and selective agents (e.g., LY301317) [54].

Neurokinin$_1$ Receptor Antagonists

The neurokinin$_1$ (NK$_1$) receptor is one of three neurokinin receptor subtypes currently identified. The preferred ligand for the NK$_1$ receptor is the undecapeptide substance P (SP). In contrast to the 5-HT$_3$ receptor, the NK$_1$ receptor is not a ligand-gated ion channel but acts via IP$_3$. A major breakthrough in identifying functional roles for NK$_1$ receptors and hence SP came from the identification of selective, potent antagonists which were not themselves peptides. The early compounds were CP-96,345 and CP-99,994 (Pfizer), but many others are now available (Table 2). Although these agents have potential clinical utility in areas other than emesis (e.g., pain, itch, migraine) their antiemetic effect in animal models is striking and presently unique.

Table 2. Preclinical spectrum of the antiemetic effects on tachykinin neurokinin$_1$ receptor antagonists

Stimulus	Species	Compound
Cisplatin (acute/delayed)	Ferret, piglet, *Suncus*	CP-99,994 [56, 64]; GR205171 [65]; CP-122,721 [66]; L-741,671 [57]; GR-203040 [67]; PD 154075 [68]
Cyclophosphamide	Ferret	GR-203040 [67]; GR205171 [69]
Nicotine	*Suncus*	CP-99,994 [70]
Morphine	Ferret	GR203040 [67]; GR205171 [69]; HSP-117 [71]
Loperamide	Ferret	CP-99,994 [56]; CP-122,721 [66]
Apomorphine	Ferret, dog	CP-99,994 [56]
Ipecacuanha	Ferret, dog	GR203040 [67]; GR205171 [65]; CP-99,994 [56]; CP-122,721 [66]
Copper sulfate	Ferret, dog	GR203040 [67]; GR205171 [65]; CP-99,994 [56]; CP-122,721 [66]; HSP-117 [71]
Radiation	Ferret	GR203040 [67]; CP-99,994 [64]; GR205171 [65]
Motion	*Suncus*, cat	GR203040 [67]; GR205171 [65]; CP-99,994 [72]
Alcohol	*Suncus*	CP-99,994 [73]
Electrical vagal afferent stimulation	Ferret/dog	CP-99,994 [56]; GR205171 [58]
Resiniferotoxin	*Suncus*	CP-99,994 [P.L.R. Andrews and N. Matsuki, unpublished observations]
Inhaled N_2O/isoflurane	*Suncus*	GR205171 [45]
Rolipram	Ferret	CP-99,994 [P.L.R. Andrews and J.W. Watson, unpublished observations]

Numbers in brackets are references

The remarkable feature of the selective NK$_1$ receptor antagonists is their broad spectrum of antiemetic action, and although the majority of studies have been performed in the ferret, more limited but consistent data are available from dog, cat, pig, and the house musk shrew (*Suncus murinus*). Results from such a range of species and numerous different agents is unique at this stage in development of an antiemetic. The studies are shown in Table 2. The results can be summarized by commenting that this class of agent is able to markedly reduce or block (depending on the species and compound) the retching and vomiting induced by both centrally (e.g., motion, morphine, loperamide, nicotine) and peripherally (copper sulfate, cisplatin, electrical stimulation of abdominal vagal afferents) acting emetic agents. This clearly differentiates them from 5-HT$_3$ receptor antagonists. The precise site of action is still a matter of debate, but there is general agreement that it is central within the brainstem and some degree of consensus that the main site is the nucleus tractus solitarius [56, 57], although a site between the nucleus tractus solitarius and emetic "central pattern generator" (see above) has also been proposed [58]. A brainstem site is supported by the observation that NK$_1$ receptor antagonists which are not centrally penetrant do not have anti-emetic activity and NK$_1$ receptor antagonists microinjected into the region of the nucleus tractus solitarius are antiemetic [57].

The remaining outstanding question regarding the NK$_1$ receptor antagonists is whether they are capable of blocking nausea as well as retching and vomiting. As discussed previously, nausea itself cannot be measured in animals' behaviors which are considered by some, but not all, to be "correlates" or "surrogates" of the sensation.

Transfer of Approaches to Man: Why Is It So Difficult?

Putting aside the issue of transferability to humans, the animal studies described previously have shown that it is possible to identify agents which are "universal" or "broad spectrum" antiemetics in the sense that they have identified agents (particularly NK_1 receptor antagonists) which can markedly reduce and often abolish retching and vomiting in several animal species. Whereas side effects have been an issue with opioid and 5-HT_{1A} agonists, this does not appear to be the case with the NK_1 receptor antagonists. The animal studies show that there are probably several key or critical pharmacologically differentiable sites at which the emetic reflex can be selectively blocked or disabled with no apparent interference with reflexes using adjacent pathways or sharing the same motor outputs [56]. The observations, particularly with the NK_1 receptor antagonists, made in several animal species suggest a strongly conserved mechanism; however, no studies have been published using non-human primates. The early clinical studies in PONV [59] and acute and delayed emesis induced by anticancer chemotherapy [60–62] are disappointing in that the efficacy against retching and vomiting does not match that in animal studies, although they do show that NK_1 receptor antagonists have antinausea as well as antivomiting effects. Although such early results should be treated with caution, they nevertheless raise the problem of the transferability of animal studies to humans. There are several possibilities which should be considered and investigated.

Receptor Isoforms

There is growing evidence for species specific isoforms of the receptor as well as isoforms in the same species [63]. Compounds have been identified which have differing degrees of selectivity for the rat, ferret, and human NK_1 receptor [57]. Whereas compounds for use in humans will have been selected for activity against the human (or perhaps ferret) NK_1 receptor, this will not necessarily reflect the selectivity or potency at the site of action relevant to antiemesis, particularly if receptor isoforms exist within the brain, as has been reported in the rat [63].

Other Neurokinin Receptors

Whereas there is a body of evidence supporting a role for substance P in emesis (e.g., presence in pathway, induction of emesis by substance P), substance P acts on $NK_1 > NK_3 > NK_2$ receptors. Thus, substance P may be a highly conserved neurotransmitter in the brainstem emetic pathway, and a difference in the critical region of the brainstem in ferret and human could explain the different efficacies. Alternatively, the animal species studied employ substance P as the major tachykinin in the brainstem, but primates including humans may use other tachykinins (e.g., NK_A, NK_B) in the same location.

Non-Tachykinin Mechanisms

Studies in the ferret, cat, dog, piglet, and shrew have shown that the involvement of NK_1 receptors and by implication substance P is a conserved mechanism; however, it is possible that in primates non-tachykinin mechanisms play a more prominent role in the central control of emesis. Other peptides identified in the dorsal brainstem include CGRP and CCK.

The Model vs the Clinic

There are marked differences between animal models of emesis and emesis in the clinic. This is best illustrated for anti-cancer chemotherapy but similar arguments apply to PONV. In animals it is the emetic effect of the chemotherapeutic agent (e.g., cisplatin, cyclophosphamide) which is being studied and not the effect of chemotherapy. The animal studies differ from the clinical situation in the following ways: the animals are naive to emetic stimuli, whereas humans usually have some "emetic history" even if they have not undergone prior chemotherapy; the animals do not have a tumor which may be releasing proemetic substances or evoking the release of proemetic substances (e.g., interleukins) as part of the response to the tumor; the animals have not had surgery, a relatively common occurrence prior to chemotherapy; the animals are not usually extensively hydrated nor are they receiving concomitant medication. Thus, the model only studies one component of the clinical environment. This should not be a problem if substance P and NK_1 receptors are at a critical point in the emetic pathway. However, if the NK_1/substance P pathway is the predominant rather than exclusive pathway, the multiplicity of inputs activated in complex clinical situations (e.g., PONV, chemotherapy) may activate additional pharmacological mechanisms. Additionally, emetic agents acting at sites distal to the site of NK_1 receptor blockade could still evoke emesis. A further possibility is that in healthy individuals the NK_1/substance P mechanism predominates but in patients this mechanism is modified or other mechanisms are induced.

Whatever the outcome of the current clinical trials, the preclinical studies with the NK_1 receptor antagonists have shown for the first time that a universal antiemetic is more than a theoretical concept. Identification of the precise site(s) of action will provide a focus for studies in man as it seems reasonable to propose that the same site could be critically involved in emesis in man even if different neurotransmitters are employed.

References

1. Tramer MR, Moore RA, Reynolds DJM, McQuay HJ (1997) A quantitative systematic review of ondansetron in treatment of established postoperative nausea and vomiting. Br Med J 314:1088–1092
2. Andrews PLR, Davis CJ (1995) The physiology of emesis induced by anti-cancer therapy. In: Reynolds DJM, Andrews PLR, Davis CJ (eds) Serotonin and the scientific basis of anti-emetic therapy. Oxford Clin Comm, Oxford, UK, pp25–49
3. Koch KL (1995) Approach to the patient with nausea and vomiting. In: Yamada T (ed) Textbook of gastroenterology, 2nd edn. Lippincott, Philadelphia, pp 731–749

4. Fox RA (1992) Current status: animal models of nausea. In: Bianchi AL, Grelot L, Miller AD, King GL (eds) Mechanism and control of emesis. Colloque INSERM/John Libbey Eurotext Ltd 223:341–350
5. Pelchat ML, Rozin P (1982) The special role of nausea in the acquisition of food dislikes by humans. Appetite 3:341–351
6. Morrow GR, Roscoe JA, Kirshner JJ, Hynes HE, Rosenbluth RJ (1998) Anticipatory nausea and vomiting in the era of 5-HT_3 antiemetics. Support Care Cancer 6:244–247
7. Allen ME, McKay C, Eaves DM, Hamilton D (1986) Naloxone enhances motion sickness: endorphins implicated. Aviation Space Environm Med 57:647–653
8. Koch KL (1997) A noxious trio: nausea, gastric dysrhythmias and vasopressin. Neurogastroenterol Motility 9:141–142
9. Andrews PLR (1999) Nausea, vomiting, and the autonomic nervous system. In: Mathias CJ, Bannister R (eds) Autonomic failure. Oxford University Press, Oxford, pp 126–235
10. Feldman M, Samson WK, O'Dorisio TM (1988) Apomorphine-induced nausea in humans: release of vasopressin and pancreatic polypeptide. Gastroenterology 95:721–726
11. Stalla GK, Doerr HG, Bidlingmaier F, Sippel WG, Restorff W von (1985) Serum levels of eleven steroid hormones following motion sickness. Aviation Space Environm Med 56:995–999
12. Midget K, Hour N, Maniac J-I, Sat R, Taken Y, Camay H-O (1998) Effects of arginine-vasopressin on neuronal interaction from the area postrema to the nucleus tractus solitarii in rat brain slices. Neurosci Lett 256:45–48
13. Nussey SS, Hawthorn J, Page SR, Ang VTY, Jenkins JS (1988) Responses of plasma oxytocin and arginine vasopressin to nausea induced by apomorphine and ipecacuanha. Clin Endocrinol 28:297–304
14. Iovino P, Azpiroz F, Domingo E, Malagelada J-R (1995) The sympathetic nervous system modulates perception and reflex responses to gut distention in humans. Gastroenterology 108:680–686
15. Miller AD, Rowley HA, Roberts TPL, Kucharczyk J (1996) Human cortical activity during vestibular- and drug-induced nausea detected using MSI. Ann NY Acad Sci 781:670–672
16. Miller AD, Grelot L (1996) The neural basis of nausea and vomiting. In: Yates BJ, Miller AD (eds) Vestibular autonomic regulation. CRC Press, Boca Raton, Florida, pp 85–94
17. Grelot L, Miller AD (1996) In: Miller AD, Bianchi AL, Bishop BP (eds) Neural control of respiratory muscle activation during vomiting. CRC Press, Boca Raton, Florida, pp 239–248
18. Andrews PLR (1992) Physiology of nausea and vomiting. Br J Anaesth 69:2s–19s
19. Ponti F de, Malagelada J-R, Azpiroz F, Yaksh TL, Thomforde GM (1990) Variations in gastric tone associated with duodenal motor events after activation of central emetic mechanisms in the dog. J Gastrointest Mot 2:1–11
20. Lang IM (1990) Digestive tract motor correlates of vomiting and nausea. Can J Physiol Pharmacol 68:242–253
21. Andrews PLR, Bhandari P, Garland S, Bingham S, Davids CJ, Hawthorn J, Davidson HIM, Roylance R, Lane S (1990) Does retching have a function?: an experimental study in the ferret. Pharmacodyn Therap (Life Sci Adv) 9:135–152
22. Fukuda H, Koga T (1993) Hypercapnia and hypoxia which developed during retching participate in the transition from retching to expulsion in dogs. Neurosci Res 17:205–215
23. Koga T, Fukuda H (1990) Characteristic behavior of the respiratory muscles, esophagus, and external anal and urethral sphincters during straining, retching, and vomiting in the decerebrate dog. Jpn J Physiol 40:789–807
24. Lang IM, Sarna SK, Dodds WJ (1993) Pharyngeal, esophageal, and proximal gastric responses associated with vomiting. Am J Physiol 265:G963–G972
25. Koga T, Qu R, Fukuda H (1998) The central pattern generator for vomiting may exist in the reticular area dorsomedial to the retrofacial nucleus in dogs. Exp Brain Res 118:139–147
26. Andrews PLR, Davis CJ, Maskell L (1990) The abdominal visceral innervation and the metic reflex: pathways, pharmacology and plasticity. Can J Physiol Pharmacol 68:325–345
27. Grundy D, Scratcherd T (1989) Sensory afferents from the gastrointestinal tract. In: Wood JD (ed) Handbook of physiology, sect 6. The gastrointestinal system, vol 1. Motility and circulation, part 1. American Physiology Society, Bethesda, Maryland, pp 593–620
28. Minami M, Endo T, Nemoto M, Hamaue N, Hirafuji M, Monama Y, Yajima T, Yoshioka M, Saito H (1995) The physiology of emesis induced by anti-cancer therapy. In: Reynolds DJM, Andrews PLR, Davis CJ (eds) Serotonin and the scientific basis of anti-emetic therapy. Oxford Clin Comm, Oxford, pp 68–83
29. Leslie RA, Reynolds DJM (1992) Functional anatomy of the emetic circuitry in the brainstem. In: Bianchi AL, Grelot L, Miller AD, King GL (eds) Mechanisms and control of emesis. Colloque INSERM/John Libbey Eurotext Ltd:19–27

30. Thompson PI, Bingham S, Andrews PLR, Patel N, Joel SP, Slevin ML (1992) Morphine 6-glucuronide: a metabolite of morphine with greater emetic potency than morphine in the ferret. Br J Pharmacol 106:3–8
31. Koch KL (1993) Motion sickness. In: Sleisenger MH (ed) The handbook of nausea and vomiting. Pathenon, New York, pp 43–60
32. Smith PF, Darlington CL (1996) Recent advances in the pharmacology of the vestibulo-ocular reflex system. TIPS 17:421–427
33. Robinson BW, Mishkin M (1968) Alimentary responses to forebrain stimulation in monkeys. Exp Brain Res 4:330–366
34. Sem-Jacobsen CW (1968) Depth electrographic stimulation of the human brain and behaviour. Thomas, Springfield, Illinois
35. Andrews PLR, Davis CJ (1993) The mechanism of emesis induced by anti-cancer therapies. In: Andrews PLR, Sanger GJ (eds) Emesis in anti-cancer therapy: mechanisms and treatment. Chapman and Hall, London, pp 113–161
36. Lucot JB (1995) 5-HT_{1A} receptor agonists as anti-emetics. In: Reynolds DJM, Andrews PLR, Davis CJ (eds) Serotonin and the scientific basis of anti-emetic therapy. Oxford Clin Comm, Oxford, pp 222–227
37. Rudd JA, Naylor RJ (1995) Opioid receptor involvement in emesis and anti-emesis. In: Reynolds DJM, Andrews PLR, Davis CJ (eds) Serotonin and the scientific basis of anti-emetic therapy. Oxford Clin Comm, Oxford, pp 208–221
38. Zabara J (1992) Neuroinhibition in the regulation of emesis. In: Bianchi AL, Grelot L, Miller AD, King GL (eds) Mechanisms and control of emesis. Colloque INSERM/John Libbey Eurotext Ltd:285–295
39. Hickok JT, Morrow GR, Roscoe JA (1999) Patients' expectations as a mechanism for the development of anticipatory nausea (AN) related to chemotherapy for cancer. Proc ASCO 18:A2287
40. Eden D, Zuk Y (1995) Seasickness as a self-fulfilling prophecy: raising self-efficacy to boost performance at sea. J Appl Psychol 80:628–635
41. Xu LH, Koch KL, Summy-Long J, Stern RM, Seaton JF, Harrison TS, Demers LM, Bingaman S (1993) Hypothalamic and gastric myoelectrical responses during vection- induced nausea in healthy Chinese subjects. Am J Physiol 265:E578–E584
42. D'Acquisto RW, Tyson LB, Gralla RJ et al. (1986) The influence of a chronic high alcohol intake on chemotherapy-induced nausea and vomiting. Proc Am Soc Clin Oncol 5:257
43. Parker RMC, Bentley KR, Barnes NM (1996) Allosteric modulation of 5-HT_3 receptors: focus on alcohols and anaesthetic agents. TIPS 17:95–99
44. Bentley KR, Barnes NM (1998) 5-hydroxytryptamine$_3$ (5-HT_3) receptor-mediated depolarisation of the rat isolated vagus nerve: modulation by trichloroethanol and related alcohols. Eur J Pharmacol 354:25–31
45. Gardner C, Perren M (1998) Inhibition of anaesthetic-induced emesis by a NK_1 or 5-HT_3 receptor antagonist in the house musk shrew, *Suncus murinus*. Neuropharmacology 37:1643–1644
46. Ueno S, Matsuki N, Saito H (1988) *Suncus murinus* as a new experimental model for motion sickness. Life Sci 43:413–420
47. Andrews PLR (1994) 5HT_3 receptor antagonists and anti-emesis. In: King FD, Sanger GJ (eds) 5HT_3 receptor antagonists. CRC Press, Boca Raton, Florida, pp 255–317
48. Costall B, Gunning SJ, Naylor RJ, Tyers MB (1987) The effect of GR38032F, novel 5-HT_3-receptor antagonist on gastric emptying in the guinea-pig. Br J Pharmacol 91:263–264
49. Amemiya N, Hatta S, Ohshika H (1997) Effects of ondansetron on electrically evoked contraction in rat stomach fundus: possible involvement of 5-HT_{2B} receptors. Eur J Pharmacol 339:173–181
50. Fu L-W, O'Neill CA, Longhurst JC (1997) Increased histamine and 5-HT in portal vein plasma and mesenteric lymph during brief ischemia and reperfusion. Am J Physiol 273:H1135–H1141
51. Hillsley K, Grundy D (1998) Sensitivity to 5-hydroxytryptamine in different afferent subpopulations within mesenteric nerves supplying the rat jejunum. J Physiol 509:717–727
52. Fu L-W, Longhurst JC (1998) Role of 5-HT_3 receptors in activation of abdominal sympathetic C fbre afferents during ischaemia in cats. J Physiol 509:729–740
53. Ladabaum U, Koshy SS, Woods ML, Hooper FG, Owyang C, Hasler WL (1998) Differential symptomatic and electrogastrographic effects of distal and proximal human gastric distension. J Physiol 275:G418–G424
54. Wolff MC, Benvenga MJ, Calligaro DO, Fuller RW, Gidda JS, Hemrick-Luecke S, Lucot JB, Nelson DL, Overshiner CD, Leander JD (1997) Pharmacological profile of LY301317, a potent and selective 5-HT_{1A} agonist. Drug Dev Res 40:17–34
55. Cubeddu LX, Alfieri AB, Hoffman IS (1995) Clinical evidence for the involvement of serotonin in acute cytotoxic-induced emesis. In: Reynolds DJM, Andrews PLR, Davis CJ (eds) Serotonin and the scientific basis of anti-emetic therapy. Oxford Clin Comm, Oxford, pp 25–49

56. Watson JW, Gonsalves SF, Fossa AA, McLean S, Seeger T, Obach S, Andrews PLR (1995) The anti-emetic effects of CP-99,994 in the ferret and the dog: role of the NK_1 receptor. Br J Pharmacol 115:84–94
57. Tattersall FD, Rycroft W, Francis B, Pearce D, Merchant K, MacLeod AM, Ladduwahetty T, Keown L, Swain C, Baker R, Cascieri M, Ber E, Metzger J, MacIntyre DE, Hill RG, Hargreaves RJ (1996) Tachykinin NK_1 receptor antagonists act centrally to inhibit emesis induced by the chemotherapeutic agent cisplatin in ferrets. Neuropharmacology 35:1121–1129
58. Fukuda H, Koga T, Furukawa N, Nakamura E, Shiroshita Y (1998) The tachykinin NK_1 receptor antagonist GR205171 prevents vagal stimulation-induced retching but not neuronal transmission from emetic vagal afferents to solitary nucleus neurons in dogs. Brain Res 802:221–231
59. Gesztesi ZS, Song D, White PF (1998) Comparison of a new NK-1 antagonist (CP122,721) to ondansetron in the prevention of postoperative nausea and vomiting. Anesth Analg 86:S32
60. Weiderpass E, Gridley G, Ekbom A, Nyren O, Hjalgrim H, Adami H-O (1997) Use of an NK_1 receptor antagonist to prevent delayed emesis after cisplatin. J Nat Cancer Inst 89:817–818
61. Navari RM, Reinhardt RR, Gralla RJ, Kris MG, Hesketh PJ, Khojasteh A, Kindler H, Grote TH, Pendergrass K, Grunberg SM, Carides AD, Gertz BJ (1999) Reduction of cisplatin-induced emesis by a selective neurokinin-1 receptor antagonist. N Engl J Med 340:190–195
62. Hesketh PJ, Gralla RJ, Webb RT, Ueno W, DelPrete S, Bachinsky ME, Dirlam NL, Stack CB, Silberman SL (1999) Randomized phase II study of the neurokinin 1 receptor antagonist CJ-11,974 in the control of cisplatin-induced emesis. J Clin Oncol 17:338–343
63. Mantyh PW, Rogers SD, Ghilardi JR, Maggio JE, Mantyh CR, Vigna SR (1995) Differential expression of two isoforms of the neurokinin-1 (substance P) receptor in vivo. Brain Res 719:8–13
64. Rudd JA, Jordan CC, Naylor RJ (1996) The action of the NK_1 tachykinin receptor antagonist, CP 99,994 in antagonizing the acute and delayed emesis induced by cisplatin in the ferret. Br J Pharmacol 119:931–936
65. Grelot L, Dapzol J, Esteve E, Frugiere A, Bianchi AL, Sheldrick RLG, Gardner CJ, Ward P (1998) Potent inhibition of both the acute and delayed emetic responses to cisplatin in piglets treated with GR205171, a novel highly selective tachykinin NK_1 receptor antagonist, in ferrets. Eur J Pharmacol 305:181–185
66. Gonsalves S, Watson J, Ashton C (1996) Broad spectrum antiemetic effects of CP-122,721, a tachykinin NK_1 receptor antagonist, in ferrets. Eur J Pharmacol 305:181–185
67. Gardner CJ, Twissell DJ, Dale TJ, Gale JD, Jordan CC, Kilpatrick GH, Bountra C, Ward P (1995) The broad-spectrum anti-emetic activity of the novel non-peptide tachykinin NK_1 receptor antagonist GR203040. Br J Pharmacol 116:3158–3163
68. Singh L, Field MJ, Hughes J, Kuo B-S, Suman-Chauhan N, Tuladhar BR, Wright DS, Naylor RJ (1997) The tachykinin NK_1 receptor antagonist PD 154075 blocks cisplatin-induced delayed emesis in the ferret. Eur J Pharmacol 321:209–216
69. Gardner CJ, Armour DR, Beattie DT, Gale JD, Hawcock AB, Kilpatrick GJ, Twissell DJ, Ward P (1996) GR205171: a novel antagonist with high affinity for the tachykinin NK_1 receptor, and potent broad-spectrum anti-emetic activity. Regul Peptides 65:45–53
70. Tattersall FD, Rycroft W, Marmont N, Cascieri M, Hill RG, Hargreaves RJ (1995) Enantiospecific inhibition of emesis induced by nicotine in the house musk shrew (*Suncus murinus*) by the Neurokinin$_1$ (NK_1) receptor antagonist CP-99,994. Neuropharmacology 34:1697–1699
71. Saito R, Suehiro Y, Ariumi H, Migita K, Hori N, Hashiguchi T, Sakai M, Saeki M, Takano Y, Kamiya H-O (1998) Anti-emetic effects of a novel NK-1 receptor antagonist HSP-117 in ferrets. Neurosci Let 254:169–172
72. Lucot JB, Obach RS, McLean S, Watson JW (1997) The effect of CP-99,994 on the responses to provocative motion in the cat. Br J Pharmacol 120:116–120
73. Chen Y, Saito H, Matsuki N (1997) Ethanol-induced emesis in the house musk shrew, *Suncus murinus*. Life Sci 60:253–261

Prediction of Postoperative Nausea and Vomiting Using Clinical Risk Factors

C. C. Apfel · N. Roewer

Abteilung für Anästhesiologie, Universität Würzburg, Josef-Schneider Strasse 2, 97080 Würzburg, Germany

Introduction

It is generally accepted that emetic sequelae, such as postoperative nausea (PN), postoperative vomiting (PV) and postoperative nausea and vomiting (PONV), are of multifactorial origin (Palazzo and Strunin 1984; Watcha and White 1992; Korttila 1992) and that the incidence of PONV after volatile anesthetics, despite the advances in the past decades, is still between 20 and 30 % (Cohen et al. 1994). Anesthetic factors, such as volatile anesthetics and opioids (Rabey and Smith 1992), the type of surgery (Watcha and White 1992), and patient-related factors (Lerman 1992), are all thought to have a major impact on PONV. Thus, it is assumed that a prediction of PONV is difficult, if not impossible, because PONV is believed to be influenced by too many factors. However, there is now increasing evidence that the risk for emetic sequelae after inhalational anesthesia can be assessed using a risk score derived from a limited number of factors (Palazzo and Evans 1993; Toner et al. 1996; Koivuranta et al. 1997; Apfel et al. 1998b), whereas numerous other risk factors are unimportant. Thus, this chapter reviews the impact of risk factors for PONV and how strongly they can contribute to its prediction.

Risk Factors of PONV

The multifactorial phenomenon of diseases or outcomes is a frequent problem in the medical field and can be handled by multivariate analyses. This is important in developing a risk score, such as the APACHE score, to predict survival in intensive care patients. The reason that such predictive models are effective is that a quantification of the relative impact of a predictor has been performed; thus, it is essential to distinguish the factors with a high predictive power from factors with low or lack of predictive power. Herein are a selection of risk factors with different levels of evidence as indicators to avoid erroneously assumed risk factors which can distort the accuracy of the few risk factors which are clinically really important (see Table 1).

M. K. Herbert et al. (Eds.), Problems of the Gastrointestinal Tract in Anesthesia...

Table 1. Risk factors for postoperative nausea and vomiting (PONV) categorized according to the level of evidence

No, flawed or negative data	Anxiety, personality of the patient, body habitus, pain, movement
Conflicting results	Menstrual cycle, site of operation, experience of the anesthetist, gastric suction, muscle relaxants, type of volatile anesthetic
Mainly positive results	Gender, history of motion sickness or PONV, non-smoking, postoperative opioids, young age, physical status, duration of anesthesia, type of anesthesia (regional vs general)

Assumed Risk Factors with No Data, Insufficient Data, or Negative Results

Numerous risk factors have been mentioned in the literature, but unfortunately no or insufficient data have been published to support their implications. One example is anxiety and psychological factors. Patients with a positive history of PONV have been shown to have an increased risk of developing PONV (Palazzo and Evans 1993; Cohen et al. 1994; Koivuranta et al. 1997; Apfel et al. 1998b). Erroneously, this has been explained by conditioning (Bardenheuer and Traut 1997), although there is no study to support this hypothesis, and a more likely explanation is the individual predisposition regardless of previous operations. Furthermore, it has been concluded that "psychological factors and experiences of the patient play a major role" (Bardenheuer and Traut 1997), and a reference has been quoted to support this hypothesis, which, in contrast, is "not in favor with this view" (Palazzo and Strunin 1984). Because "preoperative anxiety is believed to delay gastric motility (and emptying) and increase gastric fluid volume, possibly via increased circulation stress hormones" and those "hormones have been shown to induce emesis when instilled into the ventricles of cats" (Lerman 1992), preoperative anxiety may contribute to PONV, although its importance has not been established (Lerman 1992). We have investigated the impact of preoperative anxiety on PONV using Spielberger's State Trait Anxiety Inventory test on the day before the operation. Our preliminary data did not demonstrate any effect of anxiety on PONV (Lengler et al. 1998); thus, anxiety can currently not be regarded as a risk factor for PONV.

A positive correlation between body weight and postoperative emesis has been described by Smessaert (1959), whereas data of other studies at that time did not show any correlation (Burtles and Peckett 1957; Bellville et al. 1960). However, the explanation that adipose tissue acts as a reservoir for inhaled anesthetic agents from which they continue to enter the blood stream even after their administration has been discontinued was so convincing that this is still frequently quoted in reviews (Watcha and White 1992; Palazzo and Strunin 1984), although recent large prospective studies were unable to identify the body mass index as a significant risk factor (Muir et al. 1987; Cohen et al. 1994; Koivuranta et al. 1997; Apfel et al. 1998b,c). In this case it is not only a lack of evidence but evidence for a lack of effect, i.e., that there is evidence that the body habitus has no effect on the incidence of PONV.

Assumed Risk Factors with Conflicting Data

Female gender is known to be a risk factor for PONV (Bellville et al. 1959; Lerman 1992; Palazzo and Evans 1993; Koivuranta et al. 1997; Apfel et al. 1998b). One study reported that the incidence of PONV decreases after the seventh decade to the level of male patients (Purkis 1964), and it was hypothesized that this may be associated with the levels of gonadotropins (Bellville et al. 1960). In addition, an increased incidence of PONV was reported during the third or fourth week of the cycle (Bellville et al. 1960; Bellville 1961), and in animal models estrogen has been shown to increase the number of striatal dopamine receptors (Hruska and Silbergeld 1980). Because dopamine receptors play a major role in vomiting, this could be a biological basis for a relationship between hormonal changes and differences in the incidence of PONV in females. A retrospective analysis by Beattie et al. (1991) reported an increased incidence during menstruation which was confirmed in a subsequent prospective study by the same group (Beattie et al. 1993). In contrast, Honkavaara et al. (1991) confirmed the findings of Bellville et al. (1961) that the incidence of PONV is increased in the luteal phase (days 20–24). To confuse matters even further, Ramsay et al. (1994) published a prospective study to show that the periovulatory phase (days 9–15) was associated with the highest incidence. Thus, every phase of the menstrual cycle has been reported to be associated with a significantly increased incidence of PONV. Only recently, analyses of the menstrual cycle were not able to demonstrate a significant impact (Gratz et al. 1996) which is in accordance with our data of a prospective survey (Goepfert et al. 1997) and data of a randomized controlled trial (Goepfert et al. 1998); thus, the menstrual cycle cannot be regarded as a risk factor for PONV.

Certain types of surgical procedures are reported to be associated with a relatively high incidence of PONV (Andrews 1992). Those observations stem from two studies (Bonica et al. 1958; Bellville et al. 1960) in which intraabdominal surgery was reported to be associated with a higher incidence than extraabdominal surgery. Approximately 30 years later, Andrews et al. (1990) were able to identify the pathophysiological and pharmacological role of the abdominal visceral innervation for the emetic reflex; thus, abdominal surgery was assumed to be a causal risk factor for PONV (Andrews 1992). However, this is not supported by clinical data as much as it may seem. In the paper by Bonica et al. (1958) the five agents used for general anesthesia ranged in their incidence of PV between 8.3 % (thiopentone alone) and 64.2 % (ether). It is therefore conceivable that Bonica et al. (1958) wrote, "Our data suggest that inhalation anesthesia is very important, if not the most important factor". Since the anesthetic agent was not stratified throughout the operations, it is possible that the different incidences were due mainly to the anesthetic agent. This might explain the reason that Bonica et al. (1958) also wrote, "It is difficult to assign the proper role played by each of these factors in influencing the rate of these unpleasant complications". This careful interpretation appears appropriate especially in view of the data of Burtles and Peckett (1957). They reported an incidence of PV of 25 and 28 % after intra- and extraabdominal surgery and concluded that "age, sex, and duration are important", and that "the site of operation is not so important as its duration" which was entirely in accordance with previous reports (Knapp and Beecher 1956; Smessaert et al. 1959). In view of these circumstances Bellville (1961) wrote, "These results indicate that differences in technique or agents may account for the diversity and that the problem (impact of the operation itself) is not solved" which may also explain why his subsequent paper was entitled "Postanesthetic nausea and vomiting" instead of the title given 1 year previously: "Postoperative nausea and vomiting" (Bellville et al. 1960). However, the appropriate statistical method to distinguish the relative impact of anesthetic and surgical factors would have been a multivariate analysis which was not available at that time. Such analyses were applied by Cohen et al. (1994) and especially the surgical type "digestive" turned out to be not significant for postoperative nausea (relative odds 0.89; 95 % CI: 0.74, 1.06). This is in accordance with the results of our study in which intraabdominal surgery was associated with a moderate incidence of 24 % (Apfel et al. 1998c). Thus, according to previous and recent data, it is unlikely that intraabdominal surgical site can be regarded as a risk factor for PONV or PV.

Another example is the incidence of PONV after strabismus surgery, which is reported to be between 40 and 88 % (Lerman 1992). This is not surprising since most strabismus operations are performed in children. Again, a pathophysiological model was developed by van den Berg et al. (1989) assuming an "oculoemetic reflex". They reported that retrospective analysis of patients undergoing strabismus surgery showed no decreased incidence in adults as it used to be for other types of operations. However, the number of analyzed adults was low ($n < 20$) questioning the validity of the conclusion. In addition, a prospective randomized trial focusing on adults undergoing strabismus surgery revealed a low incidence of PONV (Tramer et al. 1997), which is in accordance with the results of our multivariate analysis showing only a minor and negligible effect on the incidence of PV (Apfel et al. 1998c). Thus, according to recent data, it is unlikely that strabismus surgery can be regarded as a clinically relevant risk factor for PONV or PV.

Bearing these examples in mind, it appears that as soon as a risk factor is assumed this will gain wide acceptance if a pathophysiological mechanism is found, even if there are more strong data to refute the hypothesis.

Risk Factors with a Sufficient Body of Evidence

There a basically three risk factors for PONV which constantly appear to have a major impact. These factors are female gender (Fig. 1; Burtles and Peckett 1957; Bellville et al. 1959; Palazzo and Strunin 1984; Lerman 1992; Palazzo and Evans 1993; Cohen et al. 1994; Koivuranta et al. 1997; Apfel et al. 1998b,c), a history of motion sickness, or previous PONV (Fig. 2; Burtles and Peckett 1957; Palazzo and Strunin 1984; Lerman 1992; Palazzo and Evans 1993; Cohen et al. 1994; Koivuranta et al. 1997; Apfel et al. 1998b,c) and the use of postoperative opioids (Palazzo and Strunin 1984; Lerman

Fig. 1. **a** Incidences of postoperative vomiting (PV) over 24 h according to age and gender. Data according to Burtles and Peckett (1957). **b** Incidences of PV over 2.5 h according to age and gender. Data according to Bellville et al. (1960). Note that the observation period was much shorter and thus the incidences were much lower as compared with Burtles and Peckett (1957). **c** Incidences of postoperative vomiting over 24 h after inhalational anesthesia according to age and gender (after Apfel et al. 1998a). Note that the incidences are similar compared with Burtles and Peckett (1957)

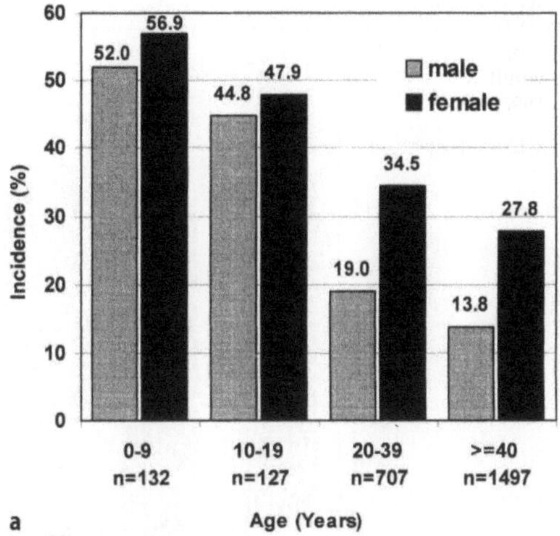

Incidence (%)
male
female
52.0
56.9
44.8
47.9
19.0
34.5
13.8
27.8
0-9 n=132
10-19 n=127
20-39 n=707
>=40 n=1497
Age (Years)

a

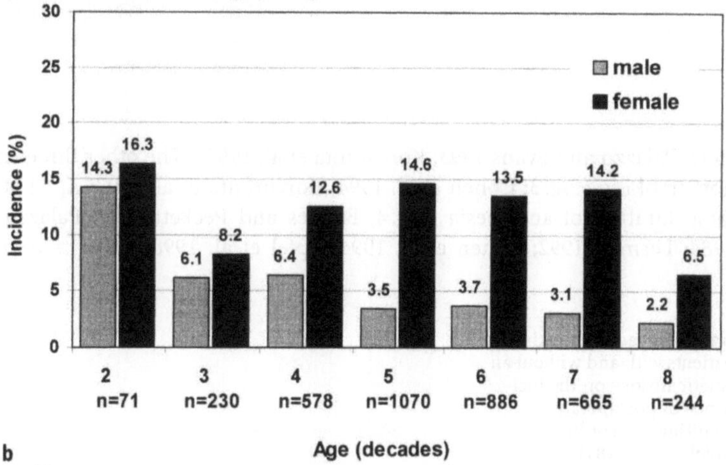

Incidence (%)
male
female
14.3
16.3
6.1
8.2
6.4
12.6
3.5
14.6
3.7
13.5
3.1
14.2
2.2
6.5
2 n=71
3 n=230
4 n=578
5 n=1070
6 n=886
7 n=665
8 n=244
Age (decades)

b

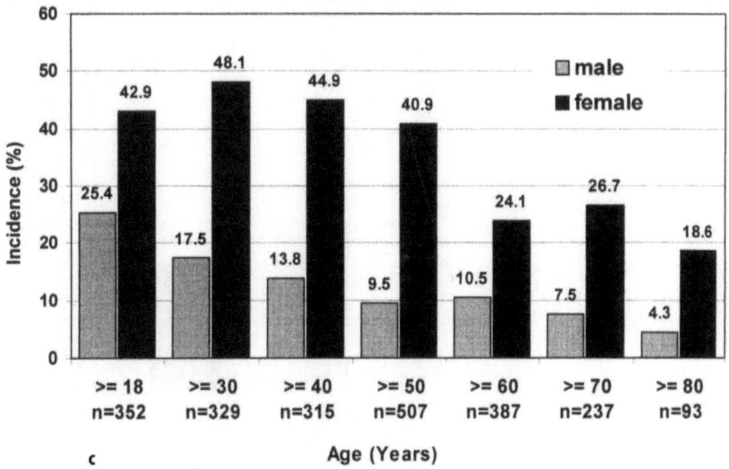

Incidence (%)
male
female
25.4
42.9
17.5
48.1
13.8
44.9
9.5
40.9
10.5
24.1
7.5
26.7
4.3
18.6
>= 18 n=352
>= 30 n=329
>= 40 n=315
>= 50 n=507
>= 60 n=387
>= 70 n=237
>= 80 n=93
Age (Years)

c

Fig. 2. Impact of the patient's history of postoperative nausea and vomiting (PONV) or motion sickness on the incidence of postoperative vomiting. (According to Apfel et al. 1998a)

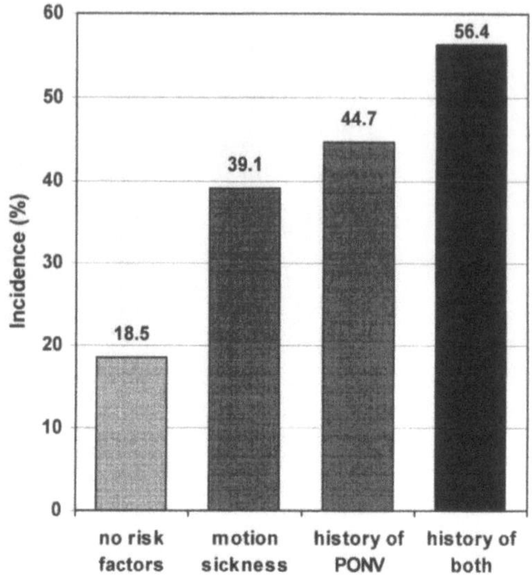

1992; Palazzo and Evans 1993; Koivuranta et al. 1997). The other three risk factors are non-smoking (Fig. 3; Cohen et al. 1994; Koivuranta et al. 1997; Apfel et al. 1998b), a long duration of anesthesia (Fig. 4; Burtles and Peckett 1957; Palazzo and Strunin 1984; Lerman 1992; Cohen et al. 1994; Apfel et al. 1998b), and a young age of the

Fig. 3. Impact of smoking in patients with and without an emetic history on the incidence of postoperative vomiting. (According to Apfel et al. 1998a)

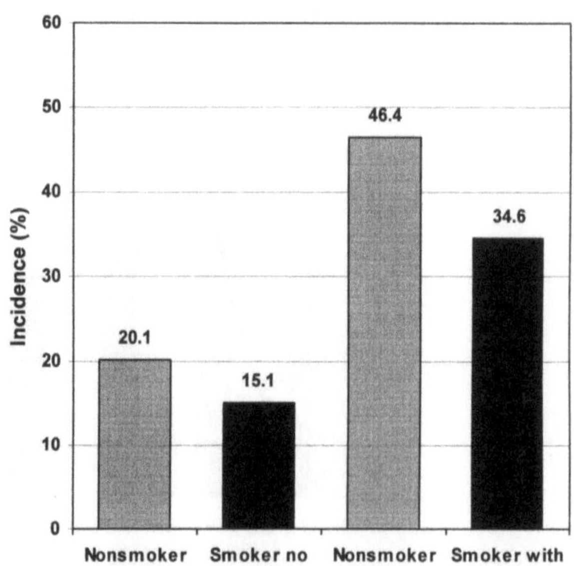

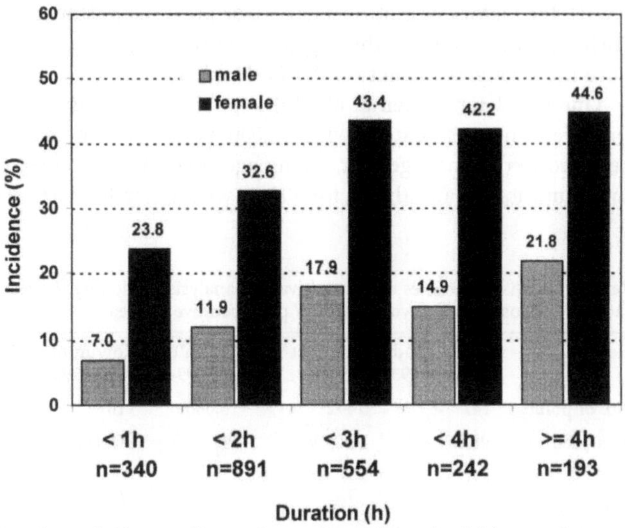

Fig. 4. Impact of the duration of anesthesia according to the gender of the patient's history of postoperative nausea and vomiting or motion sickness on the incidence of postoperative vomiting. (According to Apfel et al. 1998a)

patient (Fig. 1; Burtles and Peckett 1957; Palazzo and Strunin 1984; Lerman 1992; Cohen et al. 1994; Apfel et al. 1998b,c). Those factors have been shown to have some impact in multivariate analyses and are therefore clinically relevant even if corrected for the other factors (Cohen et al. 1994; Koivuranta et al. 1997; Apfel et al. 1998b).

Prediction of PONV Using Clinically Most Relevant Risk Factors

The identification of primary risk factors requires the use of multivariate models to quantify their relative impact in the presence of other risk factors. Therefore, only studies which used multiple logistical regression analysis to account for the relative impact of the factors included in the model could be considered.

In 1993 Palazzo and Evans were the first to apply a multivariate method to 147 patients in a well-controlled setting to assess the impact of patient-related factors on PONV (Palazzo and Evans 1993). They were able to identify female gender, a history of PONV, a history of motion sickness, and postoperative opioids as significant risk factors, and they used the coefficients to develop a risk table for PONV. The study was restricted to minor orthopedic surgery so that a potential relative impact of the operation could not be calculated (Table 2).

A few months later, a metaanalysis of factors affecting the incidence of nausea and vomiting after gynecological surgery was published in the same journal (Haigh et al. 1993). This study by Haigh et al. revealed that the most important factors for PONV were the antiemetics given (ondansetron 1, 8, or 16 mg), the type of operation and the neuromuscular blocking agents. Unfortunately, the analysis did not consider previously established risk factors such as female gender (because only females were analyzed), the history of motion sickness or previous postoperative nausea and vomiting (Bellville et al. 1959) or the length of anesthesia, so that ondansetron turned out to have the strongest impact on PONV (Table 2).

One year later, Cohen et al. (1994) published a study focusing on a postoperative interview in four centers with 16,000 patients. The main risk factors that were revealed were female gender, young age, a good physical status, non-smoking, and a long duration of anesthesia for PN as well as for PV (separate analyses). They also

Table 2. Published articles using multivariate analysis to identify the relative impact of assumed risk factors. *PV* postoperative vomiting; *PN* postoperative nausea

Reference	Pallazo and Evans (1993)	Haigh et al. (1993)	Cohen et al. (1994)	Koivuranta et al. (1997)	Apfel et al. (1998a)	Apfel et al. (1998b)
No. of points	147	1442	16,000	1107	553 and 584	542 and 549
Analyzed sequelae	PONV	PN/PV	PN	PONV/PV	PV	PV
Age	–	–/–	+	–/–	+	+
Female gender	+		+	+/+	+	+
Previous PONV	+			+/+	+	+
Motion sickness	+			+/+	+	+
Smoking			+	+/+	+	–
Weight/body mass index	–	–/–	–	–/–	–	–
Duration	–	+/–	+	+/+	+	–
Premedication		+/–				
General vs regional			+	+/+		
Volatile anesthetic		–/–			–	–
N-methyl-D-aspartate		+/+			–	–
Reversal drugs		–/+				
Postoperative opioids	+	+/–		+/–	–	–
Operation		+/+	+/–	–/–	–	+
Center/ country		+/+	+			–
Comments	Interaction of gender and previous sickness history	Important predictors (gender, smoking, PONV) are missing	Antiemetics were not recorded	Operation was not included in the multivariate analyses	For reasons of future comparability only PV was analyzed	A previously developed score predicted PV despite different risk structure

identified marked variations in the incidence of emetic sequelae across hospitals which was assigned as a "center effect". However, this may be caused by a more or less frequent use of prophylactic antiemetics, which regrettably were not recorded in the study (Table 2).

In 1996 the risk table developed by Palazzo and Evans (1993) was applied to 400 patients with different operations by a simple calibration curve of predicted and actual incidences of PONV and creation of 16 risk groups (Toner et al. 1996). It was demonstrated that the previously developed risk table may well be applicable to another hospital. Thus, it is likely that the previously described risk factors are important predictors also in other centers, and that a possible "center effect" is most likely not to be clinically relevant. Unfortunately, a multivariate recalculation was not performed which had been interesting in comparing the significance of previously described risk factors.

This has been done by Koivuranta et al. (1997) who identified female gender, non-smoking, a history of PONV, a history of motion sickness, and a long duration of anesthesia as risk factors for PV and PONV. In addition, the statistician E. Läärä of this group created a very useful and simplified risk score for PONV. Instead of using the regression coefficients of the risk factors to calculate the probability of PONV, he simply counted the number of the four most important dichotomized risk factors and a discriminating power similar to the exact method using the coefficients was reported (Table 2).

Simultaneously, another group undertook a large prospective survey in more than 1137 elective patients undergoing otolaryngological procedures (Apfel et al. 1997, 1998b). Again, patient-related factors and the duration of anesthesia were most important for the prediction of PV. In contrast to previous investigations, the type of operation was considered in the multivariate model and interestingly found to be of little importance (Apfel et al. 1998b) so that an operation-independent risk probability could be calculated using the coefficients of a logistical equation

$$\text{risk (probability of PV)} = \frac{1}{1 + e^{-z}}$$

where z = 1.28*(female gender)-0.029*(age)-0.74*(smoking) +0.63*(history of motion sickness or PONV)+0.26*(duration)-0.92, when the variables are coded as follows: gender (male = 0, female = 1), age (in years), smoking status (no = 0, yes = 1), history of motion sickness and/or PONV (no = 0, yes = 1), and duration of anesthesia (in hours).

In addition, in a consecutive study in patients undergoing general surgery, orthopedic surgery, vascular surgery and squint surgery an almost perfect calibration (Fig. 5) and a moderate discriminating power (Fig. 6) of the previously developed risk score between vomiters and non-vomiters (Apfel et al. 1998c) was demonstrated.

Thus, the developed score may be useful for the prediction of PV in patients undergoing other types of surgery, possibly because the type of operation is only a secondary but not primary risk factor for PV. A great advantage of that score is that the exact probability of PV can be calculated with the logistical equation. To ease the clinical applicability a risk table for male and female patients has been published (Apfel et al. 1998a) and is available as a "risk ruler" from the authors or Novartis Pharma.

Fig. 5. Calibration curve of predicted and actual incidence of postoperative vomiting. (According to Apfel et al. 1998a)

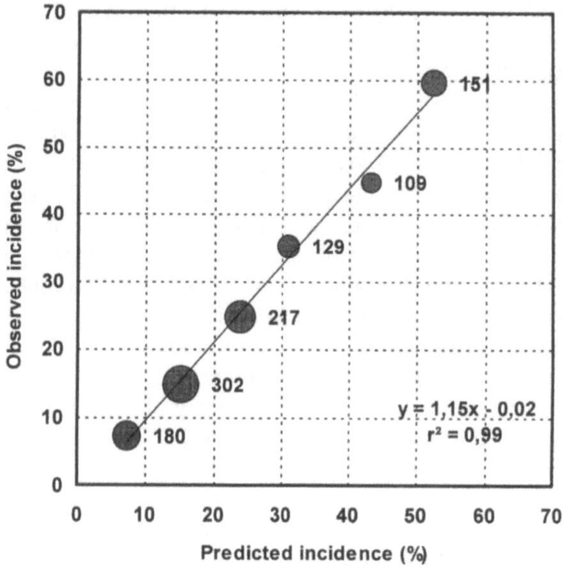

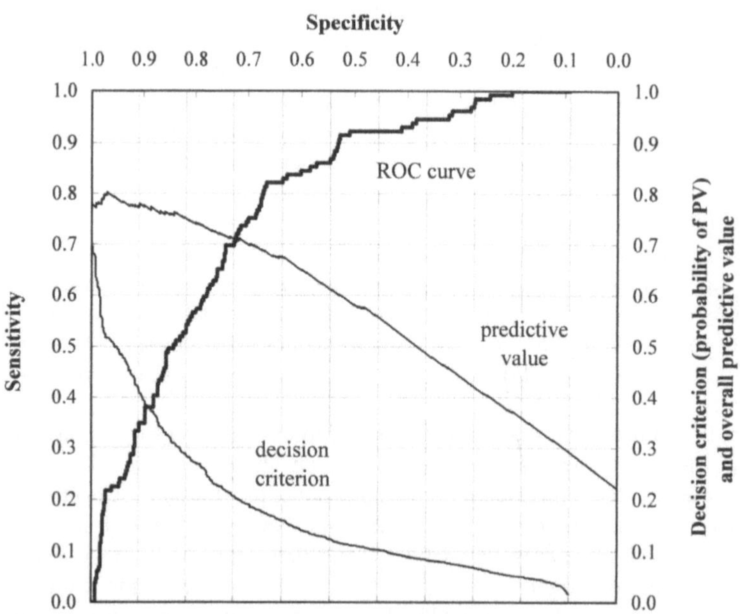

Fig. 6. A receiver-operating-characteristics curve with corresponding curves for the decision criterion and the overall predictive value. (According to Apfel et al. 1998b)

Table 3. Risk table for postoperative vomiting in percent depending on gender, age, patient history, smoking status, and duration of anesthesia. (According to Apfel et al. 1998c)

	No anamnestic emetic sequelae								With anamnestic emetic sequelae							
	Non-smoker				Smoker				Non-smoker				Smoker			
Male patients																
Duration (h)	1	2	3	4	1	2	3	4	1	2	3	4	1	2	3	4
Age (years)																
20	22	27	33	39	12	15	19	23	35	41	48	54	21	25	30	36
30	18	22	27	32	9	12	15	18	29	35	41	47	16	20	25	30
40	14	17	21	26	7	9	12	14	23	28	34	40	13	16	20	24
50	11	14	17	21	5	7	9	11	19	23	28	33	10	12	15	19
60	8	11	13	17	4	5	7	9	15	18	22	27	8	10	12	15
70	6	8	10	13	3	4	5	7	11	14	18	22	6	7	9	12
80	5	6	8	10	2	3	4	5	9	11	14	17	4	6	7	9
Female patients																
Duration (h)	1	2	3	4	1	2	3	4	1	2	3	4	1	2	3	4
Age (years)																
20	51	57	64	69	33	39	46	52	66	72	77	81	48	55	61	67
30	44	50	57	63	27	33	38	45	59	65	71	76	41	48	54	60
40	37	43	50	56	22	27	32	38	52	59	65	70	34	40	47	53
50	30	36	42	49	17	21	26	31	45	51	58	64	28	34	40	46
60	25	30	35	42	13	17	21	25	38	44	51	57	23	27	33	39
70	20	24	29	35	10	13	16	20	31	37	44	50	18	22	27	32
80	15	19	24	28	8	10	13	16	26	31	37	43	14	18	22	26

To evaluate the applicability of risk scores (see Table 3), two centers (Würzburg, Germany, and Oulu, Finland) decided to recalculate their data and to perform a "cross validation" to answer the following questions:

1. To what extent are the risk scores specific for their centers and are they applicable to a different center?
2. Can regression-based risk scores be simplified without loss of accuracy?
3. How strong is a possible center effect in a combined data set?
4. What could be the clinical consequences?

Logistical regression analyses were performed to set up risk scores for each center and for a combined data set. The discriminating power was assessed with the area under the receiver-operating-characteristics curves. The risk scores were valid for predicting PONV in patients in each center. A simplification of the scores based on equally weighted risk factors did not affect its accuracy. Although the raw data of the centers were different, the center itself did not affect the PONV in a combined data set if corrected for the relevant predictors. The final score considered four equally weighted predictors: female gender, history of motion sickness and/or PONV, non-smoking, and the use of postoperative opioids. It can therefore be concluded that the probability of PONV can accurately be estimated using a risk score, even from a different center. As the final score may have more general applicability, we recommend avoiding volatile anesthetics if two or more risk factors are present, because this will be associated with a risk of more than 30 %.

Conclusion

The risk of PV can be predicted using a risk score based on age, gender, history of previous PONV or motion sickness, non-smoking, and the duration of anesthesia (Apfel et al. 1998b) which has been proven to be applicable to a wide variety of operations (Apfel et al. 1998c). In addition, use of postoperative opioids might increase the incidence of PONV (Koivuranta et al. 1997). For all other risk factors which are claimed to be important, there is no sufficient evidence for their clinical relevance.

References

Andrews PLR (1992) Physiology of nausea and vomiting. Br J Anaesth 69:2S–19S

Andrews PL, Davis CJ, Bingham S, Davidson HI, Hawthorn J, Maskell L (1990) The abdominal visceral innervation and the emetic reflex: pathways, pharmacology, and plasticity. Can J Physiol Pharmacol 68:325–345

Apfel CC, Goepfert C, Sefrin P, Roewer N (1997) A risk score for the prediction of postoperative vomiting. Br J Anaesth 78:1–2

Apfel CC, Greim CA, Goepfert C, Grundt D, Usadel J, Sefrin P, Roewer N (1998a) Postoperatives Erbrechen. Ein Score zur Voraussage der Erbrechenswahrscheinlichkeit nach Inhalationsanaesthesien. Anaesthesist 47:732–740

Apfel CC, Greim CA, Haubitz I, Goepfert C, Usadel J, Sefrin P, Roewer N (1998b) A risk score to predict the probability of postoperative vomiting in adults. Acta Anaesthesiol Scand 42:495–501

Apfel CC, Greim CA, Haubitz I, Grundt D, Goepfert C, Sefrin P, Roewer N (1998c) The discriminating power of a risk score to predict postoperative vomiting in adults undergoing various types of surgery. Acta Anaesthesiol Scand 42:502–509

Bardenheuer HJ, Traut F (1997) Inzidenz und Pathophysiologie der postoperativen Übelkeit und des Erbrechens. Anästhesiol Intensivmed Notfallmed Schmerzther 32:617–619

Beattie WS, Lindblad T, Buckley DN, Forrest JB (1991) The incidence of postoperative nausea and vomiting in women undergoing laparoscopy is influenced by the day of menstrual cycle. Can J Anaesth 38:298–302

Beattie WS, Lindblad T, Buckley DN, Forrest JB (1993) Menstruation increases the risk of nausea and vomiting after laparoscopy. A prospective randomized study. Anesthesiology 78:272–276

Bellville JW (1961) Postanesthetic nausea and vomiting. Anesthesiology 22:773–780

Bellville JW, Bross IDJ, Howland WS (1959) A method of the clinical evaluation of antiemetic agents. Anesthesiology 20:753–760

Bellville JW, Bross IDJ, Howland S (1960) Postoperative nausea and vomiting IV: factors related to postoperative nausea and vomiting. Anesthesiology 21:186–193

Bonica JJ, Crepps W, Monk B (1958) Postoperative nausea, retching and vomiting. Anesthesiology 19:532–540

Burtles R, Peckett BW (1957) Postoperative vomiting: some factors affecting its incidence. Br J Anaesth 29:114–123

Cohen MM, Duncan PG, DeBoer DP, Tweed WA (1994) The postoperative interview: assessing risk factors for nausea and vomiting. Anesth Analg 78:7–16

Goepfert C, Apfel CC, Usadel J, Sefrin P, Roewer N (1997) Einfluss des Menstruationszyklus auf das postoperative Erbrechen in einer Evaluationsstudie. Anästhesiol Intensivmed Notfallmed Schmerzther 32:S128

Goepfert C, Apfel CC, Kranke P, Rauch S, Papenfuss T, Sefrin P, Roewer N (1998) Had der Menstruationszyklus wirklich einen Einfluss auf das postoperative Erbrechen? Anästhesiol Intensivmed Notfallmed Schmerzther 33:S166

Gratz I, Allen E, Afshar M, Joslyn AF, Buxbaum J, Prilliman B (1996) The effects of the menstrual cycle on the incidence of emesis and efficacy of ondansetron. Anesth Analg 83:565–569

Haigh CG, Kaplan LA, Durham JM, Dupeyron JP, Harmer M, Kenny GN (1993) Nausea and vomiting after gynaecological surgery: a meta-analysis of factors affecting their incidence. Br J Anaesth 71:517–522

Honkavaara P, Lehtinen AM, Hovorka J, Korttila K (1991) Nausea and vomiting after gynaecological laparoscopy depends upon the phase of the menstrual cycle. Can J Anaesth 38:876–879

Hruska RE, Silbergeld EK (1980) Increased dopamine receptor sensitivity after estrogen treatment using rat rotation model. Science 208:1466–1468

Knapp MR, Beecher HK (1956) Postanesthetic nausea, vomiting and retching. J Am Med Assoc 160:376–385
Koivuranta M, Läärä E, Snare L, Alahuhta S (1997) A survey of postoperative nausea and vomiting. Anaesthesia 52:443–449
Korttila K (1992) The study of postoperative nausea and vomiting. Br J Anaesth 69: 20S–23S
Lengler R, Apfel CC, Schäfers B, Sefrin P, Roewer N (1998) Hat präoperative Angst einen Einfluss auf postoperative Übelkeit und Erbrechen. Anästhesiol Intensivmed Notfallmed Schmerzther 33:S268
Lerman J (1992) Surgical and patient factors involved in postoperative nausea and vomiting. Br J Anaesth 69:24S–32S
Muir JJ, Warner MA, Offord KP, Buck CF, Harper JV, Kunkel SE (1987) Role of nitrous oxide and other factors in postoperative nausea and vomiting: a randomized and blinded prospective study. Anesthesiology 66:513–518
Palazzo M, Evans R (1993) Logistic regression analysis of fixed patient factors for postoperative sickness: a model for risk assessment. Br J Anaesth 70:135–140
Palazzo MG, Strunin L (1984) Anaesthesia and emesis. I. Etiology. Can Anaesth Soc J 31:178–187
Purkis IE (1964) Factors that influence postoperative vomiting. Can Anaesth Soc J 11:335–353
Rabey PG, Smith G (1992) Anaesthetic factors contributing to postoperative nausea and vomiting. Br J Anaesth 69:40S–45S
Ramsay TM, Mcdonald PF, Faragher EB (1994) The menstrual cycle and nausea or vomiting after wisdom teeth extraction. Can J Anaesth 41:798–801
Smessaert A, Schehr CA, Artusio JF (1959) Nausea and vomiting in the immediate postanesthetic period. J Am Med Assoc 170:2072–2076
Toner CC, Broomhead CJ, Littlejohn IH, Samra GS, Powney JG, Palazzo MGA, Evans SJW, Strunin L (1996) Prediction of postoperative nausea and vomiting using a logistic regression model. Br J Anaesth 76:347–351
Tramer M, Fuchs-Buder T, Sansonetti A, Rifat K (1997) Low incidence of the oculocardiac reflex and postoperative nausea and vomiting in adults undergoing strabismus surgery. Can J Anaesth 44:830–835
Van den Berg AA, Lambourne A, Clyburn PA (1989) The oculo-emetic reflex. A rationalisation of postophthalmic anaesthesia vomiting. Anaesthesia 44:110–117
Watcha MF, White PF (1992) Postoperative nausea and vomiting. Its etiology, treatment, and prevention. Anesthesiology 77:162–184

Logistical Regression Analysis of Factors Causing Postoperative Nausea or Vomiting During Different Postoperative Time Periods

T. Schröder · Ch. v. Heymann · R. Scherer · W. J. Kox

Klinik für Anästhesiologie und Intensivmedizin, Universitätsklinikum Charité Berlin,
Campus Charité Mitte, 10098-Berlin, Germany

Introduction

Postoperative nausea and vomiting (PONV) has been researched for 150 years. John Snow published in 1848 a study on this side effect of narcotism by the inhalation of vapor [12]. At the end of the twentieth century PONV remains the "big little problem" of anesthesia [5], although anesthetists are aware of the importance of PONV for patient comfort and the great number of studies that have been published. In the period from 1987 to 1997 *Anesthesia* and the *British Journal of Anesthesia* published 216 articles dealing with postoperative nausea and vomiting, i.e., 2.4 % of all articles; nevertheless, the incidence of PONV continues to be unacceptably high.

The difficulties lie in the variety of factors influencing the occurrence of postoperative nausea and vomiting. This led Palazzo and Evans [10] to the conclusion that, although most studies controlled factors regarding the anesthetic technique, they usually failed to establish strictly matched patient groups. They recommended the use of a logistical regression analysis to classify patients with the same risk for PONV.

Patients and Methods

We studied 483 patients receiving a general anesthesia for surgical procedures in different specialties. In a standardized questionnaire we collected data from the patient's history, the surgical procedure, the anesthetic technique, the use of antiemetics, and the absence or occurrence of postoperative nausea or vomiting. The applied anesthetic was not given by a study protocol but reflected the department's standard, which allowed individual variations of the procedure.

We included patients of all ages scheduled for an operation, after which an extubation in the operating room was made possible. All patients who required postoperative ventilator therapy and all emergency cases were excluded from our investigation.

Postoperative nausea was specified as no nausea, nausea without retching, and retching or vomiting, which were observed during three consecutive postoperative time periods: (a) stay at the postanesthesia care unit (PACU); (b) after discharge from PACU up to 6 h postoperatively; and (c) from 6 to 24 h postoperatively.

The collection of data was documented in a standardized questionnaire and based on the patient history, anesthetic protocol, a postoperative interview of the patient and a review of the nurse's records on the ward.

M. K. Herbert et al. (Eds.), Problems of the
Gastrointestinal Tract in Anesthesia...

Statistical analysis was done with the software package SPSS, version 6.01. For testing of statistical significance we subjected the nominal data to Student's *t*-test and categorical data to the chi-square test. Significance of results was assumed at $p < 0.05$.

Modelling the odds of PONV by means of a logistical regression was used for the analysis of the relation between risk factors and PONV:

$$P = 1/1+e^{-g(x)} \quad (1)$$

$$g(x) = \beta_1 x_1 + ... + \beta_n x_n, \quad (2)$$

where P = probability of PONV, $\beta_{(1...n)}$ = regression coefficients and $x_{(1...n)}$ = risk factors.

Tests of the hypothesis that a particular model fits the observed data were made using stepwise backward selection of the independent variables based on log-likelihood ratio criterion. Removing proceeded until no variable passed the threshold ($p > 0.1$) and then selection of variables proceeded until the log-likelihood changed less than 0.01 %.

In terms of the model equation, each risk factor weighted by the regression coefficient β contributed to the log odds of PONV. Consequently, the risk factor with the largest regression coefficient implied the greatest increase in the odds of PONV.

Results

Of 23 tested variables, 16 (Table 1) showed a significant influence on the incidence of PONV during the overall 24-h observation period or during one of the three separate time periods studied.

Table 1. Significant variables for the incidence of PONV

Variables	PACU	Up to 6 h	6–24 h	Overall 24 h
High age		↓ *		↓ *
Female	↑ **		↑ **	↑ **
Motion sickness/PONV		↑ **		↑ *
Renal failure	↑ *			
Diabetes mellitus		↑ *		
Laryngeal mask		↓ *	↓ *	
Duration of anesthesia		↑ *		↑ *
Etomidate for induction				↑ *
Intravenous anesthesia with propofol				↓ *
Nitrous oxide	↑ *			
Muscle relaxant antagonism	↑ *			
Antiemetic medication		↓ *		↓ *
Gynecological surgery		↑ **		
Postoperative opioids	↓ **		↑ **	
Eye surgery				↑ *
Tramadol			↑ **	

*$p < 0.05$; **$p < 0.01$

Risk Factors of PONV During the Stay at the PACU

For the time period until discharge from the PACU we found renal failure, the inhalation of nitrous oxide, the female gender, and the use of pyridostigmine for reversal of a neuromuscular block to increase the risk for PONV significantly. The p-values for these factors were $p< 0.05$ and $p< 0.01$ for female gender, respectively. The application of intravenous opioids in the PACU reduced the risk of PONV ($p< 0.01$).

Risk Factors of PONV up to 6 h Postoperatively

Motion sickness or PONV in the patient history, gynecological surgery ($p< 0.01$), as well as diabetes mellitus and the duration of anesthesia ($p< 0.05$) were significant proemetic factors. A lower incidence of PONV was associated with high age, an intraoperative antiemetic, and the use of a laryngeal mask airway compared with an orotracheal intubation ($p< 0.05$).

Risk Factors of PONV from 6 h to 24 h Postoperatively

The risk of PONV was elevated by female gender, intravenous administration of opioids, and tramadol postoperatively ($p< 0.01$). The incidence of PONV was reduced by the use of a laryngeal mask airway relative to an orotracheal intubation ($p< 0.05$).

Risk Factors of PONV During the 24-h Observation Period

Motion sickness and PONV in the patient history, duration of anesthesia, eye surgery, the use of etomidate for induction of anesthesia ($p< 0.05$) as well as female gender ($p< 0.01$) increased the probability of PONV. A lower risk of PONV was predicted by a high age, an intraoperative antiemetic and a propofol-maintained anesthesia ($p< 0.05$).

Regression Coefficients and Calculated Models

The logistical regression facilitates a quantitative estimation of each relevant risk factor. The impact of the individual factors can be compared by a regression coefficient β: factors with a negative calculated β reduced and a positive β increased the risk of PONV.

Table 2 shows the models for the prediction of PONV using the calculated regression coefficients β. The individual risk for PONV can be estimated by using Eqs. (1) and (2) as shown by the following example:

A 24-year-old female is scheduled for a minor gynecological operation of 30-min duration. Anesthesia is maintained by an inhalational technique using a laryngeal mask airway. The risk score for PONV in the time period up to 6 h postoperatively would be 0.15, i.e., the probability to experience nausea or vomiting is 15 %. Using an orotracheal intubation the risk would be increased to 38 %.

Table 2. Models calculated by stepwise logistical regression

	Model	Model chi-square
Total	g(x) = −1.0156−0.0138 * (age)−0.5322 (antiemetic prophylaxis) +0.6579 (motion sickness/PONV in history taking)+0.0042·(duration)+0.2575 (thiopental)+0.8105 (hypnomidate)−0.5807 (propofol maintenance)+0.7380 (eye surgery)+1.1309 (female)−1.2504 (LAMA)	$p < 0.001$
PACU	g(x) = −1.5950−1.1708 (postoperative opioids)+1.6732 (renal failure)+0.7428 (pyridostigmine)+1.4731 (nitrous oxide)+1.6533 (female)−7.8412 (LAMA)	$p < 0.001$
Up to 6 h	g(x) = −1.1088−0.0135·(age)−0.5307 (antiemetic prophylaxis)+1.1977 (motion sickness/PONV in history taking) +1.0199 (diabetes)+0.0041·(duration)+0.7960 (gynecological surgery)−1.2553 (LAMA)	$p < 0.001$
6–24 h	g(x) = −2.3878+0.8775 (postoperative opioids used)+0.8426 (tramadol)+0.7653 (female)−2.22 (LAMA)	$p < 0.001$

LAMA, Laryngeal mask

Discussion

Our results suggest that there were different risk factors for PONV in separate but consecutive postoperative time periods. These risk factors are in part different from the factors increasing the risk of PONV during the overall 24-h observation period. Renal failure, diabetes mellitus, the supplementation of nitrous oxide, gynecological operations, postoperative opioids, and the use of pyridostigmine for the reversal of a neuromuscular blockade showed no significant impact on the incidence of PONV when studied over a 24-h time period, but were identified as significant risk factors when examining the consecutive time periods separately.

Among the great number of risk factors for PONV, female gender and motion sickness/PONV in the patient history appear to be well-accepted significant risk factors throughout the literature [2, 8, 13]. According to our data, female gender was not significant for the time period after discharge from the PACU up to 6 h postoperatively and for the overall 24-h observation period. Also motion sickness/PONV in the patient history were just found to be significant up to 6 h postoperatively and over the 24-h period. Our data did not explain these findings. Further studies covering this issue are required.

The proemetic effects of nitrous oxide and the reversal of a neuromuscular block by pyridostigmine were confined to the PACU. This might have been caused by the relatively "short" pharmacokinetic of these drugs particularly in renal failure, which was a significant risk factor for this time period as well. Both factors, nitrous oxide and the reversal of a neuromuscular block by acetylcholine-esterase inhibitors (neostigmine), were supported by data from the literature [4, 6, 11].

The incidence-reducing effect of opioids given during the stay at the PACU could be explained by the proemetic properties of pain as has been published previously [1]. The increase of PONV after the application of opioids in the time period from 6 to 24 h postoperatively reflected the well-documented data from the literature [2, 8, 10, 13].

In accordance with previously published data, diabetes mellitus, the duration of anesthesia, and gynecological operations elevated the risk for PONV during the time period after discharge from PACU up to 6 h postoperatively [2, 3, 9].

Postoperative nausea or vomiting reducing factors for this time period were high age and the intraoperative application of antiemetics, as has already been described in the literature [4, 9]. We found a lower risk of PONV associated with the use of a laryngeal mask airway instead of orotracheal intubation. This finding has been the subject of debate in recent publications [7, 13].

Our data suggest the administration of tramadol for postoperative pain relief as a significant risk factor for the time period 6–24 h postoperatively. To our knowledge, this has not yet been investigated prospectively, but nausea and vomiting are described as a side effect of tramadol in the package insert.

Conclusion

The overall risk of PONV was increased by the following factors: female gender, history of PONV/motion sickness, etomidate for induction, duration of anesthesia, and eye surgery.

The overall risk of PONV was decreased by the following factors: high age, continuous propofol, laryngeal mask airway, and an antiemetic medication given intraoperatively.

There are different risk factors significantly influencing the incidence of PONV during the separate postoperative time periods studied.

References

1. Anderson R, Krohg K (1976) Pain as a major cause of postoperative nausea. Can Anaesth Soc J 23:366–369
2. Apfel CC, Greim C-A, Goepfert C, Grundt D, Usadel J, Sefrin P, Roewer N (1998) Postoperatives Erbrechen: Ein Score zur Voraussage des Erbrechensrisikos nach Inhalationsanästhesien. Anaesthesist 47:732–740
3. Beattie WS, Lindblad T, Buckley DN, Forrest JB (1993) Menstruation increases the risk of nausea after laparoscopy. Anesthesiology 78:272–278
4. Haigh CG, Kaplan LA, Durham JM, Dupeyron JP, Harmer M, Kenny GNC (1993) Nausea and vomiting after gynaecological surgery: a meta-analysis of factors affecting their incidence. Br J Anaesth 71:517–522
5. Kapur PA (1991) The big "little" problem. Anaesth Analg 73:751–755
6. King MJ, Milazakiewicz R, Carli F, Deacock AR (1988) Influence of neostigmine on postoperative vomiting. Br J Anaesth 61:403–406
7. Klockgether-Radtke A, Gerhardt D, Mühlendyck H, Braun U (1996) Einfluss der Kehlkopfmaske auf postoperatives Erbrechen und Halsschmerzen bei Kindern. Anaesthesist 44:1085–1088
8. Koivuranta M, Läärä E, Snare L, Alahuta S (1997) A survey of postoperative nausea and vomiting. Anaesthesia 52:443–449
9. Lerman J (1992) Surgical and patients factors involved in postoperative nausea and vomiting. Br J Anaesth 69:24–32
10. Palazzo M, Evans R (1993) Logistic regression analysis of fixed patient factors for postoperative sickness: a model for risk assessment. Br J Anaesth 70:135–140
11. Pandit UA, Malviya S, Lewis ICH (1995) Vomiting after outpatient tonsillectomy and adenoidectomy in children: the role of nitrous oxide. Anesth Analg 80:230–233
12. Snow J (1848) On narcotism by the inhalation of vapours, facsimile edn 1991. Royal Society of Medicine Services Ltd., London
13. Toner CC, Broomhead CJ, Littlejohn JH, Samra GS, Powney JG, Palazzo MGA, Evans SJW, Strunin L (1996) Prediction of postoperative nausea and vomiting using a logistic regression model. Br J Anaesth 76:347–351

Postoperative Nausea and Vomiting After Laparoscopy in Gynecology

S. Krüper · O.-E. Mohr

Krankenhaus Nordstadt Hannover, Anaesthesiologie und Intensivmedizin, Haltenhoffstr. 41, 30167 Hannover, Germany

Introduction

Until recently, patients' ideas of anesthesia have been dominated by the fear of postoperative nausea and vomiting (PONV). In the "ether days" this side effect occurred virtually on a regular basis.

Landerer (1898) gave a vivid description [11]:

Die Folgen der Narkose sind verschieden; je glatter und ruhiger dieselbe verläuft, je weniger Chloroform verbraucht wurde, um so geringfügiger sind sie. Kinder schlafen meist rasch wieder ein und nach einem mehrstündigen Schlaf erwachen sie munter und mit gutem Appetit. Erwachsene pflegen selten dem Chloroform-„Katzenjammer" zu entgehen. Den meisten ist es wüst im Magen oder im Kopf, Erbrechen, Abgeschlagenheit, Kopfschmerzen, heftiger Durst u.s.f. nehmen den Rest des Tages ein. Mit dem Eintreten eines guten Schlafes pflegen auch hier die Erscheinungen nachzulassen oder zu verschwinden. Manche Kranke, besonders Damen besserer Stände, habe ich dagegen zwei, selbst drei volle Tage in jämmerlichem Zustande hinbringen sehen.

Die Therapie dieser Zustände sei im Wesentlichen eine zuwartende. Werden dem Kranken viel, namentlich feste Speisen gereicht, so bricht er sie aus und ist nachher schlechter dran als vorher. Das Erbrechen wird dadurch oft erst hervorgerufen. Kaltes Selterswasser mit oder ohne Cognac, gut gekühlter herber Sect, Thee, schwarzer Kaffee, Citronenwasser werden meist am besten ertragen, daran schliesst sich Bouillon mit Ei, Thee mit Zwieback oder Cakes, ein Teller Suppe u.s.f. Gegen das Erbrechen werden von Warholm Essigeinathmungen (vor Mund und Nase gehaltene Compressen) oder eine Eisblase empfohlen."

Improvement of anesthetic equipment, technique, and the development of new drugs have achieved a considerably reduced incidence of PONV. In view of the very low rate of severe complications in current anesthetic practice, PONV is correctly termed the "big little problem" [8] for the following reasons:

1. Particularly in the context of minor ambulatory surgery, many patients consider it more debilitating than pain.
2. Apart from being distressing for the patient, vomiting can cause serious complications such as bronchial aspiration, gastric herniation, bleeding at the operation site, and increased suture tension.
3. PONV causes extra cost, not only because of longer hospital stays, but also because of extra post-anesthetic care and additional material [13].

M. K. Herbert et al. (Eds.), Problems of the Gastrointestinal Tract in Anesthesia...

Predisposing Factors for PONV

Many factors affect the incidence of PONV. Patient factors include age, gender, and history. In general, children are more likely to suffer from nausea or vomiting after anesthesia, particularly between the age of 7–14 years. However, children under 3 years of age have a remarkably low risk for PONV of approximately 3–4 %. Female gender, probably caused by the presence of sexual hormones, is a risk factor [4]. A variety of coexisting diseases of the gastrointestinal tract, history of kinetosis or migraine, obesity, and many other factors contribute to PONV.

Specific types of surgery and the length of the procedures affect the incidence of nausea and vomiting. An incidence up to 60 % is reported for intraabdominal operations. Surgery of head and neck, strabismus, inner ear, and posterior cranial fossa are other examples of increased risk for PONV, related to the type of operation. Obviously, the intensity of pain caused by the surgical manipulation contributes to PONV in the postoperative period [1]. These predisposing factors cannot be influenced by the anesthesiologist.

Anesthetic procedures affect the incidence of PONV. Regional anesthesia may trigger nausea or vomiting in less than 10 % through hypotension and bradycardia following high levels of spinal or epidural blockade [10]. Among the drugs used in general anesthesia the opioids have the highest potency to cause PONV. Opioids bind at μ-receptors in the area postrema in the medulla oblongata and exert a direct emetic effect there. Furthermore, they delay gastric emptying and sensitize the vestibular organ. The effect of nitrous oxide depends on the context of its use; some authors have found benefits in avoiding N_2O [7]. The volatile agents show no differences in their potency to cause PONV [3, 5]. Among the intravenous hypnotics, the introduction of propofol with its direct antiemetic effect has made a significant impact in reducing PONV [14]. The avoidance of long acting muscle relaxants, such as pancuronium, and thus the reduced need for antagonism also reduces the risk of PONV [6].

The findings of two clinical studies examining the contribution of two different anesthetic regimens to PONV are presented.

Studies

Study 1

Propofol/Sufentanil vs Thiopentone/Isoflurane/Sufentanil

Among the hypnotics, especially propofol is said to diminish PONV incidence after various surgical procedures. Therefore, the effect of a propofol-based transient intravenous anesthesia (TIVA) was compared with a balanced nitrous oxide-free isoflurane anesthesia for gynecological laparoscopies. These operations are usually complicated by PONV [12].

Sixty patients of the ASA classifications I and II were randomly assigned to two groups of 30 patients. All patients received an oral premedication (7.5 mg midazolam) 1 h before induction; no antiemetics or dopamine antagonists were given.

General anesthesia in group one was induced with sufentanil 0.4 $\mu g\ kg^{-1}$, thiopentone 4 $mg\ kg^{-1}$, and atracurium 0.4 $mg\ kg^{-1}$. Anesthesia was maintained with isoflurane 1.2 ± 0.3 MAC and repetitive doses of sufentanil and atracurium. Group two received propofol 1.5–2.0 $mg\ kg^{-1}$ and the same dose of sufentanil and atracurium as group one. For maintenance propofol 6–10 $mg\ kg^{-1}$ and repetitive doses of sufentanil and atracurium were given. Nitrous oxide was avoided in both groups. Postoperative nausea, vomiting, vigilance, breathing, motoric activity, and shivering were assessed with established scores [9].

A p-value less than 0.05 was regarded as statistically significant.

Both groups were identical with regard to demographic data, duration of operation, and the sufentanil doses per kilogram per hour.

No intergroup difference with respect to PONV was found (37 % vs 33 %). In each group 9 patients suffered from nausea without vomiting. In the group "balanced anesthesia" 2 patients (7 %) vomited, in group "TIVA" 1 patient (3 %). Nevertheless, the time when nausea and vomiting commenced was different. In the "balanced anesthesia group" 55 % of the patients showed first signs more than 2 h after the end of the operation, when they had already returned to their wards, compared with 40 % in the TIVA group.

Patients in the TIVA group had a higher recovery score when arriving in the postanesthetic care unit (PACU). After 30 min there was no further intergroup difference with respect to recovery.

None of both anesthetic techniques proved superior with regard to nausea, vomiting, and shivering. The difference in recovery is not of clinical importance, because it did not influence the duration of postanesthetic observation.

Under financial aspects, however, a balanced low-flow anesthesia produces lower costs.

It can be concluded that a nitrous-oxide-free isoflurane/sufentanil low-flow anesthesia for laparoscopies produces results clinically comparable to a propofol/sufentanil anesthesia, but at lower costs.

Study 2

Remifentanil vs Sufentanil to Supplement Thiopenthone/Isoflurane Anesthesia

It was the purpose of this study to assess the effects of two different opioids used to supplement a basic anesthetic regimen. Sufentanil has been our standard opioid for several years. It has the highest lipid solubility and thus offers remarkable analgesic potency. The new short-acting opioid remifentanil is rapidly hydrolyzed by nonspecific esterases in blood and tissue. The pharmacodynamic profile of remifentanil is similar to that of other μ-receptor agonists such as fentanyl. Remifentanil has a more rapid onset of action, and an analgesic potency 20–30 times higher than that of alfentanil. Available evidence suggests that neither pharmacodynamics nor pharmacokinetics of remifentanil are significantly altered by hepatic or renal dysfunction. A fast decay in plasma concentration ensures rapid recovery regardless of the duration of surgery. Particularly in laparoscopic procedures it is a problem to obtain analgesia during surgery when the intensity of surgical stimulation varies. A dose of opioid sufficient for the most intense stimuli represents an overdose at times of lesser stimulation. This results in prolonged recovery and postoperative respiratory depression. Remifentanil should allow to adjust the infusion rate according to the degree of surgical manipulation.

To evaluate this potential benefit of remifentanil we studied its effect in 64 gynecological patients (ASA classes 1 or 2). Following ethical counseling, informed consent was obtained from 64 patients presenting for elective laparoscopy. All patients were randomly allocated to one of two groups; they received an oral premedication with midazolam and 100 mg of rectal diclofenac after induction. Anesthesia was induced in group 1 (n = 32) with remifentanil 1 µg kg^{-1}, thiopentone 4 mg kg^{-1}, and atracurium 0.4 mg kg^{-1}. Anesthesia was maintained with isoflurane/air and remifentanil 0.5–2 µg kg min^{-1} via an injection pump. Muscle relaxation was maintained with atracurium and monitored with a nerve stimulator. Before skin suture all layers of tissues were infiltrated with bupivacaine 0.25 % by the surgeon. The patients in group 2 (n = 30) received sufentanil 0.4 mg kg^{-1} for induction and repetitive doses of 5–10 µg during isoflurane/air anesthesia. For postoperative examination we used a scoring system (modified from [9]) for the main parameters nausea, vomiting, shivering, recovery of respiration, consciousness, and activity; a visual analogue scale (VAS) was used to assess the intensity of pain. Postoperative status was assessed by an anesthesiologist at 30-min intervals and on the following day. Statistical analysis relied upon Mann-Whitney's U-test. A p-value less than 0.05 was considered significant.

Nausea and vomiting were observed in 56 % (n = 16) patients of the remifentanil group (R) and 30 % (n = 8) patients of the sufentanil group (S) during the entire observation period. Particularly in the early postoperative period, upon the admission to the recovery room and up to 30 min postoperatively, fewer S-patients suffered from nausea: PONV was observed in 9 % (n = 6) of R-patients compared with none in S-patients. This difference was still there 30 min postoperatively (34 % for R vs 10 % for S). After discharge from the recovery room until the visit on the next morning, no differences were observed. At least mild shivering occurred in 59 % of R-patients (n = 19) and 37 % (n = 11) of S-patients. Comparing the sums of shivering scores during the first two postoperative hours we subsequently found higher values for shivering in R-patients.

Recovery from anesthesia was assessed with a combined scoring system. On a scale from zero to ten we found the maximum score more frequently in patients who had received remifentanil: on admission to the recovery area 47 % (n = 15) R-patients achieved 10 of 10 points as compared with 3 % (n = 1) in the S-patients.

Intensity of postoperative pain was assessed using a VAS. Only upon admission to the postanesthesia care unit was a difference between the groups noted. Only 47 % (n = 15) of R-patients were completely free from pain compared with 73 % (n = 22) of S-patients. Thirty minutes later, no differences were noted. In the following course the cumulated pain scores showed no differences.

For postoperative analgesia piritramide was the rescue medication. The requirement of analgesics was the same in both groups. During the whole observation period a nearly equally sized percentage of patients received no additional analgesic drugs at all (28 %, n = 9 vs 27 %, n = 8).

Marked nausea and shivering in the early postoperative period are disadvantages of remifentanil; the more prompt return of full vigilance, in contrast, is advantageous.

This could be a significant advantage of remifentanil, particularly in 1-day surgery. However, a longer acting opioid prior to the termination of remifentanil based anesthesia is recommended.

Conclusion

Nausea and vomiting have been confirmed as an important problem following gynecological laparoscopy in both studies. There was no difference between propofol and thiopenthone/isoflurane with regard to PONV. Other authors have described an antiemetic effect of propofol in different clinical situations. In a meta-analysis of 84 studies enrolling more than 6000 patients, Tramer et al. [15] elucidated the antiemetic potency of propofol. They found a clinically relevant reduction of PONV only in the early postoperative period when propofol was given as a maintenance regimen and at an event rate for PONV between 20 and 60 %. A difference at 24 h was clinically irrelevant in most cases [15]. We found similar results in our comparison of remifentanil and sufentanil: the higher scores for nausea and vomiting in the first postoperative hour did not prevail for 24 h. We believe that it is of no concern for the patient's comfort and satisfaction whether PONV has an early or slightly later onset.

We observed that in approximately 50 % of those patients who were to suffer from PONV first signs started later than 2 h after the operation. Because at that point effects of anesthesia have largely disappeared, this reflects the contribution of other factors such as pain, transport to the wards, starvation, or first application of fluids. Only recently, Apfel et al. emphasized the impact of patient-related risk constellations on the probability of emesis [2].

We conclude that the contribution of anesthesiology to reduction of PONV following general anesthesia should not be overestimated.

References

1. Andersen R, Krogh K (1976) Pain as a major cause of postoperative nausea. Can Anaesth Soc J 23:366–369
2. Apfel CC, Greim CA, Goepfert C, Grundt D, Usadel J, Sefrin P, Roewer N (1998) Post-operatives Erbrechen. Ein Score zur Voraussage des Erbrechensrisikos nach Inhalationsanaesthesien. Anaesthesist 47:732–740
3. Apfel CC, Greim CA, Haubitz I, Goepfert C, Usadel J, Sefrin P, Roewer N (1998) A risk score to predict the probability of postoperative vomiting in adults. Acta Anaesthesiol Scand 42:495–501
4. Beattie WS, Lindblad T, Buckley DN, Forrest JB (1991) The incidence of postoperative nausea and vomiting in women undergoing laparoscopy is influenced by the day of menstrual cycle. Can J Anaesth 38:298
5. Forrest JB, Beattie WS, Goldsmith CH (1990) Risk factors for nausea and vomiting after general anesthesia. Anesthesiology 72:252–268
6. Haigh CG, Kaplan LA, Durham JM (1993) Nausea and vomiting after gynaecological surgery: a meta-analysis of factors affecting their incidence. Br J Anaesth 71:517–522
7. Jigeeshu V Divata, Jayant S Vaidya, Rajendra A Badwe, Rohini W Hawaldar (1996) Omission of nitrous oxide during anesthesia reduces the incidence of postoperative nausea and vomiting. Anaesthesiology 85:1055–1062
8. Kapur PA (1991) The big "little" problem. Anesth Analg 73:751–755
9. Klockgether-Radke A, Piorek V, Crozier T, Kettler D (1996) Nausea and vomiting after laparoscopic surgery: a comparison of propofol and thiopentone/halothane anaesthesia. Eur J Anaesthesiol 13:3–9

10. Koller C, Jakob W, Hörauf K (1994) Postoperatives Erbrechen. Anästh Intensivmed 35:137–143
11. Landerer A (1898) Die Narkose. In: Landerer (Hrsg) Allgemeine Pathologie und Therapie. Urban and Schwarzenberg, Berlin, pp 242–243
12. Marshall CA, Jones RM, Bajorek PK, Cashman JN (1992) Recovery characteristics using isoflurane or propofol for maintenance of anaesthesia: a double blind controlled trial. Anaesthesia 47:461–466
13. Norden JM, Hannallah RS, Patel RI (1995) Pharmaco-economics of vomiting: when is antiemetic prophylaxis cost effective in pediatric ambulatory surgery patients? Anesth Analg 80:346
14. Raftery S, Sherry E (1992) Total intravenous anaesthesia with propofol and alfentanil protects against postoperative nausea and vomiting. Can J Anaesth 39:37–40
15. Tramer M, Moore A, Mc Quay H (1997) Propofol anaesthesia and postoperative nausea and vomiting: quantitative systematic review of randomized controlled studies. Br J Anaesth 78:247–255

Prophylaxis and Therapy of Postoperative Nausea and Vomiting

J. Scholz · M. Steinfath

Klinik für Anästhesiologie, Universität Hamburg, Universitäts-Krankenhaus Eppendorf,
Martinistrasse 52, 20246 Hamburg, Germany

Introduction

In recent years increasing attention has been focused on a sufficient pain management following surgical and diagnostic procedures. No doubt, several convincing concepts of postoperative pain management have been introduced into clinical practice so that postoperative pain no longer should be the most common sequel after surgery. In fact, Rosen and Camu [1] recently mentioned that pain is not always the patient's prime concern in the postoperative period at present. Many patients with previous experience of surgery will rate nausea and vomiting as the most unpleasant consequences. Unfortunately, there has, to date, been little enthusiasm amongst clinicians to commit energy and expenditure to the alleviation of this distressing problem; some even question the relevance of such events to their clinical practice. Nevertheless, if patients complain about serious discomfort due to postoperative nausea and vomiting (PONV), clinicians, of course, have to think about this problem and have to develop an adequate therapeutic management of PONV.

Physiology of Nausea and Vomiting

The complex act of vomiting involves coordination of the respiratory, gastrointestinal and abdominal musculature and is controlled by the vomiting center, which is situated in the lateral reticular formation close to the tractus solitarius in the brain stem [2–4]. The evidence for such a center is based on electrical stimulation and on brain stem lesion studies [3]. Anatomic studies have shown that the parvicellular reticular formation has access to the motor pathways responsible for the visceral and somatic output involved in vomiting. Stimuli from several areas within the central nervous system can affect the vomiting center (Fig. 1). These stimuli include afferents from the pharynx, gastrointestinal tract, and mediastinum, as well as afferents from the higher cortical centers, e.g., the visual center and the vestibular portion of the eighth cranial nerve, and the chemoreceptor trigger zone in the area postrema [2–6]. The area postrema is highly vascularized, and the vessels terminate in fenestrated capillaries surrounded by large perivascular spaces. No effective blood-brain barrier exists in these areas; thus, the chemoreceptor trigger zone can be activated by chemical stimuli received through the blood as well as the cerebrospinal fluid. Furthermore, the area postrema of the brain stem is rich in dopamine, opioid, and serotonin receptors (Fig. 1) [7–9]. The nucleus tractus solitarii is rich in enkephalins and in hista-

M. K. Herbert et al. (Eds.), Problems of the
Gastrointestinal Tract in Anesthesia...

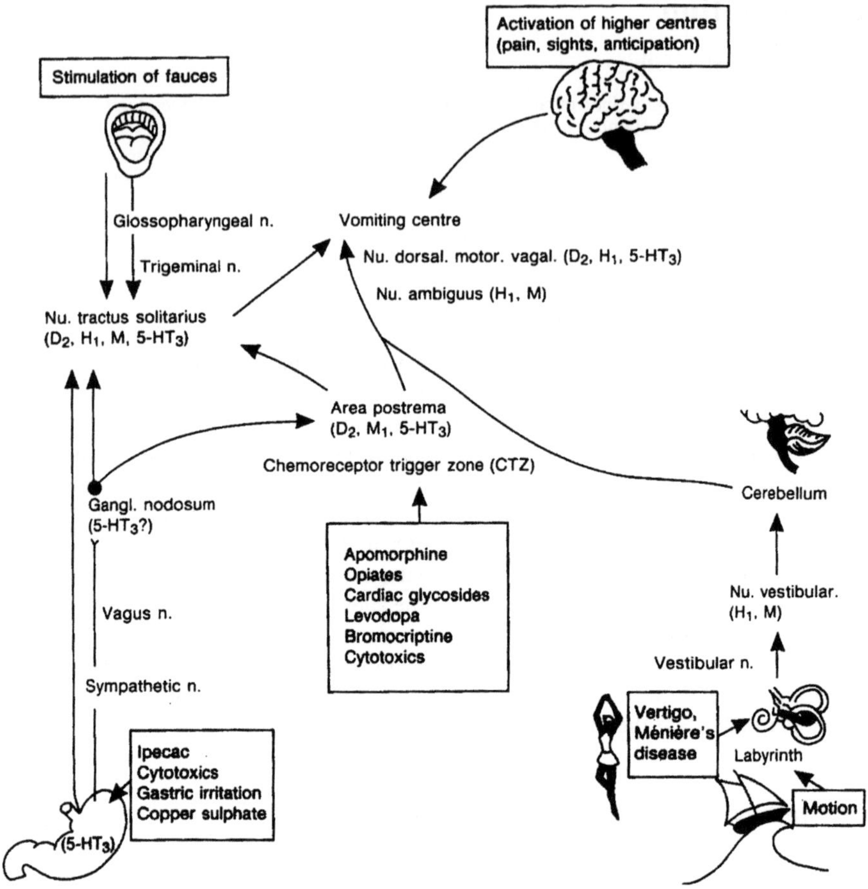

Fig. 1. Physiological pathways involved in nausea and vomiting. See text for details

minic and muscarinic cholinergic receptors (Fig. 1) [10, 11]. These receptors may play an important role in the transmission of impulses to the vomiting center.

Incidence of Postoperative Nausea and Vomiting

Worldwide approximately 80–100 million surgical procedures are performed under general anesthesia each year. Despite major advances in surgical techniques and the introduction of new anesthetic agents with reduced emetogenicity, the incidence of PONV has remained largely unchanged over the past few decades, although its severity has probably decreased [12]. Many studies have been performed to evaluate the incidence of PONV, and estimates vary from 14 to 82% [13]. This wide range might be due mainly to tremendous differences in study design. For example, some studies recorded nausea, vomiting and retching, whereas others recorded vomiting only [12].

Surgical procedure	PONV in the recovery room (%)	PONV at home (%)
Laparoscopy	22.2	44.4
Cataract	14.3	14.3
Arthroscopy	9.1	40.9
Dilatation and curettage	6.7	33.3
Hernia repair	14.3	28.6
Total (n=99)	14.1	30.3

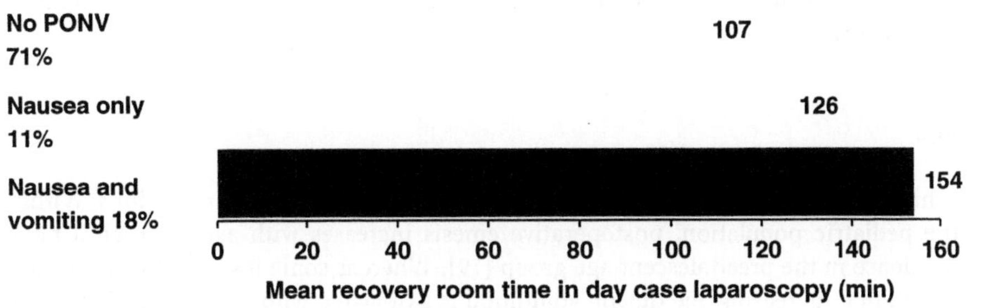

Fig. 2. Postoperative nausea and vomiting following day-case surgery

Furthermore, different anesthetic techniques including various anesthetic agents and different types of surgery or populations undergoing surgical procedures might be responsible for the wide range of PONV incidence.

From daily clinical practice it is not realistic to estimate the global occurrence of PONV markedly higher than 50 %. Without a prophylactic antiemetic therapy, the global incidence of nausea and vomiting in an adult surgical population receiving general anesthesia has been estimated with approximately 20–30 % [4]. Several investigators have studied postoperative nausea and vomiting in women undergoing laparoscopic procedures. In this particular population the incidence of postoperative emesis was found to be up to 54 % [14]. On the other hand, in patients undergoing various short surgical procedures including dental extraction, dilation and curettage of the uterus, or knee arthroscopy, the incidence of postoperative nausea and vomiting was observed in 12–22 % [4]. The difference in the occurrence of PONV depending on the type of surgery has clearly been demonstrated in a very recent multicenter trial [15]. A higher incidence in both postoperative emetic episodes and postoperative nausea was observed in patients undergoing abdominal (42 and 54 %, respectively) vs non-abdominal surgery (23 and 30 %, respectively).

Postoperative nausea and vomiting not only occurs in the recovery room but also on the ward or at home after day-case surgery. Sanchez et al. [16] demonstrated that even more patients suffered from PONV at home following different types of day-case surgery (Fig. 2), and Metter et al. [17] found that the mean recovery room time is markedly prolonged when PONV occurred after day-case surgery (Fig. 2). In addition, PONV can be associated with serious complications including tension of sutures, bleeding at the operative site, wound dehiscence, muscular fatigue, and, above all, aspiration of vomitus into the bronchial tree, which may lead to unplanned hospital admission and markedly increased cost rates [18].

The incidence of PONV can be increased significantly when different risk factors for PONV coexist in patients undergoing surgical procedures in general anesthesia.

Risk Factors for Postoperative Nausea and Vomiting

Significant factors affecting postoperative nausea and vomiting include patient characteristics, the nature of the underlying disease for which the surgical or diagnostic procedure is being performed, the anesthetic technique, as well as the type and duration of surgery.

Age

A higher risk for PONV has been reported in pediatric patients than in adults. Within the pediatric population, postoperative emesis increases with age to reach a peak incidence in the preadolescent age group [19]. Whereas some investigators have suggested that increasing age during adulthood is associated with a decreased incidence of emesis, the relationship between age and PONV is not as clear as the relationship between gender and PONV in the adult population.

Gender

Postoperative nausea and vomiting is approximately two to three times more prevalent in adult women than in men, and the severity of vomiting is greater [20, 21]. There is no significant gender difference in children [22], but the incidence of PONV increases in girls as the menarche approaches [23]. As PONV varies according to the phase of the menstrual cycle, with a fourfold increased incidence during menses [24], it has been suggested that the rising levels of estrogen, combined with decreasing levels of follicle stimulating hormone, may sensitize chemoreceptors and/or the vomiting center.

Body Weight

There is a positive correlation between body weight and PONV [4]. One of the reasons used to explain this relationship is that adipose tissue acts as a reservoir for anesthetic agents, from which they continue to enter the blood stream even after their administration has been discontinued. In other words, obesity has been linked to a higher incidence of PONV [20, 25], which has been attributed to accumulation of fat-soluble anesthetic agents in adipose tissue. On the other hand, a large retrospective analysis of clinical data failed to demonstrate a significant influence of body weight and duration of anesthesia on frequency of PONV [26].

Other explanations for an increased incidence of PONV in obese patients that have been suggested include a larger residual gastric volume and increased incidence of esophageal reflux, as well as gallbladder and other gastrointestinal diseases. In addition, compared with non-obese subjects, these patients have a higher incidence of airway difficulties, and more gastric inflation occurres during attempts to maintain an adequate airway using a face mask [4].

History of Motion Sickness

Patients with a history that suggests that they have a low threshold for vomiting are at increased risk for developing emetic symptoms. These include patients with a history of PONV after previous surgical procedures or motion sickness [4]. It has been alleged that these individuals may have a particularly well-developed reflex arc for vomiting [4].

Anxiety

Several patients have some degree of concern about the forthcoming procedure and such anxiety has been demonstrated to be a risk factor for emesis [27]. It has been suggested that PONV in anxious patients may be related to an increase in gastric fluid volume due to elevated circulating stress hormones [28] or to the anxious patient swallowing more air, thus causing gut distension and activation of mechanoreceptors [27].

Presence and Absence of Food

Patients who have had recent food or fluid intake, e.g., emergency surgery patients, are often found to be at risk for PONV [29]. This is, except the high risk for aspiration into the bronchial tree, another reason for fasting prior to elective surgery. However, prolonged fasting also tends to increase the incidence of nausea, particularly in women [12]. This may be related to hypoglycemia or acetonemia rather than to the absence of food in the stomach.

Gastroparesis

Patients with delayed gastric emptying secondary to an underlying disease may be at increased risk for PONV after surgery [4]. These disease processes include gastrointestinal obstruction, chronic cholecystitis, neuromuscular disorder, and intrinsic neuropathies. Gastric hypomotility can complicate conditions such as scleroderma, myotonic dystrophy, and progressive muscular dystrophies, amyloidosis, and familial visceral myopathies [4]. Gastroparesis also can be associated with pylorospasm, isolated antral hypomotility, and intrinsic neuropathies in patients with diabetes mellitus [4].

Type and Duration of Surgery

It has already been mentioned that PONV is more often observed in patients undergoing abdominal vs non-abdominal surgery with a markedly increased incidence in women undergoing laparoscopic procedures. The duration of surgery also has an effect on the incidence of PONV, with more frequent emesis being reported after longer operations [4]. During longer operations, the patients may receive a larger number of potentially emetic anesthetic agents.

Role of Anesthetic Agents in Postoperative Nausea and Vomiting

Nitrous Oxide and Inhalational Anesthetic Agents

Some time ago it was generally accepted that nitrous oxide is responsible for a significant degree of PONV [30]. After day-case gynecological surgery, nitrous oxide in oxygen is associated with significantly more PONV than oxygen alone (29 vs 9 %, respectively) [31]. In addition, laparoscopic procedures are associated with a high incidence of PONV, and early studies demonstrated that the addition of nitrous oxide will increase the incidence (up to 49 %) and severity of nausea and vomiting [32]. Two recent meta-analyses support the view that addition of nitrous oxide will lead to increased nausea and vomiting [33, 34].

Nitrous oxide may cause PONV through both central and peripheral mechanisms. This may involve stimulation of the sympathetic nervous system with catecholamine release, changes in middle-ear pressure with stimulation of the vestibular system, and increased distension of the gastrointestinal tract.

However, other studies found no reduction in the incidence of emesis in gynecological laparoscopy, abdominal hysterectomy, or gastrointestinal surgery when nitrous oxide was omitted [35–37]. In a recent article published by Unkel and Peters [38] the authors demonstrate that in older studies nitrous oxide appeared to increase emesis during maintenance of anesthesia with enflurane. In contrast, in newer studies the addition of nitrous oxide to an isoflurane- or enflurane-based anesthesia did not alter the incidence of postoperative emesis. Similar observations have been made with the newer, less-soluble inhalational anesthetic agents desflurane and sevoflurane. Furthermore, retrospective analysis of data from 17,201 patients in a large multicenter trial revealed no difference in the incidence of emesis between patients receiving halothane, enflurane, or isoflurane [39].

Opioid Analgesics

Opioids are well documented as powerful emetogenic agents [40]. This group of drugs is extensively used during and after anesthesia to augment the effects of the other anesthetic agents and to control pain [30]. Alfentanil infusions have been used instead of halothane for short surgical procedures in children and were associated with a higher incidence of PONV of 45 and 15 %, respectively [41]. Forrest et al. [39] found that fentanyl was associated with an incidence of approximately 25 and 18 % of nausea and vomiting, respectively, compared with incidences of around 18 and 12 % with volatile anesthetics. The more lipid-soluble agents, alfentanil and sufentanil, have also been associated with similar incidences of PONV [42, 43]. In a very recent overview Unkel and Peters [38] reported that different opioids were characterized by similar incidences of PONV.

Other Anesthetic Agents

Administration of older intravenous anesthetic agents, including barbiturates and etomidate, can also be associated with PONV [44, 45]. The association of ketamine and PONV is discussed controversially. Whereas Watcha and White [4] mentioned a high incidence of PONV following ketamine administration, Rabey and Smith [46] argued that there are no controlled data to support this contention.

The newer intravenous anesthetic agent propofol is characterized by a low incidence of PONV [47–51]. In addition, Watcha et al. [49] found that there was a lower incidence of PONV in children undergoing day-case strabismus surgery if propofol was used for both induction and maintenance of anesthesia than when administered for induction alone followed by maintenance with inhalational agents. However, although these authors concluded that propofol does not have direct antiemetic properties, other investigators believe that it does [52–55].

Therapeutic Approach

Three major groups of agents, including benzamides, butyrophenones, and 5-HT_3 receptor antagonists, are frequently used in the management of PONV in daily clinical practice.

Benzamides

The substituted benzamides, particularly metoclopramide, are widely used in chemotherapy-induced emesis and in some countries for the prevention and therapy of PONV. The efficacy of metoclopramide in preventing PONV is equivocal, with approximately 50 % of studies showing it to be no more effective than placebo [56]. At high concentrations metoclopramide has been shown to have a weak 5-HT_3 receptor antagonistic effect, which may account for some of its antiemetic properties [30], when used at high doses in chemotherapy-induced emesis. However, the doses administered for PONV and the antiemetic effects of metoclopramide are likely to reside in its ability to antagonize the action of dopamine. Side effects typical of the dopamine antagonists, such as extrapyramidal reactions and sedation, may also occur in patients receiving metoclopramide [57]. Intravenous application may be associated with significant cardiovascular side effects, which are hypotension and brady- or tachycardia [30]. Metoclopramide should not be used after gastrointestinal surgery, such as pyloroplasty or intestinal anastomosis, because it stimulates gastric motility and may delay healing.

Butyrophenones

The butyrophenones are potent neuroleptics which also have antiemetic properties mediated by their powerful D_2 receptor antagonism [30]. They were developed primarily for use in patients with schizophrenia and other psychoses, but droperidol has also been used extensively as an antiemetic in anesthesia [56]. In comparative studies, intravenous droperidol has been demonstrated to have greater prophylactic efficacy than metoclopramide [58–61]. Low doses of droperidol (0.01–0.02 mg/kg) have been used successfully in procedures associated with moderate emesis but have limited efficacy in more emetogenic procedures [4]. Other studies failed to demonstrate an efficacy of droperidol administration in preventing PONV. However, in these studies droperidol was given during induction of anesthesia, and it was suggested that the efficacy might be improved if droperidol was to be administered toward the end of surgery. Nevertheless, overall most studies found a beneficial effect of droperidol when compared with placebo in the prevention of PONV, and efficacy has been demonstrated when droperidol was administered before and at the end of surgery as well.

Butyrophenones can induce extrapyramidal side effects [4] which are not very common but extremely unpleasant. In addition, high doses of droperidol can cause hypotension, prolonged tiredness, or dysphoria [58, 62]. Anxiety and restlessness, developing after discharge, have also been reported, suggesting that droperidol may not be an appropriate prophylactic antiemetic for day-case and routine outpatient surgery [63, 64].

5-HT_3 Receptor Antagonists

The role of serotonin receptors in drug-induced emesis has recently received increased attention. Free serotonin levels showed a tendency to increase from 3 to at least 5 h following cisplatinum administration [65]. Agents such as ondansetron, granisetron, and tropisetron that competitively antagonize the effect of serotonin at 5-hydroxytryptamine subtype three (5-HT_3) receptor sites have been shown to be extremely useful antiemetics in the prevention of chemotherapy-induced nausea and vomiting [66–71]. 5-HT_3 receptor antagonists are very specific agents with almost no significant interaction with other 5-HT receptor subtypes or other specific receptor binding sites (Fig. 3) [72]. In addition, 5-HT_3 receptor antagonists represent a major advance in the management of emesis because they are highly effective and possess a low side effect profile, especially when compared with benzamides and butyrophenones.

Ondansetron was the first drug of this class, and its efficacy has been established in large studies of various patient populations (for review see [4]). In other words, ondansetron has not only been shown to be effective in chemotherapy-induced emesis but also in the prevention and therapy of PONV. Superior effects in the prevention of postoperative nausea and vomiting have been observed following administration of ondansetron in comparison with droperidol and metoclopramide [73–75]. In a "dose finding study" looking at the efficacy upon emesis, on the one hand, and side effects, on the other hand, it has been shown that ondansetron at a dose of 4 mg is associated with the lowest emesis rate along with comparable side effect profiles at various doses ranging from 1 to 8 mg (Fig. 4) [76].

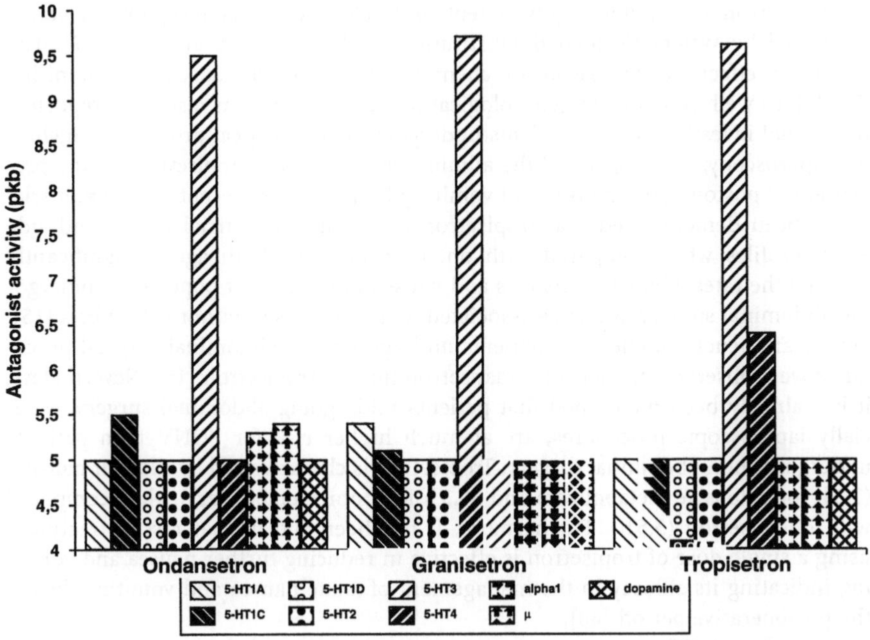

Fig. 3. Interaction of ondansetron, granisetron, and tropisetron with various receptor sites. See text for details

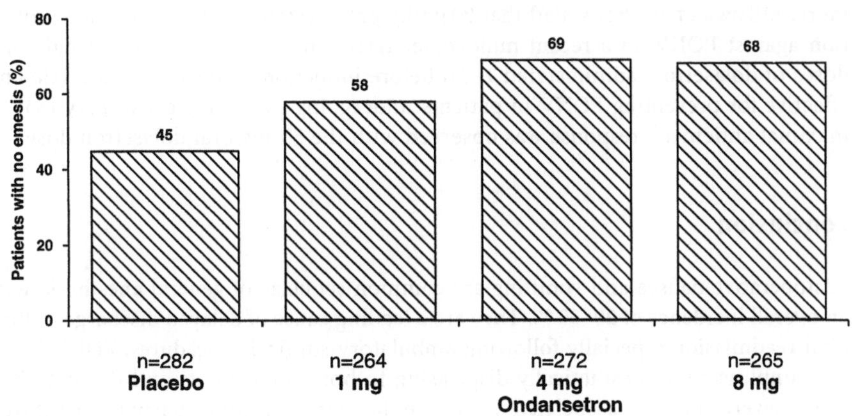

Adverse event (%)				
Headache	13	17	16	12
Dizziness	16	13	12	11
Muscle pain	11	13	13	11
Shivers	12	11	10	10
Sedation	8	13*	7	6

Fig. 4. Efficacy and side effect profile of different concentrations of ondansetron

Tropisetron is another highly potent and selective 5-HT_3 receptor antagonist developed by systematic methyl substitution of the serotonin molecule [77]. The beneficial effect of this agent in chemotherapy-induced nausea and vomiting [70, 71], as well as following gynecological procedures [78], has also been reported. Additional investigations on patients undergoing gynecological procedures, including laparoscopy, have suggested the administration of 2 mg tropisetron for the prevention of postoperative nausea and vomiting [79]. In a very recent multicenter trial it has been demonstrated that tropisetron has similar beneficial effects and side effect profiles when compared with ondansetron [15]. Both agents significantly reduced the rates of emetic episodes and nausea in the patient population undergoing abdominal surgery and were associated with low rates of minor side effects [15]. Significant beneficial effects in patients undergoing non-abdominal surgical procedures were observed neither for ondansetron nor for tropisetron [15]. Nevertheless, it has already been mentioned that patients undergoing abdominal surgery, especially laparoscopic procedures, are at much higher risk for PONV than patients undergoing non-abdominal surgery. Tropisetron is characterized by a longer half-life (7.3 h for extensive metabolizers and 30.3 h for poor metabolizers) when compared with ondansetron (3.5 h). Furthermore, it has been shown that rescue treatment using a single dose of tropisetron is effective in reducing further nausea and vomiting indicating its efficacy in the management of acute nausea and vomiting during the postoperative period [80].

Two other 5-HT_3 receptor antagonists, granisetron and dolasetron, have been demonstrated to reveal beneficial effects in the management of PONV. In a dose-ranging study performed by Fujii et al. [81] 40 μg/kg granisetron was as effective as 60 μg/kg and both doses were better than placebo or 20 mg/kg granisetron. Furthermore, Mikawa et al. [82] stated that 20 μg/kg granisetron provided adequate protection against PONV. In a recent multicenter trial it has been shown that single oral doses of dolasetron, administered 1–2 h before induction of anesthesia, are safe and effective for preventing PONV in patients undergoing gynecological surgery [83]. A maximal antiemetic response was observed with the 50-mg oral dolasetron dose.

Conclusion

Postoperative nausea and vomiting are common sequelae of general anesthesia with an overall incidence of 20–30 %. They are a leading cause of delayed discharge or hospital readmission especially following ambulatory surgical procedures. PONV is not only unpleasant and esthetically displeasing to both the patients and the staff, but, when severe, may be associated with complications including tension on sutures, bleeding at the operative site, wound dehiscence, muscular fatigue, and, above all, aspiration of vomitus into the bronchial tree [18]. 5-HT_3 receptor antagonists are very attractive because of their long-term prophylactic effect on PONV. In addition, they are usually superior to other agents used for the prevention and therapy of PONV. However, it has to be mentioned that prophylactic therapy with 5-HT_3 receptor antagonists is very expensive and not always wise when, for example, looking at the efficacy of these agents depending on the type of surgery, but it is justified in high-risk patients, particularly in those with a history of nausea and vomiting undergoing long-term abdominal surgery. On the other hand, postoperative nausea and vomiting are of greatest concern after day-case surgery as they may delay discharge and result in unanticipated hospital admission which very likely is more expensive than prophylactic therapy with 5-HT_3 receptor antagonists. Thus, it seems to be reasonable to administer agents such as ondansetron and tropisetron in patients at higher risk and a history of postoperative nausea and vomiting, especially in light of day-case surgery. Nevertheless, other potent agents, such as droperidol, should still be considered in the management of postoperative nausea and vomiting, especially when realizing the fact that single prophylactic 5-HT_3 receptor antagonist administration failed to reveal a significant antiemetic effect in patients undergoing non-abdominal surgery. A very recent review of the literature suggests that the best results might be obtained by using a combined regimen in the prophylaxis of PONV [84]. For patients who have a high risk of PONV, the use of propofol for induction and maintenance and a small dose of droperidol (0.5–1.0 mg) plus ondansetron (4 mg) or tropisetron (2 mg) administered intravenously toward the end of surgery has been recommended. In addition, it has to be mentioned that when different drugs that cause similar effects but act via distinct receptor mechanisms are combined in therapy, synergistic effects are often demonstrated. Thus, it is reasonable to postulate that the combination of 5-HT_3 receptor antagonists and droperidol or metoclopramide, or other agents such as transdermal scopolamine, in antiemetic therapy may produce efficacy of a magnitude not seen with any of the drugs administered alone [85].

References

1. Rosen M, Camu F (1994) Postoperative nausea and vomiting. Anaesthesia 49:1
2. Andrews PLR, Davis CJ, Binham S et al. (1990) The abdominal visceral innervation and the emetic refex: pathways, pharmacology and plasticity. Can J Physiol Pharmacol 68:325–345
3. Borison HL (1989) Area postrema: chemoreceptor circumventricular organ of the medulla oblongata. Prog Neurobiol 32:351–390
4. Watcha MF, White PF (1992) Postoperative nausea and vomiting. Anesthesiology 77:162–184
5. Borison HL, McCarthy LE (1983) Neuropharmacology of chemotherapy-induced emesis. Drugs 25:8–17
6. Davis CJ, Harding RK, Leslie RA et al. (1986) The organization of vomiting as a protective reflex. In: Davis CJ et al. (eds) Nausea and vomiting: mechanisms and treatment. Springer, Berlin Heidelberg New York pp 65–75
7. Stefanini E, Clement-Cormier Y (1981) Detection of receptors in the area postrema. Eur J Pharmacol 74:257–260
8. Atweh SF, Kuhar MJ (1977) Autoradiographic localization of opiate receptors in the rat brain. II. The brain stem. Brain Res 129:1–12
9. Waeber C, Dixon K, Hoyer D et al. (1988) Localisation by autoradiography of neuronal 5-HT3 receptors in the mouse. Eur J Pharmacol 151:351–352
10. Palacios JM, Wamsley JK, Kuhar MJ (1981) The distribution of histamine H1-receptors in the rat brain: an autoradiographic study. Neuroscience 6:15–17
11. Wamsley JK, Lewis MS, Young WS III et al. (1981) Autoradiographic localization of muscarinic cholinergic receptors in rat brainstem. J Neurosci 1:176–191
12. Palazzo MGA, Strunin L (1984) Anaesthesia and emesis. I. Etiology. Can Anaesth Soc J 31:178–187
13. Aitkenhead AR, Smith G (eds) (1990) Textbook of anaesthesia. Churchill Livingstone, Edinburgh
14. Patasky AO, Kitz DS, Andrews RW, Lecky JH (1988) Nausea and vomiting following ambulatory surgery: Are all procedures created equal? Anesth Analg 67:S163
15. Scholz J, Hennes HJ, Steinfath M, Färber L, Schweiger C, Dick W, Schulte AM, Esch J (1998) Tropisetron or ondansetron compared with placebo for prevention of post-operative nausea and vomiting. Eur J Anaesthesiol 15:676–685

16. Sanchez AG (1985) Pharmacoeconomics for postoperative nausea and vomiting. Am J Hosp Pharm 27:121–125
17. Metter SE, Kitz DS, Young ML et al. (1987) Nausea and vomiting after outpatient laparoscopy: incidence, impact on recovery room stay and cost. Anesth Analg 66:S116
18. Watcha MF, White PF (1995) New anti-emetic drugs. Int Anesthesiol Clin 33:1–20
19. Rowley MP, Brown TCK (1982) Postoperative vomiting in children. Anaesth Intensive Care 10:309–313
20. Belville JW, Bross IDJ, Howland WS (1960) Postoperative nausea and vomiting IV: factors related to postoperative nausea and vomiting. Anesthesiology 21:186–193
21. Cookson RF (1986) Mechanisms and treatment of post-operative nausea and vomiting. In: Davis CJ et al. (eds) Nausea and vomiting: mechanisms and treatment. Springer, Berlin Heidelberg New York, pp 130–150
22. Vance JP, Neill RS, Norris W (1973) The incidence and aetiology of nausea and vomiting in a plastic surgical unit. Br J Plast Surg 26:336–339
23. Rita L, Goodarzi M, Seleny F (1981) Effects of low dose droperidol on postoperative vomiting in children. Can Anaesth Soc J 28:259–262
24. Beattie WS, Lindblad T, Buckley DN et al. (1991) The incidence of postoperative nausea and vomiting in women undergoing laparoscopy is influenced by the day of the menstrual cycle. Can J Anaesth 38:298–302
25. Editorial (1989) Nausea and vomiting after general anaesthesia. Lancet 1:651–652
26. Haigh CG, Kaplan LA, Durham JM et al. (1993) Nausea and vomiting after gynaecological surgery: a meta-analysis of factors affecting their incidence. Br J Anaesth 71:517–522
27. Andrews PLR (1992) Physiology of nausea and vomiting. Br J Anaesth 69:2S–19S
28. Ong BY, Palahniuk RJ, Cumming M (1978) Gastric volume and pH in out-patients. Can Anaesth Soc J 25:36–39
29. Kapur PA (1991) The big "Little Problem". Anesth Analg 73:751–755
30. Kenny GNC (1994) Risk factors for postoperative nausea and vomiting. Anaesthesia 49:6–10
31. Felts J, Poler SM, Spitznagel EL (1990) Nitrous oxide, nausea and vomiting after outpatient gynecologic surgery. J Clin Anesth 2:168–171
32. Lonie DS, Harper NJ (1986) Nitrous oxide anaesthesia and vomiting. The effect of nitrous oxide anaesthesia on the incidence of vomiting following gynaecological laparoscopy. Anaesthesia 41:703–707
33. Tramer MR (1996) Omitting nitrous oxide in general anaesthesia: metaanalysis of intraoperative awareness and postoperative emesis in randomized controlled trials. Br J Anaesth 76:186–193
34. Divatia JV (1996) Omission of nitrous oxide during anesthesia reduces the incidence of postoperative nausea and vomiting. A meta-analysis. Anesthesiology 85:1055–1062
35. Kortilla K, Hovorka J, Erkola O (1987) Nitrous oxide does not increase the incidence of nausea and vomiting after isoflurane anesthesia. Anesth Analg 66:761–765
36. Hovorka J, Kortilla K, Erkola O (1989) Nitrous oxide does not increase nausea and vomiting following gynaecological laparoscopy. Can J Anaesth 36:145–148
37. Ranta P, Nuutinen I, Laitinen J (1991) The role of nitrous oxide in postoperative nausea and recovery in patients undergoing upper abdominal surgery. Acta Anaesth Scand 35:339–341
38. Unkel W, Peters J (1998) Postoperative Nausea und Vomiting: Mechanismen und Behandlung. AINS 33:533
39. Forrest JB, Cahalan MK, Rehder K et al. (1990) Multicenter study of general anesthesia. II. Results. Anesthesiology 72:262–268
40. Clarke RSJ (1991) Post-operative gastrointestinal complications. Curr Anaesth Crit Care 2:20–24
41. Davis PJ, Chopyk JB, Nazif M et al. (1991) Continuous alfentanil infusion in paediatric patients undergoing general anaesthesia for complete oral restoration. J Clin Anesth 3:125–130
42. White PF, Sung ML, Doze VA (1995) Use of sufentanil in outpatient anesthesia: determining an optimal preinduction dose. Anesthesiology 63:A202
43. White PF, Coe V, Shafer A et al. (1986) Comparison of alfentanil with fentanyl for outpatient anesthesia. Anesthesiology 64:99–106
44. Smessaert A, Schehr CA, Artusio JF (1959) Nausea and vomiting in the immediate postanesthetic period. J Am Med Assoc 170:2072–2076
45. Clarke RSJ (1984) Nausea and vomiting. Br J Anaesth 56:19–27
46. Rabey PG, Smith G (1992) Anaesthetic factors contributing to postoperative nausea and vomiting. Br J Anaesth 69:40S–45S
47. Gunawardene RD, White DC (1988) Propofol and emesis. Anaesthesia 43:65–67
48. Kortilla K, Faure E, Apfelbaum J et al. (1988) Less nausea and vomiting after propofol than after enflurane or isoflurane anesthesia. Anesthesiology 69:A578
49. Watcha MF, Simeon RM, White PF (1991) Effect of propofol on the incidence of postoperative vomiting after strabismus surgery in pediatric outpatients. Anesthesiology 75:204–207

50. Jobila N, Mathieu A (1994) A meta-analysis of published studies confirm decreased postoperative nausea and vomiting with propofol. Anesthesiology 81:A33
51. Sneyd JR, Carr A, Byrom WD et al. (1998) A meta-analysis of nausea and vomiting following maintenance of anaesthesia with propofol or inhalational agents. Eur J Anaesth 15:433–445
52. McCollum JSC, Milligan KR, Dundee JW (1988) The antiemetic action of propofol. Anaesthesia 43:239–240
53. Borgeat A, Wilder-Smith OH, Wilder-Smith CH et al. (1992a) Adjuvant propofol for refractory cisplatin-associated nausea and vomiting. Lancet 340:679–680
54. Borgeat A, Wilder-Smith OH, Saiah M et al. (1992b) Subhypnotic doses of propofol possess direct antiemetic properties. Anesth Analg 74:539–541
55. Raftery S, Sherry E (1992) Total intravenous anaesthesia with propofol and alfentanil protects against postoperative nausea and vomiting. Can J Anaesth 39:37–40
56. Rowbothan DJ (1992) Current management of postoperative nausea and vomiting. Br J Anaesth 69:46S–59S
57. Allen RW (1990) Metoclopramide: a safe anti-emetic? S Afr Med J 77:219
58. Kortilla K, Kauste A, Auvinen J (1979) Comparison of domperidone, droperidol, and metoclopramide in the prevention and treatment of nausea and vomiting after balanced general anesthesia. Anesth Analg 66:761–765
59. Cohen SE, Woods WA, Wyner J (1984) Anti-emetic efficacy of droperidol and metoclopramide. Anesthesiology 60:67–69
60. Kauste A, Tuominen M, Heikkinen H et al. (1986) Droperidol, alizapride and metoclopramide in the prevention and treatment of postoperative emetic sequelae. Eur J Anaesth 3:1–9
61. Pandit SJ, Kothary SP, Pandit UA et al. (1989) Dose-response study of droperidol and metoclopramide as antiemetics for outpatient anesthesia. Anesth Analg 68:798–802
62. Loeser EA, Bennett G, Stanley TH et al. (1979) Comparison of droperidol, haloperidol and prochlorperazine as postoperative anti-emetics. Can Anaesth Soc J 26:125–127
63. Melnick B, Sawyer R, Karambelkar D et al. (1989) Delayed side effects of droperidol after ambulatory general anesthesia. Anesth Analg 69:748–751
64. Foster PN, Stickle BR, Laurence AS (1996) Akathisia following low-dose droperidol for antiemesis in day-case patients. Anaesthesia 51:491–494
65. Cubeddu LX, Hoffmann IS, Fuenmayor NT et al. (1992) Changes in serotonin metabolism in cancer patients: its relationship to nausea and vomiting induced by chemotherapeutic drugs. Br J Cancer 66:198–203
66. Editorial (1987) 5-HT3 receptor antagonists: a new class of antiemetics. Lancet i:1470–1471
67. Hesketh PJ, Murphy WK, Lester EP et al. (1989) GR 38032F (GR-C507/75): a novel compound effective in the prevention of acute cisplatin-induced emesis. J Clin Oncol 7:700–705
68. Cubeddu LX, Hoffman IS, Fuenmayer NT, Finn AL (1990) Efficacy of ondansetron (GR 38032F) and the role of serotonin in cisplatin-induced nausea and vomiting. N Engl J Med 322:810–816
69. Marty M, Ponillart P, Scholl S et al. (1990) Comparison of 5-hydroxytryptamine3 (serotonin) antagonist ondansetron (GR 38032F) with high-dose metoclopramide in the control of cisplatin-induced emesis. N Engl J Med 322:816–821
70. Sorbe BG, Högberg T, Glimelius B et al. (1994) A randomized, multicenter study comparing the efficacy and tolerability of tropisetron, a new 5-HT3 receptor antagonist, with a metoclopramide-containing antiemetic cocktail in the prevention of cisplatin-induced emesis. Cancer 73:445–454
71. Sorbe B, Högberg T, Himmelmann A et al. (1994) Efficacy and tolerability of tropisetron in comparison with a combination of tropisetron and dexamethasone in the control of nausea and vomiting induced by cisplatin-containing chemotherapy. Eur J Cancer 30:629–634
72. Naylor RJ, Inall FC (1994) The physiology and pharmacology of postoperative nausea and vomiting. Anaesthesia 49:2–5
73. Alon E, Himmelseher S (1992) Ondansetron in the treatment of postoperative vomiting: a randomized, double-blind comparison with droperidol and metoclopramid. Anesth Analg 75:561–565
74. Diemunsch P, Conseiller C, Clyti N et al. (1997) Ondansetron compared with metoclopramide in the treatment of established postoperative nausea and vomiting. Br J Anaesth 79:322–326
75. Polați E, Verlato G, Finco G et al. (1997) Ondansetron versus metoclopramide in the treatment of postoperative nausea and vomiting. Anesth Analg 85:395–399
76. Pearman MH (1994) Single dose intravenous ondansetron in the prevention of postoperative nausea and vomiting. Anaesthesia 49:11–15
77. Richardson BP, Engel G, Donatsch P et al. (1985) Identification of serotonin M-receptor subtypes and their specific blockade by a new class of drugs. Nature 316:126
78. Zomers PJW, Langenberg CJM, DeBruijn KM (1993) Tropisetron for postoperative nausea and vomiting in patients after gynaecological surgery. Br J Anaesth 71:677–680

79. Capouet V, Depauw C, Vernet B et al. (1996) Single dose i.v. tropisetron in the prevention of postoperative nausea and vomiting after gynaecological surgery. Br J Anaesth 76:54–60
80. Alon E, Buchser E, Herrera E et al. (1998) Troisetron for treating established postoperative nausea and vomiting: a randomized, double-blind, placebo-controlled study. Anesth Analg 86:617–623
81. Fujii Y, Tanaka H, Toyooka H (1994) Optimal anti-emetic dose of ganisetron for prevention of postoperative nausea and vomiting. Can J Anaesth 41:794–797
82. Mikawa K, Takao Y, Nishina K et al. (1995) The antiemetic efficacy of prophylactic ganisetron in gynecologic surgery. Anesth Analg 80:970–974
83. Diemunsch P, Kortilla K, Leeser J et al. (1998) Oral dolasetron mesylate for prevention of postoperative nausea and vomiting: a multicenter, double-blind, placebo-controlled study. J Clin Anesth 10:145–152
84. Eriksson H, Kortilla K (1997) Prevention of postoperative pain and emesis. Curr Opin Anaesthesiol 10:438–444
85. Dershwitz M (1994) Advances in antiemetic therapy. Anesthesiol Clin North Am 12:119–132

PART VI

Update – Gastric, Duodenal, and Stress Ulcer, Etiology, Pathophysiology, Treatment

Gastric Acid Backdiffusion and Neural Alarm System

P. Holzer · I. T. Lippe · M. Jocić · Á. Heinemann

Department of Experimental and Clinical Pharmacology, University of Graz, Universitätsplatz 4, 8010 Graz, Austria

Introduction

The pathophysiological concept that gastroduodenal ulcer is caused by aggressive factors including acid, pepsin, and *Helicobacter pylori* is met by the current medical treatment involving proton pump inhibitors and antibiotics. Since the time when prostaglandins were discovered to be protective factors, with their deficiency being responsible for the mucosal lesions caused by nonsteroidal anti-inflammatory drugs, attention has also been paid to the defensive forces of the gastroduodenal mucosa. However, the possibility that nociceptive neurons participate in gastric mucosal protection from injury was not thought of until recently. This article summarizes the experimental evidence for afferent neurons being a neural emergency system (Holzer 1998) that alarms protective mechanisms in the stomach in the face of pending acid injury. There is good reason to postulate that a malfunction of this alarm system is an etiological factor in certain forms of gastroduodenal ulcer disease.

The implications of nociceptive afferent neurons in gastroduodenal mucosal defense were discovered with the help of capsaicin, the pungent ingredient in red peppers such as paprika or chili. Capsaicin is a pharmacological tool with which the activity of primary afferent neurons with unmyelinated or thinly myelinated nerve fibers can selectively be manipulated (Holzer 1991; Wood 1993). In terms of its action, capsaicin is an excitotoxin which acutely stimulates a group of unmyelinated and thinly myelinated afferents (C- and A fibers) and, depending on the dose and route of administration, causes a long-lasting defunctionalization of, and depletion of transmitter substances from, these neurons. In contrast, afferent neurons with thick myelin sheaths are not sensitive to capsaicin (Holzer 1991). The selectivity of capsaicin's excitotoxic action on afferent neurons derives from the fact that only these neurons express receptor binding sites ("vanilloid receptors") for capsaicin and structurally related ligands (Szallasi 1994; Caterina et al. 1997; Helliwell et al. 1998). By taking use of the neurotoxic action of capsaicin it is possible to ablate afferent neurons without severing efferent autonomic neurons which unavoidably are cut by nerve transection.

Innervation of the Stomach by Extrinsic Afferents

The concept that gastric mucosal integrity is surveyed by nociceptive afferent neurons which alarm protective mechanisms in emergency situations is supported by the presence of extrinsic sensory nerve fibers in the mucosal lamina propria behind the

M. K. Herbert et al. (Eds.), Problems of the Gastrointestinal Tract in Anesthesia...

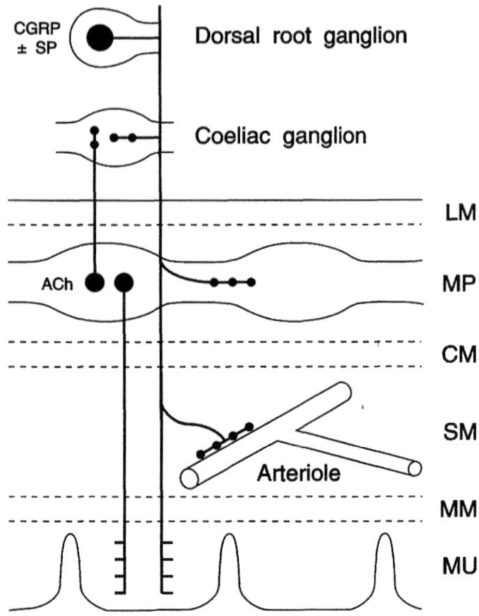

Fig. 1. Innervation of the rodent gastric mucosa by extrinsic afferent neurons originating from dorsal root ganglia and by intrinsic afferent neurons of the myenteric plexus. *ACh* acetylcholine; *CGRP* calcitonin gene-related peptide; *CM* circular muscle; *LM* longitudinal muscle; *MM* muscularis mucosae; *MP* myenteric plexus; *MU* mucosa; *SM* submucosa; *SP* substance P

epithelium (Fig. 1). Many of these fibers originate from dorsal root ganglia, contain bioactive peptides such as calcitonin gene-related peptide (CGRP) and the tachykinins substance P (SP) and neurokinin A (NKA) as messenger molecules, and are sensitive to the excitotoxic action of capsaicin (Furness et al. 1982; Su et al. 1987; Green and Dockray 1988; Sternini 1992). It is particularly worth noting that CGRP is an almost exclusive marker of spinal afferents in the distal rat stomach (Green and Dockray 1988; Sternini 1992) and that approximately 98 % of the spinal afferents supplying the rat gut contain CGRP (Perry and Lawson 1998). Some vagal afferent nerve fibers also contribute to the gastric content of SP and CGRP (Hayashi et al. 1982; Bäck et al. 1994; Suzuki et al. 1997) especially in the proximal part of the stomach (Holzer 1998).

The extrinsic spinal afferents expressing CGRP run in the sympathetic (splanchnic) nerves and on their way from the dorsal root ganglia to the stomach pass through the celiac ganglion (Fig. 1) where they give off collaterals to form axodendritic and axosomatic synapses with the sympathetic ganglion cells (Green and Dockray 1988; Lindh et al. 1988). In addition, intestinofugal myenteric neurons containing acetylcholine and, in part, nitric oxide (NO) also project to the celiac ganglion (Fig. 1) and, in cooperation with intrinsic sensory neurons, serve as an additional afferent system to the prevertebral ganglia (Furness and Anderson 1994; Domoto et al. 1995; Ma and Szurszewski 1996). Within the gastric wall it is particularly the arterial and arteriolar system that receives a dense supply by spinal afferent nerve fibers expressing CGRP, SP, and NKA, whereas the venous system is sparsely innervated (Furness et al. 1982; Su et al. 1987; Green and Dockray 1988; Sternini 1992). The peptide-containing axons run primarily in the connective tissue (tunica adventitia) surrounding the vessels and at the border between adventitia and muscle (media). In addition, some peptide-containing afferent nerve fibers supply the myenteric plexus, the circular muscle layer and the mucosa of the gut (Furness et al. 1982; Green and Dockray 1988; Sternini 1992).

Gastric Blood Flow Regulation by Afferent Neurons

The possibility that perivascular afferent nerve fibers control vascular functions in the stomach went unrecognized for a long time, as these axons were considered to subserve only sensory but not effector functions. However, with the advent of capsaicin it became feasible to prove that sensory neurons containing CGRP participate in the regulation of the rat gastric circulation (Holzer 1998). Afferent nerve stimulation by intragastric administration of capsaicin leads to a marked increase in gastric mucosal blood flow, which is brought about by dilatation of submucosal arterioles, but not venules (Chen et al. 1992; Chen and Guth 1995). The vasodilator effect of capsaicin depends on the extrinsic innervation of the stomach (Holzer et al. 1991b), because defunctionalization of afferent neurons with a neurotoxic dose of capsaicin abolishes the hyperemic response to acute sensory nerve stimulation. Nerve-selective ablation of afferent neurons has shown that only spinal afferents passing through the celiac ganglion, but not vagal afferents, contribute to the capsaicin-evoked increment of gastric mucosal blood flow (Li et al. 1991). However, the course and relays of the neural pathway responsible for the capsaicin-induced vasodilatation, which involves ganglionic transmission through nicotinic acetylcholine receptors (Leung 1993), remain to be elucidated.

Since the $CGRP_1$ receptor antagonist $CGRP_{8-37}$ prevents the vasodilatation caused by intragastric capsaicin (Li et al. 1991; Chen et al. 1992), it follows that CGRP is an important mediator, an implication which is consistent with the ability of capsaicin to release CGRP within the rat stomach (Holzer et al. 1990) and with the vascular pharmacology of the peptide. Calcitonin gene-related peptide fails to affect gastric venules but potently dilates submucosal arterioles (Chen et al. 1992; Chen and Guth 1995) and enhances blood flow through the rat stomach (Lippe et al. 1989; Holzer and Guth 1991; Li et al. 1991; Holzer et al. 1993). The vasodilator action of both capsaicin and CGRP depends on NO (Whittle et al. 1992; Holzer et al. 1993; Chen and Guth 1995), and the localization of CGRP receptors in the stomach (Gates et al. 1989; Sternini 1992) suggests that CGRP increases the formation of NO in endothelial cells. However, the gastric vasodilator response to CGRP is only partly NO dependent (Holzer et al. 1993) and less susceptible to inhibition by an NO synthase blocker than the vasodilator response to capsaicin (Chen and Guth 1995). It is evident, therefore, that the sequential components of the capsaicin-induced hyperemia still await identification and that it is not clear whether CGRP and NO are the final vasodilator messengers.

Substance P and NKA are two further peptides released from afferent nerve fibers but, unlike CGRP, do not contribute to the afferent nerve-mediated rise of gastric mucosal blood flow (Holzer and Guth 1991; Katori et al. 1993; Grønbech and Lacy 1994; Holzer et al. 1994; Heinemann et al. 1996; Stroff et al. 1996). On the contrary, SP constricts gastric submucosal venules (Katori et al. 1993), which is consistent with the ability of tachykinins to decrease the vascular perfusion of the rat stomach (Heinemann et al. 1996; Stroff et al. 1996; Lippe et al. 1997). In addition, SP blocks the capsaicin-induced hyperemia through liberation of mast cell proteases that may degrade CGRP (Grønbech and Lacy 1994).

Gastric Mucosal Protection Afforded by Capsaicin-sensitive Afferents

The available evidence indicates that afferent nerve fibers do not regulate blood flow under basal conditions but come into play under emergency situations in which they improve the circulatory situation and support the protective forces of the gastric mucosa (Holzer 1998). This concept is supported by experimental findings showing that intragastric administration of capsaicin prevents experimental injury induced by factors such as stress, hemorrhagic shock, acid, acidified taurocholate, aspirin, indomethacin, and ethanol (Holzer 1998). The protective effect of capsaicin is shared by chili as examined in the rat (Kang et al. 1995a) and human (Yeoh et al. 1995) gastric mucosa.

Like the vasodilator response, the protective effect of intragastric capsaicin is prevented by defunctionalization of extrinsic afferent neurons, the $CGRP_1$ receptor antagonist $CGRP_{8-37}$, immunoneutralization of CGRP and inhibition of NO synthesis (Holzer et al. 1991b; Lambrecht et al. 1993; Peskar et al. 1993; Whittle 1993; Merchant et al. 1994). Tachykinins acting via NK_2 receptors are also involved in the capsaicin-induced protection, but not hyperemia, of the rat stomach (Stroff et al. 1996). The participation of CGRP and NO in the protective and vasodilator effects of capsaicin on the stomach points to a close relationship between the two processes but does not prove it. There is in fact evidence that mechanisms other than vasodilatation play a significant part in the gastroprotective action of sensory nerve stimulation (Stroff et al. 1996; Holzer 1998). The hyperemia-independent modes of action include inhibition of gastric emptying, dilution of injurious agents by gastric fluid secretion, inhibition of gastric acid secretion, and stimulation of bicarbonate and mucus output (Holzer 1998).

It is not only the acute defense against pending injury but also the repair of the injured gastric mucosa which are facilitated by sensory nerve stimulation. Whereas the process of rapid restitution of the surface epithelium is not directly governed by afferent neurons (Pabst et al. 1993), the healing of gastric ulcers induced by hydrochloric acid, acetic acid, or ethanol is delayed after sensory nerve ablation (Takeuchi et al. 1994; Tramontana et al. 1994; Peskar et al. 1995). Conversely, sensory nerve stimulation with low-dose capsaicin promotes the healing of acetic acid-induced ulcers (Kang et al. 1996).

Gastric Vasodilatation Evoked by Acid Backdiffusion

The implications of afferent neurons in the regulation of gastric mucosal blood flow and gastric mucosal resistance to injury are put into pathophysiological perspective if their role in the gastric response to acid challenge is considered. Acid backdiffusion, which ensues when the gastric mucosal barrier is disrupted with ethanol (Holzer et al. 1991a) or taurocholate (Takeuchi et al. 1993) in the presence of luminal acid, causes a quick rise of blood flow through the left gastric artery (Fig. 2) and gastric

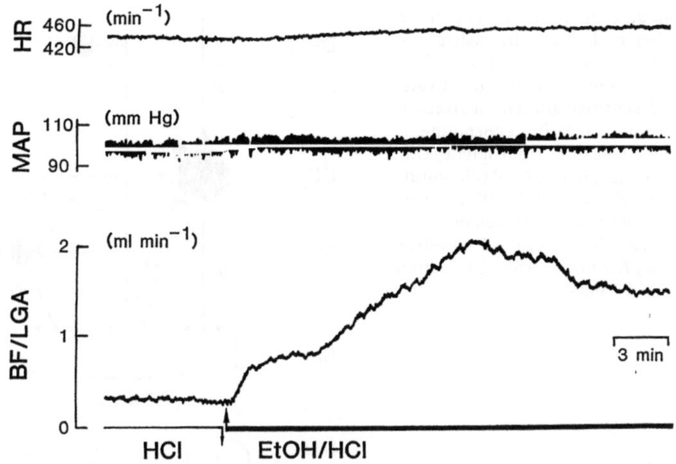

Fig. 2. Recording of the acid-evoked hyperemia in the left gastric artery of a urethane-anesthetized rat. The response was elicited by disruption of the gastric mucosal barrier with ethanol (EtOH, 15 %) in the presence of luminal acid (HCl, 0.15 M). The traces from the top to the bottom show heart rate (*HR*), mean arterial blood pressure (*MAP*), and blood flow in the left gastric artery (*BF/LGA*). Data from Holzer et al. (1994)

mucosa (Holzer et al. 1991a). This prompt response requires rapid signaling between the acid-threatened surface of the mucosa and the gastric resistance vessels, which is accomplished by neurons since the acid-evoked rise of gastric blood flow is inhibited by tetrodotoxin or pretreatment of rats with a neurotoxic dose of capsaicin (Holzer et al. 1991a, 1994).

The nerve fibers involved in the acid-induced hyperemia pass through the celiac ganglion and hence originate from spinal ganglia (Raybould et al. 1992). The inhibitory effects of tetrodotoxin (Holzer et al. 1991a) and the autonomic ganglion blocking drug hexamethonium (Holzer and Lippe 1992; Wachter et al. 1995) suggest that the acid-evoked hyperemia arises from a reflex-like mechanism the individual arcs and relays of which have not yet been identified. It is known, however, that the acid-evoked rise of gastric blood flow relies on intact pathways in the splanchnic nerves and through the celiac ganglion (Holzer and Lippe 1992; Wachter et al. 1995), whereas a contribution from noradrenergic neurons (Holzer and Lippe 1992) and postganglionic cholinergic neurons (Bruggeman et al. 1979; Holzer et al. 1991a) has been ruled out.

The involvement of ganglionic transmission and pathways running in the splanchnic nerves and through the celiac ganglion negates the originally proposed concept (Holzer et al. 1991a) that the gastric hyperemic response to acid backdiffusion results from an axon reflex between mucosal and submucosal collaterals of afferent neurons (Holzer and Lippe 1992; Holzer 1998). The main support for this conjecture came from the findings that acidification is able to cause a calcium-dependent release of CGRP from rat gastric tissue (Geppetti et al. 1991; Manela et al. 1995), that both CGRP and NO participate in the acid-evoked gastric hyperemia (Li et al. 1992; Lippe and Holzer 1992; Holzer et al. 1994; Merchant et al. 1995), and that in the rat stomach

Fig. 3. Diagram of the neural circuitry underlying the gastric hyperemia evoked by acid backdiffusion, which is likely to activate acid-sensitive afferent neurons in the mucosa. *ACh* acetylcholine; *ATP* adenosine triphosphate; *CG* celiac ganglion; *CGRP* calcitonin gene-related peptide; *DRG* dorsal root ganglion; *MP* myenteric plexus; *MU* mucosa; *NA* noradrenaline; *NO* nitric oxide; *SM* submucosa; *SP* substance P

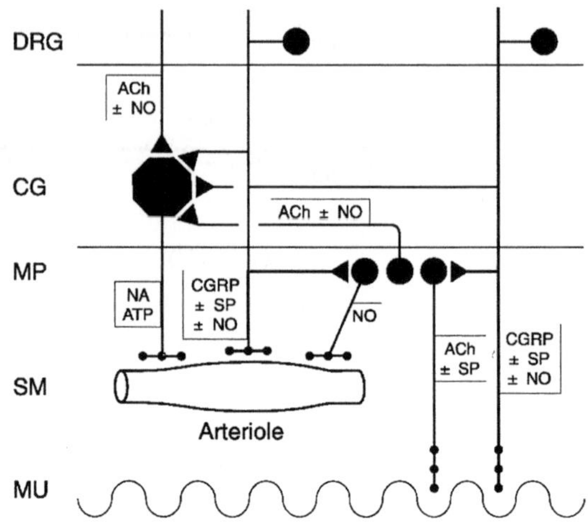

CGRP occurs in extrinsic afferents only (Green and Dockray 1988). However, there is no conclusive proof that CGRP and NO are in fact the final vasodilator messengers of the reflex pathways behind the acid-evoked hyperemia.

Since gastric acid backdiffusion does not appear to activate afferent pathways in the spinal cord (Schuligoi et al. 1996), it is proposed that the acid-induced rise of gastric blood flow is mediated by a peripheral reflex circuitry that is relayed in the celiac ganglion (Fig. 3). This hypothesis takes into account that prevertebral ganglia are important reflex centers in which sympathetic efferent, primary afferent, and intestinofugal enteric neurons interact in the regulation of gastrointestinal functions (Miolan and Niel 1996). In view of the available information it is postulated that CGRP and NO can operate at multiple sites within the vasodilator reflex arc (Fig. 3). Calcitonin gene-related peptide may act as messenger of primary afferents in the celiac ganglion and in the gastric resistance vessels. Nitric oxide may be released from preganglionic sympathetic, primary afferent, and intestinofugal enteric nerve fibers in the celiac ganglion (Furness and Anderson 1994; Domoto et al. 1995; Morales et al. 1995), from enteric (Ekblad et al. 1994; Reiche and Schemann 1998) and primary afferent (Domoto et al. 1995) nerve fibers around gastric resistance vessels, and from vascular endothelial cells.

Tachykinin NK_1 or NK_2 receptor antagonists do not alter the hyperemic response to gastric acid backdiffusion, whereas SP and NKA inhibit the acid-evoked rise of blood flow via activation of NK_2 receptors (Holzer et al. 1994; Heinemann et al. 1996, 1997). Since endogenous tachykinins released by acid backdiffusion depress the concomitant gastric vasodilatation, it seems that SP and/or NKA function as negative control factors (Heinemann et al. 1997). As with CGRP, it is not clear at which level tachykinins participate in the acid-evoked hyperemia, at the level of the celiac ganglion, or at the level of the gastric circulation. Histamine acting via histamine H_1 receptors (Holzer et al. 1991a) and H_2 receptors (unpublished observation), vasodilator prostanoids (Lippe and Holzer 1992), acetylcholine acting via muscarinic receptors (Holzer et al. 1991a), and noradrenaline (Holzer and Lippe 1992) have been ruled out as mediators of the hyperemic reaction to acid challenge of the rat stomach. Bradykinin plays some role, given that the bradykinin B_2 receptor antagonist HOE-140 attenuates the hyperemia elicited by barrier disruption in the presence of a high concentration of luminal acid (Pethö et al. 1994). It remains to be examined, though, whether bradykinin causes vasodilatation by its own or by stimulating the vasodilator reflex.

The physiological role of the hyperemic response to acid backdiffusion is to protect the mucosa from the formation of deep erosions and ulcers due to influxing acid and pepsin. The defensive nature of the vascular reaction is confirmed by the observation that inhibition of the acid-induced vasodilatation by tetrodotoxin, capsaicin pretreatment, morphine (Holzer et al. 1991a), $CGRP_{8-37}$ (Li et al. 1992), the bradykinin antagonist HOE-140 (Pethö et al. 1994), and NKA or SP (Heinemann et al. 1996) is associated with aggravation of gross and histological damage to the mucosa. By facilitating the disposal of acid, this rise of mucosal blood flow prevents the build-up of an injurious concentration of H^+ ions in the tissue and thus limits acid damage to the surface of the mucosa. The afferent nerve-mediated response to acid challenge thus reflects a neural emergency system which is called into operation when there is pending or actual injury to the stomach. In addition, the rise of gastric blood flow creates favorable conditions for rapid restitution and healing of the wounded mucosa (Takeuchi et al. 1994; Grønbech and Lacy 1996).

Somatic Vasoconstriction Evoked by Gastric Acid Backdiffusion

Gastric hyperemia in response to acid backdiffusion through a disrupted gastric mucosal barrier is aided by a reduction of blood flow to somatic vascular beds, e.g., those of the femoral artery (Wachter et al. 1995, 1998). Somatic vasoconstriction and gastric vasodilatation peak at different times and represent different entities with regard to pathways, mechanisms, and mediators. Further analysis has shown that it is the acid-induced gastric injury which gives rise to femoral vasoconstriction, because the gastric hyperemia evoked by intragastric capsaicin, which does not injure the mucosa, is not accompanied by a reduction of femoral blood flow (Wachter et al. 1995). Although in part dependent on the extrinsic innervation of the stomach, the gastric acid-evoked constriction of the femoral artery does not involve capsaicin-sensitive afferent neurons and remains unaltered after blockade of ganglionic transmission with hexamethonium, blockade of noradrenergic transmission with guanethidine, and ligation of the vascular supply to the adrenal glands (Wachter et al. 1995). Further experiments have shown that acid injury of the rat gastric mucosa is associated with luminal release of 5-hydroxytryptamine, that the femoral vasoconstrictor response to gastric acid injury is significantly attenuated by methiothepin, and that hence the neural and/or endocrine pathway leading to constriction of the femoral artery involves 5-hydroxytryptamine acting via 5-HT_1, 5-HT_2, and/or 5-HT_7 receptors (Wachter et al. 1998).

Pathophysiological Implications of Capsaicin-sensitive Afferents in Gastric Mucosal Homeostasis

The findings reviewed here prove the existence of a neural emergency system in the stomach, which is called into operation in the face of pending injury to the tissue but is not tonically active. In case of alarm, blood flow to the stomach is greatly augmented, an effect that facilitates the delivery of bicarbonate to the surface epithelium and overlying mucus layer, adds to the removal of injurious factors from the mucosa, and promotes a wide range of processes that either reduce the vulnerability, or aid the repair, of the gastric mucosa. Apart from facilitation of gastric blood flow, augmentation of bicarbonate and mucus secretion, and, under certain conditions, inhibition of acid output and motor activity also contribute to the overall protective role of afferent neurons (Holzer 1998). This neural emergency system acts in concert with other mechanisms of protection (Whittle 1993).

With the gastroprotective role of afferent neurons in mind it is logical to assume that improper functioning of this neural emergency system is liable to weaken the resistance of the tissue to injurious stimuli and thus may be an etiological factor in gastroduodenal ulcer disease (Fig. 4). Evidence in favor of this conjecture is indeed accumulating (Holzer 1998), as there are reports that either a prejunctional dysfunction of the afferent nerve fibers (sensory neuropathy) or a postjunctional defect in the effector mechanisms disturbs gastric mucosal homeostasis. It need be emphasized, though, that sensory neuropathies resulting from excessive intake of capsaicin-containing peppers are not known. On the contrary, it seems as if dietary chili intake is actually a factor that protects from peptic ulcer disease (Kang et al. 1995b).

The conjecture that sensory neuropathies weaken the defensive forces of the stomach is mirrored by the observation that defunctionalization of afferent neurons by a neurotoxic dose of capsaicin in experimental animals weakens the resistance of the gastric mucosa to injury and disturbs gastric mucosal homeostasis (Holzer 1998). Clinically relevant instances of sensory neuropathies affecting the stomach may be associated with bile reflux, aging, and diabetes (Fig. 4). Thus, chronic treatment of rats with oral taurocholate, to mimic chronic bile reflux, attenuates the capsaicin-evoked CGRP release and hyperemia in the gastric mucosa and weakens mucosal resistance to injury (Narita et al. 1995). Aging causes periarteriolar axons containing

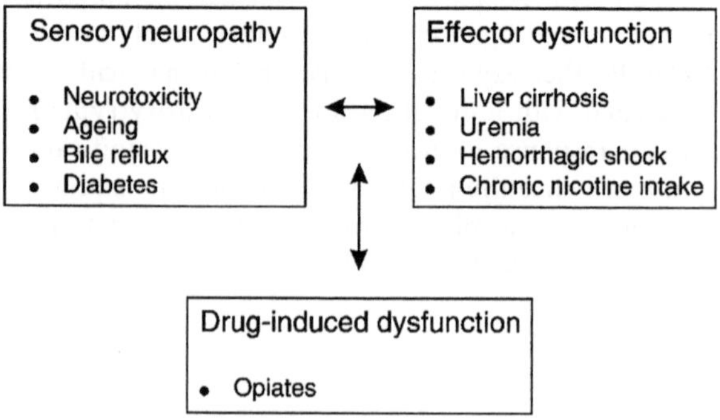

Fig. 4. Pathophysiological conditions associated with a malfunction of the neural alarm system in the gastric mucosa

CGRP to disappear from the rat stomach, which is associated with a decline in the capsaicin- and acid-evoked increase in mucosal blood flow and an impairment of gastric mucosal defense (Grønbech and Lacy 1995; Miyake et al. 1996). Sensory neuropathies arising from experimental diabetes also diminish CGRP release from nociceptive afferents in the rat stomach and lessen the ability of the gastric mucosa to defend itself against injury (Tashima et al. 1998).

Effector dysfunctions that prevent the neural emergency system from becoming operative have been observed in experimental situations involving chronic nicotine intake, cirrhosis, uremia, and hemorrhagic shock (Fig. 4). For instance, chronic intake of nicotine by rats suppresses the increase in mucosal blood flow due to gastric acid backdiffusion, possibly because the formation of vasoconstrictor leukotrienes in the rat stomach is considerably upregulated (Battistel et al. 1993). The gastropathy arising from experimental cirrhosis (Ferraz et al. 1995; Nishizaki et al. 1996) and uremia (Quintero et al. 1992) is associated with an inadequate rise of gastric mucosal blood flow in response to capsaicin or acid backdiffusion through a leaky gastric mucosal barrier. Since the supply of gastric submucosal arterioles by CGRP-containing nerve fibers is unchanged in experimental cirrhosis (Ferraz et al. 1995; Nishizaki et al. 1996) and uremia (Quintero et al. 1992) it is evident that the gastric circulatory dysregulation arises from an effector defect, possibly in the vascular NO/guanosine 3',5'-cyclic monophosphate signaling pathway (Ferraz et al. 1995).

The concept that a derangement of nociceptive neuron function contributes to ulcer disease is in keeping with the emerging role of sensory neurons in functional bowel disorders. From a medical point of view it is important to consider that drugs influencing the release, action, and metabolism of CGRP, NKA, and NO will interfere with the homeostatic function of afferent neurons in the stomach (Fig. 4). For instance, opioid receptor agonists such as morphine inhibit the release of peptide transmitters from afferent nerve fibers and in this way enhance the vulnerability of the gastric mucosa (Esplugues and Whittle 1990; Holzer 1998). From a therapeutic perspective it is obvious that future strategies to manage ulcer disease will need to take account of measures that secure and strengthen the neural alarm system in the gastric mucosa.

References

Bäck N, Ahonen M, Häppölä O, Kivilaakso E, Kiviluoto T (1994) Effect of vagotomy on expression of neuropeptides and histamine in rat oxyntic mucosa. Digest Dis Sci 39:353–361

Battistel M, Plebani M, Di Mario F, Joci M, Lippe IT, Holzer P (1993) Chronic nicotine intake causes vascular dysregulation in the rat gastric mucosa. Gut 34:1688–1692

Bruggeman TM, Wood JG, Davenport HW (1979) Local control of blood flow in the dog's stomach: vasodilatation caused by acid backdiffusion following topical application of salicylic acid. Gastroenterology 77:736–744

Caterina MJ, Schumacher MA, Tominaga M, Rosen TA, Levine JD, Julius D (1997) The capsaicin receptor: a heat-activated ion channel in the pain pathway. Nature 389:816–824

Chen RYZ, Guth PH (1995) Interaction of endogenous nitric oxide and CGRP in sensory neuron-induced gastric vasodilation. Am J Physiol 268:G791–G796

Chen RYZ, Li D-S, Guth PH (1992) Role of calcitonin gene-related peptide in capsaicin-induced gastric submucosal arteriolar dilation. Am J Physiol 262: H1350–H1355

Domoto T, Teramoto M, Tanigawa K, Tamura K, Yasui Y (1995) Origins of nerve fibers containing nitric oxide synthase in the rat celiac-superior mesenteric ganglion. Cell Tissue Res 281:215–221

Ekblad E, Mulder H, Uddman R, Sundler F (1994) NOS-containing neurons in the rat gut and coeliac ganglia. Neuropharmacology 33:1323–1331
Esplugues JV, Whittle BJR (1990) Morphine potentiation of ethanol-induced gastric mucosal damage in the rat. Role of local sensory afferent neurons. Gastroenterology 98:82–89
Ferraz JGP, McKnight W, Sharkey KA, Wallace JL (1995) Impaired vasodilatory responses in the gastric microcirculation of anesthetized rats with secondary biliary cirrhosis. Gastroenterology 108:1183–1191
Furness JB, Anderson CR (1994) Origins of nerve terminals containing nitric oxide synthase in the guinea-pig coeliac ganglion. J Auton Nerv Syst 46:47–54
Furness JB, Papka RE, Della NG, Costa M, Eskay RL (1982) Substance P-like immunoreactivity in nerves associated with the vascular system of guinea-pigs. Neuroscience 7:447–459
Gates TS, Zimmerman RP, Mantyh CR, Vigna SR, Mantyh PW (1989) Calcitonin gene-related peptide-receptor binding sites in the gastrointestinal tract. Neuroscience 31:757–770
Geppetti P, Tramontana M, Evangelista S, Renzi D, Maggi CA, Fusco BM, Del Bianco E (1991) Differential effect on neuropeptide release of different concentrations of hydrogen ions on afferent and intrinsic neurons of the rat stomach. Gastroenterology 101:1505–1511
Green T, Dockray GJ (1988) Characterization of the peptidergic afferent innervation of the stomach in the rat, mouse, and guinea-pig. Neuroscience 25:181–193
Grønbech JE, Lacy ER (1994) Substance P attenuates gastric mucosal hyperemia after stimulation of sensory neurons in the rat stomach. Gastroenterology 106:440–449
Grønbech JE, Lacy ER (1995) Role of gastric blood flow in impaired defense and repair of aged rat stomachs. Am J Physiol 269:G737–G744
Grønbech JE, Lacy ER (1996) Role of sensory afferent neurons in hypertonic damage and restitution of the rat gastric mucosa. Gastroenterology 111:1474–1483
Hayashi H, Ohsumi K, Ueda N, Fujiwara M, Mizuno N (1982) Effect of spinal ganglionectomy on substance P-like immunoreactivity in the gastroduodenal tract of cats. Brain Res 232:227–230
Heinemann Á, Joci M, Herzeg G, Holzer P (1996) Tachykinin inhibition of acid-induced gastric hyperaemia in the rat. Br J Pharmacol 119:1525–1532
Heinemann Á, Sattler V, Joci M, Holzer P (1997) Inhibition of acid-induced hyperaemia in the rat stomach by endogenous NK_2 receptor ligands. Neurosci Lett 237:133–135
Helliwell RJA, McLatchie LM, Clarke M, Winter J, Bevan S, McIntyre P (1998) Capsaicin sensitivity is associated with the expression of the vanilloid (capsaicin) receptor (VR1) mRNA in adult rat sensory ganglia. Neurosci Lett 250:177–180
Holzer P (1991) Capsaicin: cellular targets, mechanisms of action, and selectivity for thin sensory neurons. Pharmacol Rev 43:143–201
Holzer P (1998) Neural emergency system in the stomach. Gastroenterology 114:823–839
Holzer P, Guth PH (1991) Neuropeptide control of rat gastric mucosal blood flow. Increase by calcitonin gene-related peptide and vasoactive intestinal polypeptide, but not substance P and neurokinin A. Circ Res 68:100–105
Holzer P, Lippe IT (1992) Gastric mucosal hyperemia due to acid backdiffusion depends on splanchnic nerve activity. Am J Physiol 262:G505–G509
Holzer P, Peskar BM, Peskar BA, Amann R (1990) Release of calcitonin gene-related peptide induced by capsaicin in the vascularly perfused rat stomach. Neurosci Lett 108:195–200
Holzer P, Livingston EH, Guth PH (1991a) Sensory neurons signal for an increase in rat gastric mucosal blood flow in the face of pending acid injury. Gastroenterology 101:416–423
Holzer P, Livingston EH, Saria A, Guth PH (1991b) Sensory neurons mediate protective vasodilatation in rat gastric mucosa. Am J Physiol 260:G363–G370
Holzer P, Lippe IT, Joci M, Wachter C, Erb R, Heinemann Á (1993) Nitric oxide-dependent and -independent hyperaemia due to calcitonin gene-related peptide in the rat stomach. Br J Pharmacol 110:404–410
Holzer P, Wachter C, Joci M, Heinemann Á (1994) Vascular bed-dependent roles of the peptide CGRP and nitric oxide in acid-evoked hyperaemia of the rat stomach. J Physiol Lond 480:575–585
Kang JY, Teng CH, Chen FC (1996) Effect of capsaicin and cimetidine on the healing of acetic acid induced gastric ulceration in the rat. Gut 38:832–836
Kang JY, Teng CH, Wee A, Chen FC (1995a) Effect of capsaicin and chilli on ethanol induced gastric mucosal injury in the rat. Gut 36:664–669
Kang JY, Yeoh KG, Chia HP, Lee HP, Chia YW, Guan R, Yap I (1995b) Chili: protective factor against peptic ulcer? Dig Dis Sci 40:576–579
Katori M, Ohno T, Nishiyama K (1993) Interaction of substance P and leukotriene C_4 in ethanol-induced mucosal injury of rat stomach. Regul Pept 46:241–243
Lambrecht N, Burchert M, Respondek M, Müller KM, Peskar BM (1993) Role of calcitonin gene-related peptide and nitric oxide in the gastroprotective effect of capsaicin in the rat. Gastroenterology 104:1371–1380

Leung FW (1993) Inhibition of spinal afferent nerve-mediated gastric hyperemia by nicotine: role of ganglionic blockade. Am J Physiol 264:H1087–H1092
Li D-S, Raybould HE, Quintero E, Guth PH (1991) Role of calcitonin gene-related peptide in gastric hyperemic response to intragastric capsaicin. Am J Physiol 261:G657–G661
Li D-S, Raybould HE, Quintero E, Guth PH (1992) Calcitonin gene-related peptide mediates the gastric hyperemic response to acid backdiffusion. Gastroenterology 102:1124–1128
Lindh B, Hökfelt T, Elfvin L-G (1988) Distribution and origin of peptide-containing nerve fibers in the celiac superior mesenteric ganglion of the guinea-pig. Neuroscience 26:1037–1071
Lippe IT, Holzer P (1992) Participation of endothelium-derived nitric oxide but not prostacyclin in the gastric mucosal hyperaemia due to acid backdiffusion. Br J Pharmacol 105:708–714
Lippe IT, Lorbach M, Holzer P (1989) Close arterial infusion of calcitonin gene-related peptide into the rat stomach inhibits aspirin- and ethanol-induced hemorrhagic damage. Regul Pept 26:35–46
Lippe IT, Wachter CH, Holzer P (1997) Neurokinin A-induced vasoconstriction and muscular contraction in the rat isolated stomach: mediation by distinct and unusual neurokinin$_2$ receptors. J Pharmacol Exp Ther 281:1294–1302
Ma RC, Szurszewski JH (1996) Modulation by opioid peptides of mechanosensory pathways supplying the guinea-pig inferior mesenteric ganglion. J Physiol Lond 491:435–445
Manela FD, Ren J, Gao J, McGuigan JE, Harty RF (1995) Calcitonin gene-related peptide modulates acid-mediated regulation of somatostatin and gastrin release from rat antrum. Gastroenterology 109:701–706
Merchant NB, Dempsey DT, Grabowski MW, Rizzo M, Ritchie WP (1994) Capsaicin-induced gastric mucosal hyperemia and protection: the role of calcitonin gene-related peptide. Surgery 116:419–425
Merchant NB, Goodman J, Dempsey DT, Milner RE, Ritchie WP (1995) The role of calcitonin gene-related peptide and nitric oxide in gastric mucosal hyperemia and protection. J Surg Res 58:344–350
Miolan JP, Niel JP (1996) The mammalian sympathetic prevertebral ganglia: integrative properties and role in the nervous control of digestive tract motility. J Auton Nerv Syst 58:125–138
Miyake H, Inaba N, Kato S, Takeuchi K (1996) Increased susceptibility of rat gastric mucosa to ulcerogenic stimulation with aging: role of capsaicin-sensitive sensory neurons. Dig Dis Sci 41:339–345
Morales MA, Holmberg K, Xu ZQ, Cozzari C, Hartman BK, Emson P, Goldstein M, Elfvin LG, Hökfelt T (1995) Localization of choline acetyltransferase in rat peripheral sympathetic neurons and its coexistence with nitric oxide synthase and neuropeptides. Proc Natl Acad Sci USA 92:11819–11823
Narita M, Takahashi S, Takeuchi K, Okabe S (1995) Desensitization of capsaicin-sensitive sensory neurons in rat stomachs on chronic treatment with sodium taurocholate. Jap J Pharmacol 67:321–328
Nishizaki Y, Guth PH, Sternini C, Kaunitz JD (1996) Impairment of the gastric hyperemic response to luminal acid in cirrhotic rats. Am J Physiol 270:G71-G78
Pabst MA, Schöninkle E, Holzer P (1993) Ablation of capsaicin-sensitive afferent nerves impairs defence but not rapid repair of rat gastric mucosa. Gut 34:897–903
Perry MJ, Lawson SN (1998) Differences in expression of oligosaccharides, neuropeptides, carbonic anhydrase and neurofilament in rat primary afferent neurons retrogradely labelled via skin, muscle or visceral nerves. Neuroscience 85:293–310
Peskar BM, Lambrecht N, Stroff T, Respondek M, Müller K-M (1995) Functional ablation of sensory neurons impairs healing of acute gastric mucosal damage in rats. Dig Dis Sci 40:2460–2464
Peskar BM, Wong HC, Walsh JH, Holzer P (1993) A monoclonal antibody to calcitonin gene-related peptide abolishes capsaicin-induced gastroprotection. Eur J Pharmacol 250:201–203
Pethö G, Joci M, Holzer P (1994) Role of bradykinin in the hyperaemia following acid challenge of the rat gastric mucosa. Br J Pharmacol 113:1036–1042
Quintero E, Kaunitz J, Nishizaki Y, Giorgio R de, Sternini C, Guth PH (1992) Uremia increases gastric mucosal permeability and acid backdiffusion injury in the rat. Gastroenterology 103:1762–1768
Raybould HE, Sternini C, Eysselein VE, Yoneda M, Holzer P (1992) Selective ablation of spinal afferent neurons containing CGRP attenuates gastric hyperemic response to acid. Peptides 13:249–254
Reiche D, Schemann M (1998) Ascending choline acetyltransferase and descending nitric oxide synthase immunoreactive neurones of the myenteric plexus project to the mucosa of the guinea pig gastric corpus. Neurosci Lett 241:61–64
Schuligoi R, Herzeg G, Wachter C, Joci M, Holzer P (1996) Differential expression of c-fos messenger RNA in the rat spinal cord after mucosal and serosal irritation of the stomach. Neuroscience 72:535–544
Sternini C (1992) Enteric and visceral afferent CGRP neurons. Targets of innervation and differential expression patterns. Ann NY Acad Sci 657:170–186
Stroff T, Plate S, Seyed Ebrahim J, Ehrlich K-H, Respondek M, Peskar BM (1996) Tachykinin-induced increase in gastric mucosal resistance: role of primary afferent neurons, CGRP, and NO. Am J Physiol 271:G1017–G1027

Su HC, Bishop AE, Power RF, Hamada Y, Polak JM (1987) Dual intrinsic and extrinsic origins of CGRP- and NPY-immunoreactive nerves of rat gut and pancreas. J Neurosci 7:2674–2687
Suzuki T, Kagoshima M, Shibata M, Inaba N, Onodera S, Yamaura T, Shimada H (1997) Effects of several denervation procedures on distribution of calcitonin gene-related peptide and substance P immunoreactive fibers in rat stomach. Dig Dis Sci 42:1242–1254
Szallasi A (1994) The vanilloid (capsaicin) receptor: receptor types and species differences. Gen Pharmacol 25:223–243
Takeuchi K, Ohuchi T, Narita M, Okabe S (1993) Capsaicin-sensitive sensory nerves in recovery of gastric mucosal integrity after damage by sodium taurocholate in rats. Jap J Pharmacol 63:479–485
Takeuchi K, Ueshima K, Ohuchi T, Okabe S (1994) The role of capsaicin-sensitive sensory neurons in healing of HCl-induced gastric mucosal lesions in rats. Gastroenterology 106:1524–1532
Tashima K, Korolkiewicz R, Kubomi M, Takeuchi K (1998) Increased susceptibility of gastric mucosa to ulcerogenic stimulation in diabetic rats: role of capsaicin-sensitive sensory neurons. Br J Pharmacol 124:1395–1402
Tramontana M, Renzi D, Calabro A, Panerai C, Milani S, Surrenti C, Evangelista S (1994) Influence of capsaicin-sensitive afferent fibers on acetic acid-induced chronic gastric ulcers in rats. Scand J Gastroenterol 29:406–413
Wachter C, Heinemann Á, Joci M, Holzer P (1995) Visceral vasodilatation and somatic vasoconstriction evoked by acid challenge of the rat gastric mucosa:diversity of mechanisms. J Physiol Lond 486:505–516
Wachter CH, Heinemann Á, Donnerer J, Pabst MA, Holzer P (1998) Mediation by 5-hydroxytryptamine of the femoral vasoconstriction induced by acid challenge of the rat gastric mucosa. J Physiol Lond 509:541–550
Whittle BJR (1993) Neuronal and endothelium-derived mediators in the modulation of the gastric microcirculation: integrity in the balance. Br J Pharmacol 110:3–17
Whittle BJR, Lopez-Belmonte J, Moncada S (1992) Nitric oxide mediates rat mucosal vasodilatation induced by intragastric capsaicin. Eur J Pharmacol 218:339–341
Wood J (1993) Capsaicin in the study of pain. Academic Press, London
Yeoh KG, Kang JY, Yap I, Guan R, Tan CC, Wee A, Teng CH (1995) Chili protects against aspirin-induced gastroduodenal mucosal injury in humans. Dig Dis Sci 40:580–583

INVITED ARTICLE

Intensive Care Pharmacotherapy: Stress Ulcer Prophylaxis and Mucosecretolysis

B. M. W. Schmidt · M. Wehling

Institute for Clinical Pharmacology, Faculty for Clinical Medicine Mannheim, Ruprecht-Karls-University Heidelberg, Theodor-Kutzer-Ufer 1–3, 68135 Mannheim, Germany

Abstract. Drugs to prevent stress ulcers and secretolytics belong to the standard therapy in intensive care units (ICUs). Despite their wide use, evidence from clinical trials for both interventions is inconclusive or missing. Evidence of a mortality or at least morbidity lowering potency is mandatory for therapies in evidence based medicine; the latter should be assessed not only by the incidence of a specific complication, e.g., upper gastrointestinal bleeding or pneumonia, but by the integral outcome as measured by shortening of the stay on the ICU.

Stress Ulcer Prophylaxis. As natural-history studies have shown that the incidence of upper gastrointestinal bleeding is very low in an overall population of critically ill patients, it has been suggested that prophylaxis should be focused on patients at high risk only, i.e., patients on mechanical ventilation who additionally suffer from coagulopathies or sustained shock. This is underlined by a recent meta-analysis which showed no benefit regarding mortality either for H_2 antagonists, sucralfate, or antacids in comparison with placebo in ICU patients in general. Stress ulcer prophylaxis with the H_2 antagonist ranitidine has been shown to prevent more clinically relevant upper gastrointestinal bleedings than sucralfate in a very recent randomized double-blinded study in approximately 1000 patients requiring mechanical ventilation; however, the median duration of the stay in the intensive care unit was equal in both study groups and mortality was even slightly higher in the ranitidine group. The study was lacking a placebo control. At the moment there is no clear evidence as to who requires stress ulcer prophylaxis and which drug should be used. Further studies are necessary to elucidate the subgroup of patients on the ICU who might benefit from stress ulcer prophylaxis and which drug should be used. At present, sucralfate appears to be favorable solely on the grounds of costs being lower than for H_2 antagonists.

Mucosecretolysis. Mucosecretolysis by N-acetylcysteine (NAC) and ambroxol is widely used in ICUs under prophylactic aspects. In addition, NAC is used in patients suffering from septic shock and/or acute respiratory distress syndrome (ARDS) under curative auspices. However, as most studies did not show either positive effects in preventive use or in the use in patients suffering from ARDS or septic shock, the use of both drugs cannot be recommended, despite the low profile of side effects. It may be appropriate to use ambroxol per inhalationem which has been clearly shown to liquefy mucous plugs and help expectoration. In conclusion, both stress ulcer prophylaxis and secretolysis in the ICU should be used restrictively, as no unequivocal evidence of beneficial effects has been provided up to now, and subgroup identification of high-risk patients may be essential for its proper use.

M. K. Herbert et al. (Eds.), Problems of the Gastrointestinal Tract in Anesthesia...

Stress-related Upper Gastrointestinal Bleeding

Incidence of Stress-related Upper Gastrointestinal Bleeding

Over the past decades the incidence of stress-related upper gastrointestinal bleeding (SRUGB) in hospitalized patients has decreased markedly (Navab and Steingrub 1995). In previous studies the incidence of SRUGB was up to 30 %. Studies in the 1990s have shown incidences around 1 %. Cook et al. (1994) studied 2252 patients (674 receiving stress ulcer prophylaxis) admitted to ICUs. Of these patients 33 (1.5 %) had clinically relevant bleeding, which was defined as an overt bleeding with either hypotension or the need for blood transfusion. In contrast, Zandstra and Stoutenbeek (1994) studied patients treated with mechanical ventilation ($n = 183$) without stress ulcer prophylaxis, representing a group at even higher risk for SRUGB, and reported an incidence of 0.6 %, which is surprisingly low (potential reasons are discussed later).

In fact, the low incidence of SRGUB makes it necessary to define further risk factors to sufficiently justify the requirements of sufficient prophylaxis and the economic needs.

Risk Factors of SRUGB

Multiple risk factors for SRGUB have been proposed:
1. Recent history of peptic ulcer
2. Sustained shock
3. Sepsis
4. Multiple trauma
5. Burns over more than 30 % of body surface
6. Head injury and central nervous disorders
7. Mechanical ventilation
8. Coagulopathy

Mechanical ventilation and coagulopathy have been defined as the major risk factors by multiple regression analysis (Cook et al. 1994). However, in this study approximately 50 % of the patients had cardiovascular surgery. Therefore, these results might not be representative, e.g., for trauma patients or patients with major burns. Scores which have been developed to characterize patients at high risk for SRUGB remain questionable concerning their usefulness (Navab and Steingrub 1995).

Characteristics of the Drugs Used for Prophylaxis

The drugs most frequently used for prophylaxis of SRUGB are antacids, H_2 antagonists (ranitidine, famotidine, and others), and sucralfate. Despite the recent observation that proton pump inhibitors are feasible for prophylaxis (Phillips et al. 1996), they have not yet been used extensively. This is probably due to their high costs.

Table 1. Antacids

Substance(s)	Trade name	Acid-binding capacity (g/50 mmol)
Aluminum hydroxide	Amphojel, Aludrox (Wyeth, Münster, Germany)	28
Aluminum phosphate	Phosphalugel (Yamanouchi, Heidelberg, Germany)	325
Aluminum hydroxide + magnesium hydroxide	Maalox, Maaloxan (Natterman, Cologne, Germany)	19
Magaldrat ($Al_5Mg_{10}OHSO_4$)	Riopan (Byk-Gulden, Konstanz, Germany)	25
Hydrotalcit [$Mg_6Al_2(OH)_{16}$*CO_3]	Talcid (Bayer Vital, Leverkusen, Germany	37

Antacids

Antacids are weak basic substances which form insoluble salts with hydrochloric acids. They consist of an anionic (hydroxide, phosphate, silicate, or carbonate) and of a cationic part (calcium, magnesium, or aluminum). The main mechanism of action is the elevation of the pH of gastric juice to levels which do not cause peptic injury to the mucosa and prevent activation of pepsinogen. Furthermore, antacids bind pepsin and biliary acids. Table 1 shows the relative efficacy of different antacids. Dosage depends on the antacid used. It is important to choose very narrow dosing intervals, e.g., every 2 h. This and potential side effects (constipation) limit the use of these compounds.

H_2 Antagonists

Histamine is the major messenger in the final common pathway of all stimulants of acid secretion. H_2 antagonists, which block the H_2 receptors of parietal cells, are effective in inhibiting gastric acid secretion. This is true for the basal, nocturnal, food- and pentagastrin-stimulated acid secretion. The H_2 antagonist most widely used is ranitidine. Ranitidine shows less side effects especially with regard to drug interactions and antiandrogen properties than cimetidine, the first available member of this class of drugs. Ranitidine is approximately four to five times as potent as cimetidine. Famotidine (20 times more potent than cimetidine) also shows a favorable pattern of side effects and has been used for prophylaxis of SRUGB. The recommended dosages for prophylaxis of SRUGB for ranitidine are 50 mg b.i.d. or t.i.d. or 0.125–0.25 mg/kg body weight as continuous infusion or 20 mg b.i.d. for famotidine (Gramatté and Hinrichsen 1996). Other H_2 antagonists are nizatidine and roxatidine, which are comparable to ranitidine and famotidine, but are not commonly used. The pharmacokinetic parameters of H_2 antagonists are provided in Table 2. Side effects of H_2 antagonists relevant in the setting of an ICU are skin rash, constipation, and diarrhea. In the case of famotidine mental confusion has been observed occasionally, especially in elderly patients (Piper et al. 1997).

Table 2. Pharmacokinetic parameters of H_2 antagonists

Drug	Half-life of terminal elimination (h)	Protein binding (%)	Volume of distribution (L per 70 kg)	Renal elimination (%)
Cimetidine	2	20	91	70
Ranitidine	2	15	105	70
Famotidine	3	16	84	80
Nizatidine	1.4	30	91	60
Roxatidine	6[a]	6	1190[a]	60

[a]Data are for active metabolite (parent drug not detectable) adapted from Taeschner and Vozeh (1997)

Sucralfate

Sucralfate is a basic aluminum salt of sulfated sucrose. At an acidic pH it forms a viscous paste, which adheres to the gastric mucosa, especially at ulcer surfaces, thereby inhibiting further peptic damage. Sucralfate decreases pepsin activity and absorbs bile acids. Furthermore, cytoprotective effects have been suggested, i.e., increasing of mucosal prostaglandin E_2 synthesis with an increase in bicarbonate and mucus secretion (Ligumsky et al. 1984). Sucralfate has no acid-binding properties and acts locally. Approximately 90 % is excreted in the faces and only 2 % is excreted in the urine. Side effects include urticaria and constipation. The occurrence of bezoars has been reported, especially when nasogastric tubes are used (Schneider and Ouellette 1984). The recommended dosages for prophylaxis of SRUGB is 1 g every 4 h (Gramatté and Hinrichsen, 1996), while in a very recent study an interval of 6 h was chosen (Cook et al. 1998).

Results of Clinical Studies on Prophylaxis of SRUGB

A large number of clinical studies have been conducted dealing with prophylaxis of SRUGB. A major problem of these trials is the definition of gastrointestinal bleeding and, looking at the possible complications of gastric pH-altering prophylaxis, nosocomial pneumonia.

Efficacy of Prophylaxis

The problems in interpreting these studies have been documented by the conflicting results of meta-analyses by Cook et al. (1991a,b) and Tryba (1991). This uncertainty has led to an integrated meta-analysis published more recently (Cook et al 1996), which aimed to sort out the problems of the former meta-analyses. The endpoints focused on in this meta-analysis were (a) overt bleeding, (b) clinically important bleeding, (c) pneumonia, and (d) mortality.

Overt bleeding was defined as hematemesis, melena, bloody gastric aspirate, or hematochezia. Bleeding was assessed to be "clinically important" if a drop in blood pressure of 20 mmHg within 24 h or a drop in blood pressure of 10 mmHg accompa-

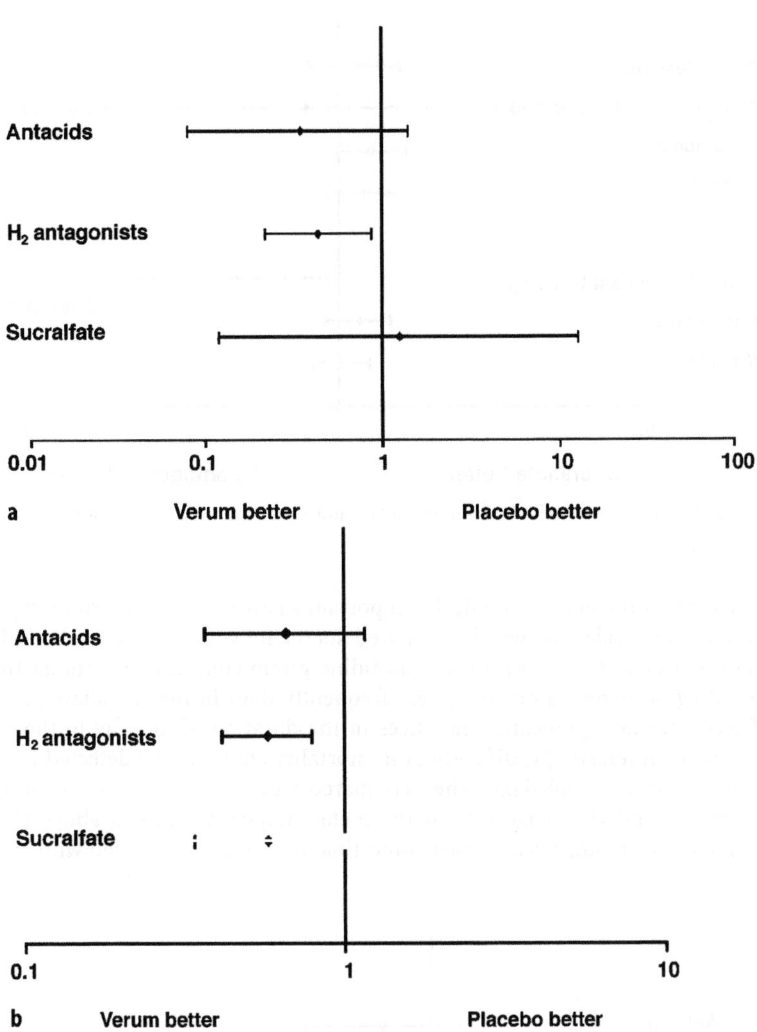

Fig. 1. **a** Incidence of clinically important gastrointestinal bleeding (after Cook et al. 1996). **b** Incidence of overt bleeding (after Cook et al. 1996)

nied by a rise in heart rate by 20 bpm on orthostasis occurred, or if hemoglobin decreased by 20 g/L or blood transfusion or surgery were required.

Figure 1 shows the results for the endpoint "clinically important gastrointestinal bleeding" and "overt bleeding" when the active drug (either antacid, H_2 antagonist or sucralfate) was compared with placebo. Only in the case of H_2 antagonists was a significant lower odds ratio observed in the endpoint "clinically important gastrointestinal bleeding". However, only one study was analyzed which compared sucralfate and placebo. Comparison of sucralfate and H_2 antagonists in this meta-analysis revealed a tendency to a lower incidence of overt bleeding under prophylaxis with sucralfate

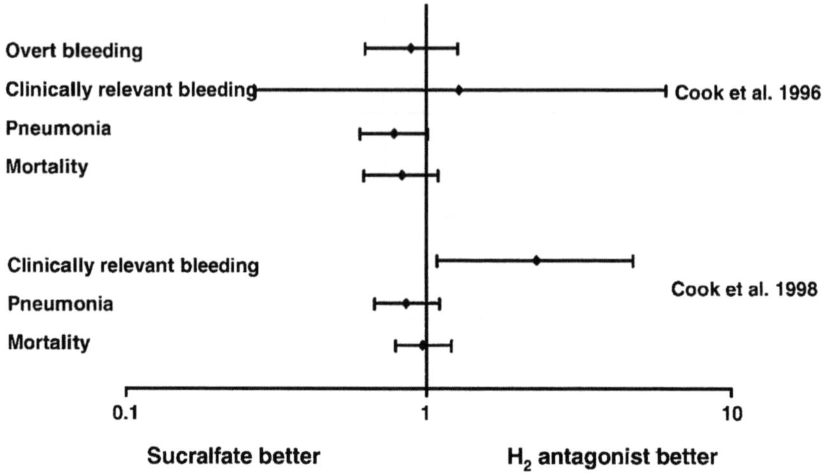

Fig. 2. Comparison of the efficacy of sucralfate and H_2 antagonists. (After Cook et al. 1996, 1998)

but a higher incidence of clinically important gastrointestinal bleeding (Fig. 2). A very recent large-scale trial which compared sucralfate with ranitidine showed divergent results (Cook et al. 1998). In the ranitidine group clinically relevant gastrointestinal bleeding occurred significantly less frequently than in the sucralfate group (Fig. 2). There were no significant differences in the duration of the stay in the ICU and in mortality. Interestingly, differences in mortality could not be detected for any of the drugs used for prophylaxis when compared with placebo or for the comparison of sucralfate and H_2 antagonists in the meta-analysis mentioned above (Fig. 3). This might be surprising because gastrointestinal bleeding is associated with an high mor-

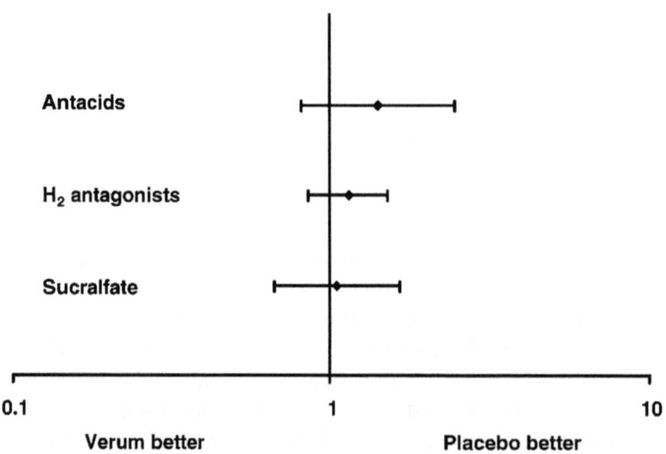

Fig. 3. Mortality of critically ill patients as measure for efficacy of prophylaxis of stress-related upper gastrointestinal bleeding (SRUGB). (After Cook et al. 1996)

tality in critically ill patients. Obviously the high mortality is not a consequence of gastrointestinal bleeding, but gastrointestinal bleeding is the result of the severity of the illness leading to death.

Late-onset Pneumonia

In the early 1980s there was rising evidence for a higher incidence of nosocomial pneumonia in patients treated with drugs lowering gastric pH. In a controlled study Prod'hom et al (1994) assessed prophylaxis with an antacid (aluminum hydroxide + magnesium hydroxide), sucralfate and ranitidine for the incidence of early- and late-onset pneumonia, gastrointestinal bleeding and gastric bacterial colonization. They showed that among the patients observed for more than 4 days pneumonia developed significantly less often in the sucralfate group. Furthermore, 84 % of the patients suffering from late-onset pneumonia were found to have gastric colonization with the same bacteria causing pneumonia. This finding was consistent with the theory that increasing gastric pH leads to gastric colonization with pathogenic, predominantly gram-negative bacteria, which then cause pneumonia via tracheal colonization. The connection between high gastric pH and late-onset nosocomial pneumonia is supported by the finding that patients on sucralfate who develop a rise in gastric pH above pH 4, due to "gastric exocrine failure", were at the same risk as the patients in the other groups.

In the meta-analysis mentioned above (Cook et al. 1996) the comparison of sucralfate and H_2 antagonists revealed also a tendency towards a lower incidence of pneumonia with sucralfate, but a recent study by the same group (Cook et al. 1998) did not confirm this effect (Fig. 2).

Cost-effectiveness of Prophylaxis

Taking into consideration that mortality is not influenced by prophylaxis of SRUGB, the question arises of whether prophylactic therapy might be cost-effective, i.e., whether the potential shortening of the stay in the ICU can outweigh the costs of therapy. This issue has been addressed in some studies.

There are three factors influencing the result of cost-effectiveness analyses for any drug used in prophylaxis of SRUGB: (a) the cost of the therapy itself; (b) the incidence of SRUGB and the costs of its treatment; and (c) the incidence of nosocomial pneumonia and the costs of its treatment.

An intervention is inexpensive if the net costs of the medication are low, the effect in lowering the incidence of SRUGB is high, and the induction of nosocomial pneumonia is rare. The most important factor is the natural incidence of SRUGB (Ben-Menachem et al. 1996). In low-risk patients prophylaxis is expensive because the costs per bleeding period averted are high. The opposite is true in patients at high risk. In the analysis of Ben-Menachem et al. (1996) costs ranged from US$ 521 005 per bleeding period averted assuming a 10 % reduction of an underlying risk of 0.1 % down to a saving of US$ 419 assuming a 90 % reduction of an underlying risk of 33 % for sucralfate (Fig. 4). In this study the costs of ranitidine were estimated to be 6.5 times higher than those of sucralfate.

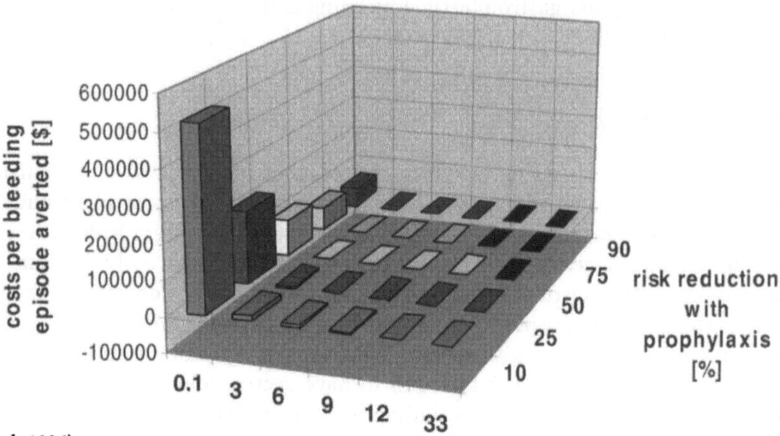

ıachem et al. 1996)

Another analysis was to estimate the cost-effectiveness of different drugs by using pooled data of efficacy from the literature (Schumock et al. 1996). This study estimates the costs per acute gastrointestinal bleeding averted ranging from savings of $7373 and $4321 in the case of sucralfate and antacids, respectively, to expenditures of $7374 for cimetidine. The major problem of this analysis is that a very small effect of H_2 antagonists is used for the calculation. Thus, the costs of prophylaxis with H_2 antagonists are overestimated. It is very important to perform a cost-effectiveness analysis based on the very recent study by Cook et al. (1998). Until such an analysis is available, sucralfate seems to be the more appropriate drug based on costs.

Other Factors Influencing Incidence of SRUGB

Early Enteric Feeding

Early enteric feeding has been shown to be effective in preventing SRUGB in severely burned patients, who are at the highest risk for the development of SRUGB (Raff et al. 1997). Therefore, early enteric feeding should be a major goal in each critically ill patient, thus reducing the need for prophylaxis.

Intensive Care Therapy

The surprising results of the study by Zandstra and Stoutenbeek (1994) have already been mentioned. There have been some explanations for the very low incidence of SRUGB in the high-risk group of mechanically ventilated ICU patients. One important therapeutic element might have been corticosteroid therapy, which was routinely delivered in this study. The positive effect of the steroids might be due to their protective effects against the membrane-destroying effects of hypoxia (Tryba 1994). Furthermore, the early use of vasodilators and adequate volume replacement may have contributed to the low incidence of SRUGB by shortening the time of hypoperfusion and shock.

In the future the achievements of intensive care medicine might further reduce the need for prophylaxis against SRUGB.

Conclusion

At the moment there is no clear evidence as to who requires stress ulcer prophylaxis and which drug should be used. Further studies are necessary to elucidate the subgroup of patients on the ICU who might benefit from stress ulcer prophylaxis and which drug should be used. At present, sucralfate appears to be favorable on the grounds of costs being lower than for H_2 antagonists. On the basis of the current knowledge clinical practice guidelines have been developed which aim at providing adequate therapy at reasonable costs (Fig. 5; Pitimana-aree et al. 1998). We suggest slight modifications of this algorithm by defining two groups of underlying conditions: severe and non-severe. Severe conditions would be a current history of ulcer disease, brain injury, more than three conditions, and any protracted course of the individual conditions given in the algorithm. In the presence of severe conditions we prefer H_2 antagonists, and in the presence of non-severe conditions prophylaxis should be performed with sucralfate. These guidelines should be under current

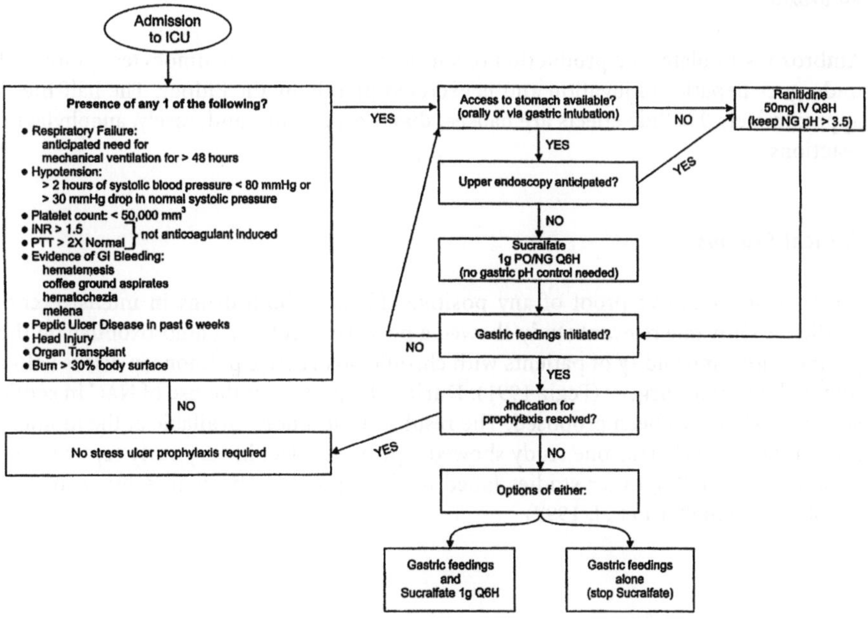

Fig. 5. Algorithm of a practice guideline for SRUGB prophylaxis. *INR* international normalized ratio; *PTT* partial thromboplastin time; *PO* by mouth; *NG* nasogastric. (From Pitimana-aree et al. 1998)

review and the results of further studies must be implemented. Furthermore, one should be aware that adequate and sufficient intensive therapy of shock and other serious conditions is the best prophylaxis of SRUGB.

Mucosecretolysis

Mucosecretolysis with N-acetylcysteine (NAC) and ambroxol is widely used in ICUs under prophylactic aspects. In addition, NAC is used in patients suffering from septic shock and/or ARDS under curative auspices.

Characteristics of the Drugs Used for Prophylaxis

N-Acetylcysteine

N-Acetylcysteine acts as a mucolytic by splitting disulfide bonds. Furthermore, it acts directly as a free radical scavenger, restores glutathione stores, and inhibits neutrophil aggregation and tumor necrosis factor production. The terminal half-life is approximately 6 h, NAC being excreted mainly renally in the form of inactive metabolites. Side effects are nausea, diarrhea, stomatitis, allergic reactions, and anaphylaxis. Inhalative use of NAC in asthma may precipitate bronchospasm.

Ambroxol

Ambroxol stimulates the production of surfactant in type-II pneumocytes. Ambroxol undergoes hepatic conjugation and is excreted mainly by the kidney. The half-life is approximately 9 h. Side effects are nausea, diarrhea, eczema, and, rarely, anaphylactic reactions.

Clinical Studies

There is no definitive proof of any positive effects of both drugs in intensive care medicine. Only one relevant study showed a positive effect of 1 g ambroxol/day on the postoperative morbidity of patients with chronic obstructive pulmonary disease after upper abdominal surgery (Fegiz 1991). During the past years the use of NAC in septic shock or ARDS has been proposed. The results of the studies available at the moment are conflicting: Whereas one study showed a positive effect in very early septic shock (Spapen et al. 1998), other studies failed to show positive effects in septic shock or ARDS (Domenighetti et al. 1997).

Conclusion

At the moment there is no evidence to support the prophylactic use of NAC or ambroxol in critically ill patients. It may be appropriate to use ambroxol per inhalationem, which has been clearly shown to liquefy mucous plugs and help expectoration.

References

Ben-Menachem T, McCarthy BD, Fogel R, Schiffman RM, Patel RV, Zarowitz BJ, Nerenz DR, Bresalier RS (1996) Prophylaxis for stress-related gastrointestinal hemorrhage: a cost effectiveness analysis. Crit Care Med 24:338–345

Cook DJ, Laine LA, Guyatt GH, Raffin TA (1991a) Nosocomial pneumonia and the role of gastric pH: a meta-analysis. Chest 100:7–13

Cook DJ, Witt LG, Cook RJ, Guyatt GH (1991b) Stress ulcer prophylaxis in the critical ill: a meta-analysis. Am J Med 91:519–527

Cook DJ, Fuller HD, Guyatt GH, Marshall JC, Leasa D, Hall R, Winton TL, Rutledge F, Todd TJR, Roy P, Lacroix J, Griffith L, Willian A for the Canadian Critical Care Trials Group (1994) Risk factors for gastrointestinal bleeding in critically ill patients. N Engl J Med 330:377–381

Cook DJ, Reeve BK, Guyatt GH, Heyland DK, Griffith LE, Buckingham L, Tryba M (1996) Stress ulcer prophylaxis in critical ill patients: resolving discordant meta-analyses. J Am Med Assoc 275:308–314

Cook D, Guyatt G, Marshall J, Leasa D, Fuller H, Hall R, Peters S, Rutlede F, Griffith L, McLellan A, Wood G, Kirby A, for the Canadian Critical Care Trials Group (1998) A comparison of sucralfate and ranitidine for the prevention of upper gastrointestinal bleeding in patients requiring mechanical ventilation. N Engl J Med 338:791–797

Domenighetti G, Suter PM, Schaller M-D, Ritz R, Perret C (1997) Treatment with N-acetylcyteine during acute respiratory distress syndrome: a randomized, double-blind, placebo-controlled clinical study. J Crit Care 12:177–182

Fegiz G (1991) Prevention by ambroxol of bronchopulmonary complications after upper abdominal surgery: double-blind Italian multicenter clinical study versus placebo. Lung 169:69–76

Gramatté T, Hinrichsen H (1996) Therapie gastrointestinaler Erkrankungen. In: Frölich JC, Kirch W (eds) Praktische Arzneitherapie. Fischer, Stuttgart

Ligumsky M, Karmeli F, Rachmilewitz D (1984) Sucralfate protection against gastrointestinal damage: possible role of prostanoids. Isr J Med Sci 22:801–806

Navab F, Steingrub J (1995) Stress ulcer: Is routine prophylaxis necessary? Am J Gastroenterol 90:708–712

Phillips JO, Metzler MH, Palmieri MTL, Huckfeldt RE, Dahl NG (1996) A prospective study of simplified omeprazole suspension for the prophylaxis of stress-related mucosal damage. Crit Care Med 24:1793–1800

Piper DW, de Carle DJ, Talley NJ, Gallagher ND, Wilson JS, Powell LW, Crawford D, Gibson PR, Sorrell TC, Kellow JE, Roberts RK (1997) Gastrointestinal and hepatic diseases In: Spapen H, Zhang H, Demanet C, Vleminckx W, Vincent JL Huyghens L (1998) Does N-acetyl-l-cyteine influence cytokine responses during early human septic shock? Chest 113:1616–1624

Pitimana-aree S, Forrest D, Brown G, Anis A, Wang XH, Dodek P (1998) Implementation of a clinical practice guideline for stress ulcer prophylaxis inceases appropriateness and decreases cost of care. Intensive Care Med 24:217–223

Prod'hom G, Leuenberger P, Koerfer J, Blum A, Chiolero R, Schaller M-D, Perret C, Spinnler O, Blondel J, Siegrist H, Saghafi L, Blanc D, Francioli P (1994) Nosocomial pneumonia in mechanically ventilated patients receiving antacid, ranitidine, or sucralfate as prophylaxis for stress ulcer: a randomized controlled trial. Ann Intern Med 120:653–662

Schneider JS, Ouellette SM (1984) Sucralfate administration via nasogastric tube. N Engl J Med 310: 990

Schumock GT, Lam NP, Winkler SR, Kong SX (1996) Pharmacoeconomic analysis of stress ulcer prophylaxis for critically ill patients. Pharmacoeconomics 9:455–465

Taeschner W, Vozeh S (1997) Pharmakokinetic drug data. In: Speight TM, Holford NHG (eds) Avery's drug treatment. Adis International, Auckland, p 1657

Tryba M (1991) Prophylaxis of stress ulcer bleeding: a meta-analysis. J Clin Gastroenterol 13 (Suppl 2):544–555

Tryba M (1994) Stress ulcer prophylaxis – quo vadis? Intensive Care Med 20:311–313
Zandstra DF, Stoutenbeek CP (1994) The virtual absence of stress-ulceration related bleeding in ICU patients receiving prolonged mechanical ventilation without any prophylaxis: a prospective cohort study. Intensive Care Med 20:335–340

Pneumonia Prophylaxis Under Ulcer Therapy

G. Stöhr[1] · M. Kunze[1, 2] · C. Ohmann[1, 3] · H. D. Röher[1, 3] · J. Piek[1, 4]
W. Sandmann[1, 5] · H. Becker[1]

[1] Department of General Surgery, University of Göttingen, Robert-Koch-Strasse 40, 37075 Göttingen, Germany
[2] Department of Anaesthesiology, University of Essen, Essen, Germany
[3] Department of General and Accident Surgery, University of Duesseldorf, Duesseldorf, Germany
[4] Department of Neurosurgery, University of Greifswald, Greifswald, Germany
[5] Department of Vascular Surgery and Kidney Transplantation, University of Duesseldorf, Duesseldorf, Germany

Introduction

Even under modern intensive care conditions surgical high-risk patients are endangered mainly by stress ulcer bleeding (SB) and nosocomial pneumonia (NP) [8, 13, 34]. Stress ulcer prophylaxis by elevation of the gastric pH is effective against upper gastrointestinal bleeding [6, 17, 35, 38]; on the other hand, a gastric pH over 3.5 with a potential consecutive contamination of stomach juice seems to play an important role in endogenous infections and NP [2, 14, 18]. Several studies show that in high-risk patients a prophylaxis is important [16, 28].

Sucralfate is a complex salt of sucrose sulfate and aluminum hydroxide, and its effect against upper gastrointestinal bleeding is comparable to antacids or H_2 antagonists [11, 36]; however, sucralfate seems to have advantages compared with other common agents. Several studies showed less incidence and less proliferation of gastric contamination with gram-negative germs compared with antacids and H_2 blockers [11, 21, 22, 36], but the benefit of NP is discussed controversially [31, 39].

If microaspiration of contaminated gastric juice should be the main reason for NP, the drainage of the subglottic area should decrease the risk of pneumonia.

The aim of this study is the comparison of different bleeding prophylaxes (ranitidine vs sucralfate) regarding endoscopic controlled SB and NP and to define the effect of subglottic lavage in the incidence of NP.

Materials and Methods

One hundred critically ill and mechanically ventilated surgical patients with an expected risk of 20 % for SB under placebo medication [25] were randomized into three therapy groups before starting treatment. Patient allocation was performed with block randomization. Block size was 30. A certification was not performed because a comparable stress ulcer risk was assumed for all diagnoses. Criteria of inclusion were obligatory mechanical ventilation and at least one severe disease or trauma (Table 1). Exclusion criteria were as follows: pregnancy, earlier operations of duodenum or stomach, ulcer anamnesis, active upper gastrointestinal bleeding or pneumonia, treatment with antacids, H_2 blockers, sucralfate, omeprazole, and pirenzepine within the past year, treatment with non-steroidal antiphlogistic drugs, and cumarine during the preceding 7 days, primary disease of blood coagulation system, and expected ventilation period less than 3 days.

M. K. Herbert et al. (Eds.), Problems of the Gastrointestinal Tract in Anesthesia...

Table 1. Criteria of inclusion

Mechanical ventilation obligatory, and:
Polytrauma (injury severity score ISS >25)
Sepsis (four of the seven criteria of The Veterans Administration Systemic Sepsis Cooperative Study Group [40]: fever, tachypnea, tachycardia, hypotonia, leukocytosis, thrombocytopenia, local infection, or surgical treatment within the past 48 h)
Hemorrhagic shock (systolic pressure <90 mm Hg more than 30 min, perforated aortic aneurysm, severe operations with serious bleeding complications, and transfusion of at least 2000 ml blood)
Respiratory insufficiency (lung injury score <1.3 [29], hypoxemia, PEEP score, atelectasis, reduced compliance)
Renal insufficiency (anuria, creatinine level >200 μmol/l for at least 24 h)
Coma II–III (craniocerebral trauma, spontaneous intracerebral bleeding)

Table 2. Stress ulcer prophylaxis

Treatment group	Prophylaxis
A	Ranitidine (200 mg/24 h, i.v.) with subglottic lavage
B	Sucralfate (6·1 g/24 h) with subglottic lavage
C	Sucralfate (6·1 g/24 h) without subglottic lavage

All patients were randomized into the following three therapy groups: A = ranitidine (200 mg/d) as a continuous intravenous infusion with subglottic lavage (SL); every 4 h the subglottic area was flushed and drained over a specific endotracheal tube; B = sucralfate, 1 g every 4 h with SL; and C = sucralfate without SL (Table 2). Once a day, germ investigations of stomach, oropharynx, and trachea were performed and the APACHE II score was defined. The acid concentration of stomach juice was also controlled every 4 h.

An obligatory special nasogastric tube with an integrated pH meter in its distal end (Zinetics Medical, Salt Lake City, Utah) was used, and every 4 h before stomach flushing the gastric pH was investigated.

The subglottic lavage was performed with a special endotracheal tube (HI-LO EVAC tube, Mallinckrodt Medical, St. Louis, Mo.), which incorporates a separate lumen ending dorsally in the subglottic area directly above the cuff (Fig. 1).

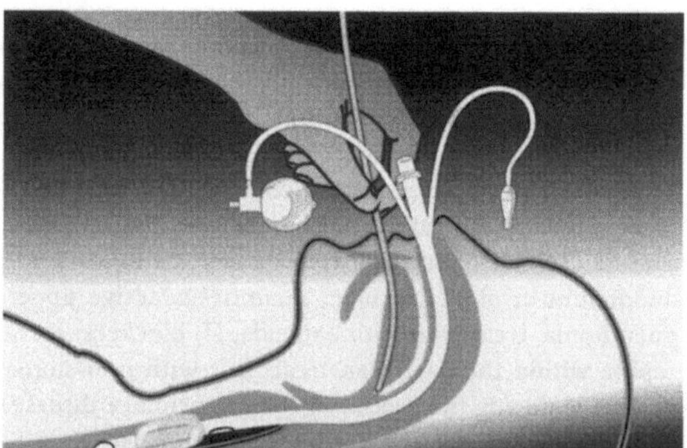

Fig. 1. The HI-LO Evac tracheal tube

The subglottic space has an average volume of 4 ml and is usually filled with contaminated mucus of the oropharynx. The SL took place as follows: every 4 h through the incorporated separate lumen the subglottic area was flushed with 200 ml 0.9 % sterile sodium chloride solution and was aspirated out of the oropharynx under laryngoscopic control. The probe was investigated for germs and fungi, and after the 4th day of ventilation the oropharynx was treated six times per day with topic antifungal solution (amphotericin B). During the stay in the ICU and for another 7 days after ICU treatment the patients were observed.

In case of an upper gastrointestinal bleeding an endoscopic investigation of esophagus, stomach, and duodenum was performed within the first 12 h to identify the localization and kind of bleeding (cancer, ulcer, lesion by nasogastric tube). Criteria of bleeding are hematemesis, blood in the gastric tube, Hb decrease of at least 2 gram percent within 24 h.

The nosocomial pneumonia is defined as follows: purulent tracheal aspirate, colonization of tracheal secretion, leukocytosis (> 10,000/mm^3), fever (> 38.5 °C), and a new and persistent infiltrate on chest X-ray, judged by an independent radiologist. Qualitative and quantitative cultures of aerobic pathogens were performed on each aspirate (stomach, oropharynx, trachea, subglottic lavage).

Data of the main criteria of investigation (SB and NP) were statistically analyzed by using the chi-square test and Fisher's exact test. This study conforms to the declarations of Helsinki (1964), Venice (1983), and the statutes of the ethical committee of the University of Düsseldorf, Germany.

Results

One hundred patients were randomly distributed into the three therapy groups. Table 3 gives details on the patients studied. The average period of mechanical ventilation was 11.9 days (range 3–58 days), group A = 12 days (range 3–58 days), B = 13 days (range 3–35 days), C = 11 days (range 3–32 days), the mean time of ICU treatment and observation was 15.0 days, A = 14 days (range 3–60 days), B = 13 days (3–37 days), C = 18 days (3–37 days). The mean age of the patients was 43.4 years (A = 46.5 years, range 18–79 years; B = 34 years, range 18–77 years, C = 49 years, range 19–78 years). With regard to age, gender, APACHE II score, period of mechanical ventilation and ICU treatment, and accompanying diseases, there were no significant differences between the three groups observed. Mainly accompanying diseases were

Table 3. Patient diagnoses and randomization

Diagnosis	Ranitidine with SL (A)	Sucralfate with SL (B)	Sucralfate without SL (C)	Total
Polytrauma	16	15	17	48
Brain coma	11	10	9	30
Respiratory insufficiency	4	2	4	10
Hemorrhagic shock	2	4	2	8
Sepsis	1	–	1	2
Renal failure	–	1	1	2
Total	34	32	34	100

Table 4. Incidence of complications in the therapy collectives

Criteria	Ranitidine with SL (A)	Sucralfate with SL (B)	Sucralfate without SL (C)	Total
Stress ulcer bleeding (%)	2 (5.9 %)	1 (3.1 %)	–	3
Pneumonia (%)	1 (2.9 %)	1 (3.1 %)	4 (11.8 %)	6
Death	3	1	2	6

noticed. The median gastric pH was in both sucralfate groups 1.2 points lower (pH 4.2, 0.8–6.2) than in the ranitidine collective (pH 5.4, 0.8–7.8) and showed a more continuous curve.

Three stress ulcer bleedings appeared, two in group A (5.9 %; Table 4): A 37-year-old woman with severe polytrauma, injury severity score (ISS) = 50, developed at the 20th day of mechanical ventilation a stress ulcer bleeding with Hb decrease of 2.4 g%. The pH range was between 0.8 and 7.5; five blood transfusions were necessary without operative or interventional management. She died of multiorgan failure after 26 days. In a 68-year-old polytraumatized woman, ISS = 25, pH range 1.0–1.7, an endoscopic stress ulcer bleeding was documented at the 6th day of treatment. Two blood transfusions were administered and the patient died from multiorgan failure during the 9th day. One patient (65 years) of group B (3.1 %) died on the 4th day of a perforated mycotic aneurysm of the common iliac artery, after he developed an SB on the 3rd day of treatment. The average gastric pH was 3.1, 20 % of tests were under pH 1.5. In every case of SB no surgical treatment was necessary.

In six cases a pneumonia by clinical and radiological criteria was observed, 1 in group A (1 of 34, 2.9 %), 1 in B (1 of 32, 3.1 %), and four in C (4 of 34, 11.8 %). The first patient (45 years) with an intracerebral hemorrhage developed an NP on the fourth day of *Pseudomonas aeruginosa,* and he died of cerebral complications on the fifth day. The average gastric pH was between 6.3 and 7.3. The female patient in group B (34 years) suffered severe polytrauma (ISS = 36) with rib fractures, unstable thorax, and hemorrhagic lung contusions. On the 14th day we noticed a pneumonia caused by *Escherichia coli;* 75 % of the gastric pH values were between 2 and 3, 25 % between 4 and 6. The four patients in group C were all endangered by polytrauma and severe thorax injuries on both sides and showed the following development: the first (22 years, polytrauma ISS 25, mechanical ventilation 7 days), had NP on the 12th day of *Pseudomonas aeruginosa.* In the second patient (33 years, polytrauma ISS = 42, death through ARDS after 22 days) pneumonia was observed on the 17th day, and *Pseudomonas aeruginosa* and *E. coli* were isolated (gastric pH 5.2–7.6). In another patient (64 years, polytrauma ISS 38) an NP was defined on day 13 (*Enterobacter*), with a gastric pH 1.4–6.5. The last male patient (58 years, polytrauma ISS = 48) developed an NP on the 17th day by *E. coli* and *Enterobacter;* the median pH was 4.8 (range 3.0–6.2), and he died from sepsis after the 21st day of treatment.

In all six cases of NP the origin of infection was not the stomach, but the oropharynx, where germs were isolated 1–3 days earlier than in the trachea and stomach (Table 5); thus, subglottic lavage seems to be a causal therapy regarding NP. In no patient did a germ migration from the stomach over the oropharynx into the trachea take place.

Table 5. Characteristics of nosocomial pneumonias. *R* ranitidine; *S* sucralfate

Patient no.	Age (years)	Therapy	Duration of therapy	Germ	Migration
3	46	R with SL	4	*Pseudomonas*	no
19	36	S with SL	14	*E. coli*	no
20	25	S without SL	12	*Pseudomonas*	no
67	32	S without SL	17	*Pseudomonas*	no
68	64	S without SL	13	*Enterobacter*	no
84	52	S without SL	14	*Enterobacter*	no

With regard to SB, NP, gastric pH, and mortality (average 27 %, A = 23.5 %, B = 18.8 %, C = 38.2 %) no significant differences between the three therapy groups were observed. The most frequent causes of death were brain complications (40.7 %), multiorgan failure (33.3 %), and septic shock (18.5 %). In SB the rate of mortality was 100 % and in NP 50 %. No patient died directly from gastrointestinal bleeding or pneumonia; however, both organ failures increased morbidity and mortality.

Discussion

Results of placebo-controlled trials [16, 28], where SBs were observed in up to 33 % without any prophylaxis and average bleeding rates under current medication are between 0 % [30] and 31 % [23], call for stress ulcer prophylaxis in the well-defined group of surgical high-risk patients with obligatory mechanical ventilation. Presently, stress bleeding prophylaxis is accepted worldwide. Most of the randomized prospective studies show good effectiveness for all common drugs without statistically significant differences regarding mucosal lesion bleedings [7, 21, 30–33]. However, time of assistance, quantity of agents, kind and number of applications, cost-effectiveness ratio [3, 27] and mainly the side effects distinguish antacids and H_2 receptor blockers, which induce a gastric pH elevation, and sucralfate from each other. Alkalinization of the gastric juice is effective against SB, but an acidic stomach environment is the best prophylaxis regarding gastric colonization with gram-negative germs. While raising gastric pH over 3.5, the contamination of the stomach content increases rapidly. This effect is reversible when the gastric juice becomes acidic again [11]. Many trials over the past years have postulated that a passive chronic reflux of contaminated duodenal and stomach content via the esophagus and oropharynx into the trachea may lead to tracheal colonization and pneumonia [22, 26, 27, 33]. Some authors have shown a coherence of gastric colonization and NP in some cases [27, 37]. Other nosocomial infections up to septic complications and hematogenous distribution of bacteria may be induced by the contaminated upper gastrointestinal tract [1, 4, 10, 18].

According to a multicenter study [8] risk factors for upper gastrointestinal bleeding are respiratory insufficiency and irritation of the blood coagulation system with a mortality of 48.5 % and an incidence of 3.7 %. However, study designs and methodological differences of the comparative trials yield controversial results [5, 23]. The main problems are non-defined criteria of inclusion, small patient groups, short observation periods, no endoscopic investigation in case of gastrointestinal bleeding, no mechanical ventilation, low-risk patients for NP, and additional enteral nutrition. Further problems are combination and individual dosage of agents against SB or NP, no random distribution into therapy groups, large number of units within multicenter studies and insufficient definition of pneumonia [5, 20, 24].

In our opinion, the following two mechanisms are important to decrease the risk of NP under appropriate stress ulcer prophylaxis: agents without elevating the gastric pH and an effective barrier between throat and trachea to stop the potential germ microaspiration.

Sucralfate has, compared with other common drugs, a lot of advantages: no relevant pharmacological influence on gastric pH, an antibacterial effect, stimulation of mucosal perfusion and prostaglandin E_2 synthesis, an increase in viscosity and amount of gastric mucus, and absorption of bile acid, pepsin, and trypsin. Especially the duodeno-gastric reflux, which leads to an intermittent gastric pH elevation and reflux of intestinal germs, is not at all treated with other agents. In in vitro measurements the antibacterial activity of sucralfate is documented [11], except for *Pseudomonas aeruginosa* and *Candida albicans*. Two meta-analyses found lower mortality rates under sucralfate [9, 33].

In our study we demonstrated that in both sucralfate collectives the average gastric pH was lower, although without statistical significance. Furthermore, there is a trend toward a lower gastric colonization rate compared with the ranitidine group, which has also been confirmed by other authors [5, 31]. However, all three cases of gastric bleeding, two of which were in patients with ranitidine treatment (group A), developed under low gastric pH conditions (pH 0.8–3.4). Compared with results from the literature the stress ulcer bleeding incidence was very low in our trial.

Pneumonias are, among nosocomial infections, the most frequent cause of death [7, 31] and the second most common nosocomial infection [18], as the pneumonia rate in mechanically ventilated patients under H_2-receptor blocker prophylaxis is documented in up to 36 % [15, 17, 33] with an elevated mortality rate. On the other hand, lower pneumonia rates [7, 31, 35] and reduced mortality under sucralfate are documented. Nosocomial pneumonias are presently a more relevant danger for high-risk patients than SB. Their origin, however, is controversial [4, 5, 18, 19, 22, 35, 31]. The gastro-esophageal reflux of contaminated gastric juice, supported by the horizontal position of patients, complete relaxation, and naso-gastric tubes were considered as the main reason for NP. Some authors have documented, by microbiological measurements, silent aspiration rates into the trachea in up to 31.6 % [12, 37], mostly with gram-negative bacilli.

Intubation and artificial ventilation destroy the defense mechanisms of the nose and the lymphatic systems of the throat, and reduce the lock effect of the epiglottis and the ciliar function in the bronchioli. Furthermore, elevated oxygen concentrations reduce the activity of alveolar macrophages [12]. Exogenous infections in the form of contaminated ventilation gas are no longer relevant.

Our results identify the oropharynx as a primary contaminated organ. One to three days after microbiological identification of germs in the throat, identical species were found in the trachea during development of an NP; gastric reflux was in no case responsible for the infection. Pneumonias appearing within the first days (early-onset NP) seem to be induced by primary or iatrogenic infection.

In our opinion, an NP is a multifactorial event, consisting of microaspiration, contamination of body fluids, lung injury with primary infection, reduced local defense mechanisms, and hematogenous or lymphogenous germ distribution. The tube's cuff is no effective barrier between oropharynx and trachea; however, the microaspiration from oropharynx or stomach may induce an NP. Both high-risk patient collectives, treated with the HI-LO EVAC tube with intermittent lavage, show an extremely low incidence of NP. Even in the ranitidine group with elevated gastric contamination only one early-onset and no late-onset pneumonia appeared. The NP in patients treated with sucralfate without subglottic lavage had its origin in the oropharynx, and the low-grade contaminated gastric juice was in no case responsible for the pulmonary infection.

Conclusion

Between the three therapy groups there is no significant difference with regard to SB, nosocomial pneumonia, and mortality; however, the incidence of SB and NP is extremely low, compared with data from the literature. Of NPs, 83 % are late-onset pneumonias, i.e., they appear after the tenth day of mechanical ventilation, and their origin is not the stomach, but the oropharynx. The subglottic lavage is an effective barrier for germ migration into the trachea, and it supports prevention of NP and prolongation of the infect-free interval even under H_2-blocker therapy. The main advantages of sucralfate are effective local protection of the gastric mucosa, no modulation of gastric pH, no increase of gastric juice contamination, no interactions with parenterally applied drugs and no systemic side effects. Both subglottic lavage and sucralfate are recommended therapies in severely ill surgical patients under intensive care conditions, because NP and SB are complications with a high mortality rate. Stomach bleeding and NPs are symptoms of multiorgan failure.

References

1. Abele-Horn M, Dauber A, Bauernfeind A, Russwurm W, Seyfarth-Metzger I, Gleich P, Ruckdeschel G: Decrease in nosocomial pneumonia in ventilated patients by selective oropharyngeal decontamination (SOD). Intensive Care Med 1997; 23: 187–195
2. American Thoracic Society: Hospital-aquired pneumonia in adults: diagnosis, assessment of severity, initial antimicrobial therapy and preventative strategies. A consensus statement. Am J Respir Crit Care Med 1995; 153:1711–1725
3. Ben-Menachem T, McCarthy BD, Fogel R, Schiffman RM, Patel RV, Zarowitz BJ, Nerenz DR, Bresalier RS: Prophylaxis for stress-related gastrointestinal hemorrhage: a cost effectiveness analysis. Crit Care Med 1996; 24:338–353
4. Bert F, Lambert-Zechovsky N: Sinusitis in mechanically ventilated patients and its role in the pathogenesis of nosocomial pneumonia. Eur J Clin Microbiol Infect Dis 1996; 15:533–544
5. Bonten MJ, Gaillard CA, van der Geest S, van Tiel FH, Beysens AJ, Smeets HG, Stobberingh EE: The role of intragastric acidity and stress ulcus prophylaxis on colonization and infection in mechanically ventilated ICU patients. A stratified, randomized, double-blind study of sucralfate versus antacids. Am J Respir Crit Care Med 1995; 152:1825–1834
6. Cannon LA, Heiselman D, Gardner W et al.: Prophylaxis of upper gastrointestinal tract bleeding in mechanical ventilated patients. A randomized study comparing the efficacy of sucralfate, cimetidine and antacids. Arch Intern Med 1987; 147:2101–2106
7. Cook DJ: Stress ulcer prophylaxis: gastrointestinal bleeding and nosocomial pneumonia. Best evidence synthesis. Scand J Gastroenterol Suppl 1995; 210:48–52
8. Cook DJ, Fuller HD, Guyatt GH et al.: Risk factors for gastrointestinal bleeding in critically ill patients. N Engl J Med 1994; 330:377–381

9. Cook DJ, Reeve BK, Guyatt GH, Heyland DK, Griffith LE, Buckingham L, Tryba M: Stress ulcer prophylaxis in critically ill patients. Resolving discordant meta-analyses. J Am Med Assoc 1996; 275:308–314
10. Craven DE, Steger KA: Nosocomial pneumonia in mechanically ventilated adult patients: epidemiology and prevention in 1996. Semin Respir Infect 1996; 11:32–53
11. Daschner F, Kappstein I, Engels I: Antibakterielle Aktivität von Sucralfat in künstlichem Magensaft. Intensivmed 1987; 24:163–166
12. Daschner F, Reuschenbach K, Pfisterer J, Kappstein I, Vogel W, Krieg N, Just H: The influence of stress ulcer prophylaxis on the incidence of pneumonia in artifically ventilated patients. Anaesthesist 1987; 36:9–18
13. Driks M, Craven DE, Celli BR et al.: Nosocomial pneumonia in intubated patients given sucralfate as compared with antacids or histamine type 2 blockers. The role of gastric colonization. N Engl J Med 1987; 317:1376–1382
14. Du Moulin GC () Tracheobronchial colonisation. Klin Wochenschr 1991; 69 (Suppl 27):6–11
15. Eddleston JM, Vohra A, Scott P et al.: A comparison of the frequency of stress ulceration and secondary pneumonia in sucralfate- or ranitidine-treated intensive care unit patients. Crit Care Med 1991; 19:1491–1496
16. Eddleston JM, Pearson RC, Holland J, Tooth JA, Vohra A, Doran BH: Prospective endoscopic study of stress erosions and ulcers in critically ill adult patients treated with either sucralfate or placebo. Crit Care Med 1994; 22:1949–1954
17. Fabian TC, Boucher BA, Croce MA et al.: Pneumonia and stress ulceration in severely injured patients: a prospective evaluation of the effects of stress ulcer prophylaxis. Arch Surg 1993; 128:185–192
18. Guidelines for prevention of nosocomial pneumonia. Centers for Disease Control and Prevention. Morb Mortal Wkly Rep 1997; 46:1–79
19. Hauer T, Lacour M, Gastmeier P, Schulgen G, Schumacher M, Ruden H, Daschner F: Nosocomial infections intensive care units. A nation-wide prevalence study. Anaesthesist 1996; 45:1184–1191
20. Jourdain B, Joly-Guillou ML, Dombret MC, Calvat S, Trouillet JL, Gibert C, Chastre J: Usefulness of quantitative cultures of BAL fluid for diagnosing nosocomial pneumonia in ventilated patients. Chest 1997; 11:411–418
21. Labattut AG, Santolalla PM, Andres AP de et al.: Efficacy of sucralfate in the prevention of upper gastrointestinal stress bleeding in intensive care patients: comparison versus a control group. Clin Intensive Care 1992; 3 (Suppl):19–25
22. Laggner AN, Tryba M, Georgopoulos A, Lenz K, Grimm G, Graninger W, Schneeweiss B, Druml W: Oropharyngeal decontamination with gentamicin for long-term ventilated patients on stress ulcer prophylaxis with sucralfate? Wien Klin Wochenschr 1994; 106:15–19
23. Levy MJ, Seelig CB, Robinson NJ, Ranney JE: Comparison of omeprazole and ranitidine for stress ulcer prophylaxis. Dig Dis Sci 1997; 42:1255–1259
24. Lipchik RJ, Kuzo RS: Nosocomial pneumonia. Radiol Clin North Am 1996; 34:47–58
25. Lorenz W, Fischer M, Rohde H et al.: Histamine and stress ulcer: new components in organizing a sequential trial on cimetidine prophylaxis in seriously ill patients and definition of a special group at risk (severe polytrauma). Klin Wochenschr 1980; 58:653–665
26. Mahul P, Auboyer C, Jospe R et al.: Prevention of nosocomial pneumonia in intubated patients: respective role of mechanical subglottic secretions drainage and stress ulcer prophylaxis. Intensive Care Med 1992; 18:20–25
27. Maier RV, Mitchell D, Gentilello L: Optimal therapy for stress gastritis. Ann Surg 1994; 220:353–363
28. Martin LF, Booth V, Karlstadt RG et al.: Continuous intravenous cimetidine decreases stress-related upper gastrointestinal hemorrhage without promoting pneumonia. Crit Care Med 1993; 21:19–30
29. Murray JF, Matthay MA, Luce JM et al.: An expanded definition of the adult respiratory distress syndrome. Am Rev Respir Dis 1988; 138:720–724
30. Pickworth KK, Falcone RE, Hoogeboom JE, Santanello SA: Occurrence of nosocomial pneumonia in mechanically ventilated trauma patients: a comparison of sucralfate and ranitidine [see comments]. Crit Care Med 1993; 2:1856–1862
31. Prod'hom G, Leuenberger P, Koerfer J, Blum A, Chiolero R, Schaller MD, Perret C, Spinnler O, Blondel J, Siegrist H et al.: Nosocomial pneumonia in mechanically ventilated patients receiving antacid, ranitidine, or sucralfate as prophylaxis for stress ulcer. A randomized controlled trial. Ann Intern Med 1994; 120:653–662
32. Rello J, Ausina V, Ricart M et al.: Risk factors for infection by *Pseudomonas aeruginosa* in patients with ventilator-associated pneumonia. Intensive Care Med 1994; 20:193–198
33. Ryan P, Dawson J, Teres D: Nosocomial pneumonia during stress ulcer prophylaxis with cimetidine and sucralfate. Arch Surg 1993; 128:1353–1357

34. Schaberg T, Lode H: Diagnostik der nosokomialen Pneumonie. Dtsch Med Wschr 1997; 122:61–64
35. Sirvent JM, Verdaguer R, Ferrer MJ, Avila FJ, Diaz Prieto A, Carratala J: Mechanical ventilation-associated pneumonia and the prevention of stress ulcer. A randomized clinical trial of antacids and ranitidine versus sucralfate. Med Clin Barc 1994; 102:407–411
36. Tarnawski A, Hollander D, Gergely H.: The mechanism of protective, therapeutic and prophylactic actions of sucralfate. Scand J Gastroenterol 1987; 22 (Suppl 140):7–13
37. Thomason MH, Payseur ES, Hakenewerth AM, Norton HJ, Mehta B, Reeves TR, Moore-Swartz MW, Robbins PI: Nosocomial pneumonia in ventilated trauma patients during stress ulcer prophylaxis with sucralfate, antacid, and ranitidine. J Trauma 1996; 41:503–508
38. Tryba M: Sucralfate versus antacids or H_2-antagonists for stress ulcer prophylaxis: a meta-analysis on efficacy and pneumonia rate. Crit Care Med 1991; 19:942–949
39. Tryba M, Cook DJ: Gastric alkalinization, pneumonia, and systemic infections: the controversy. Scand J Gastroenterol 1995 (Suppl); 210:53–59
40. Veterans Administration Systemic Sepsis Cooperative Study Group: Effect of high-dose glucocorticoid therapy on mortality in patients with clinical signs of systemic sepsis. N Engl J Med 1987; 317:659–665

Subject Index

P

R

MIX
Papier aus verantwortungsvollen Quellen
Paper from responsible sources
FSC® C105338

If you have any concerns about our products,
you can contact us on
ProductSafety@springernature.com

In case Publisher is established outside the EU,
the EU authorized representative is:
Springer Nature Customer Service Center GmbH
Europaplatz 3, 69115 Heidelberg, Germany

Printed by Libri Plureos GmbH
in Hamburg, Germany